ANNUAL REVIEW OF NURSING RESEARCH

Volume 21, 2003

ANNUAL REVIEW OF NURSING RESEARCH

Volume 21, 2003

Research on Child Health and Pediatric Issues

Joyce J. Fitzpatrick, PhD, RN, FAAN
Series Editor

Margaret Shandor Miles, PhD, RN, FAAN
Diane Holditch-Davis, PhD, RN, FAAN
Volume Editors

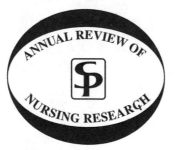

 SPRINGER PUBLISHING COMPANY

Order ANNUAL REVIEW OF NURSING RESEARCH, Volume 22, 2004, prior to publication and receive a 10% discount. An order coupon can be found at the back of this volume.

Springer Publishing Company, Inc.
536 Broadway
New York, NY 10012-3955

03 04 05 06 07 / 5 4 3 2 1

ISBN-0-8261-4133-1
ISSN-0739-6686

ANNUAL REVIEW OF NURSING RESEARCH is indexed in *Cumulative Index to Nursing and Allied Health Literature* and *Index Medicus*.

Printed in the United States of America by Maple-Vail.

This volume of ARNR is dedicated to the memory of Robert B. Cairns, Cary C. Boshamer Professor of Psychology and Director of the Center for Developmental Science at the University of North Carolina at Chapel Hill from its inception until his untimely death in 1999.

Contents

Part III: Parents and Families

Part IV: Looking Back: The Last 10 Years

Preface

In September 2002 at the State of the Science Conference held in Washington DC, we celebrated the publication of the 20th volume of the Annual Review of Nursing Research (ARNR) series. The concluding chapter in this 21st volume is a review of the content of Volumes 11 through 20, the second decade of the ARNR Series. As senior editor for the Series, I have coauthored this chapter. Joanne Stevenson, author of the review of the first decade of the ARNR Series, published in Volume 10, is the second author of this review chapter. The format of the review chapter follows the model originally developed by Stevenson in her review of Volumes 1 through 10. We are particularly indebted to the staff of the National Institute of Nursing Research (NINR), in particular, Daniel O'Neal, for their input and review of this chapter, with particular attention to the historical facts related to research development and support through NINR.

This 21st volume follows the pattern established in Volume 18, i.e., the entire volume is devoted to one area of nursing research. In this volume the focus is child health research from a developmental science perspective. Drs. Margaret Miles and Diane Holditch Davis from the University of North Carolina Chapel Hill, well-known scientists in developmental research, have served as volume editors. They selected the content themes and the authors, and edited the chapters for this comprehensive volume.

Drs. Miles and Holditch-Davis set the tone for the volume in their introductory chapter, "Enhancing nursing research with children and families using a developmental science perspective." The developmental science content for this volume is then organized into three sections: Preterm infants, children with health problems, and parents and families.

Part I, Preterm Infants, includes two chapters. The first chapter by Diane Holditch-Davis and Beth Black includes a comprehensive review of the programs of research on care of preterm infants and analyzes these from a developmental science perspective. The second preterm infant chapter, written by Suzanne Thoyre, is focused specifically on research on the transition from gavage to oral feeding in the preterm infant.

Part II, Children with Health Problems, includes five chapters. Hyekyun Rhee critiques research on physical symptoms in children and adolescents, and Sharron Docherty reviews research on symptom experiences of children and adolescents with cancer. Becky Christian critiques research on the psychosocial adjustment of children and adolescents with cystic fibrosis, Judith Vessey reviews the research focused on children's psychological responses to hospitalization, and Janet Stewart critiques the research on the stressors, coping responses and health outcomes of children living with chronic illness.

Part III, Parents and Families, includes three chapters. In the first of these three chapters, Margaret Miles reviews the research programs focused on parents of children with chronic health problems. The second chapter, with a family focus, includes a review by Marcia Van Riper in which she critiques the research on the experiences of the siblings of children with chronic illness or disability. Then in the final chapter in this section, Linda Beeber and Margaret Miles critique the research focused on maternal mental health and parenting in poverty.

As with previous volumes, there is a significant debt to the scientists who contributed to the writing of the chapters and those who reviewed the various drafts while the volume was in process. Also, we wish to recognize the many nurse researchers whom the authors cite in their reviews; they continue to build the foundation for the future of nursing research. ARNR Advisory Board members have been loyal supporters of our continuing efforts to describe the "state of the science" in the selected content areas. We wish to recognize the contributions of the ARNR Advisory Board in the critical review of the series, both in the content focus of the chapters and volume themes and in the overall scientific direction of the ARNR series. Especially, we wish to acknowledge the Advisory Board members who have completed their five-year terms of appointment to the Board.

And, lastly, all of us involved in the ARNR Series, publishers, editors, authors, reviewers, and Advisory Board members, owe a significant debt to Dr. Harriet H. Werley, the founding editor and first senior editor of the ARNR Series. On October 14, 2002, two days after her 88th birthday, Harriet died a peaceful and quiet death. Her legacy for nursing research is reflected not only in the ARNR Series, but also in a series of other projects and activities that she launched and nourished throughout her career in nursing research. She was one of our research pioneers, a dedicated scientist who was not afraid to take risks, and who encouraged the scientific community not to veer from the road to quality in all that we do and claim. Harriet was the leader upon whose shoulders many of us stood in our career development, and we will not forget the lessons learned at the many meetings and gatherings with her. Thank you, Harriet.

JOYCE J. FITZPATRICK, PhD, RN, FAAN
Series Editor

Contributors

Linda S. Beeber, PhD, RN
Professor
School of Nursing
The University of North Carolina
   at Chapel Hill
Chapel Hill, NC

Beth Perry Black, MSN
Clinical Assistant Professor
School of Nursing
The University of North Carolina
   at Chapel Hill
Chapel Hill, NC

Becky Christian, PhD, RN
Associate Professor
School of Nursing
The University of North Carolina
   at Chapel Hill
Chapel Hill, NC

**Sharron L. Docherty, PhD,
   CPNP**
Assistant Professor
School of Nursing
Duke University Medical Center
Durham, NC

Hyekyun Rhee, PhD, PNP
Assistant Professor
Theresa A. Thomas Faculty
School of Nursing
University of Virginia
Charlottesville, VA

Janet L. Stewart, PhD, RN
School of Nursing
The University of North Carolina
   at Chapel Hill
Chapel Hill, NC

Suzanne M. Thoyre, PhD, RN
Assistant Professor
School of Nursing
The University of North Carolina
   at Chapel Hill
Chapel Hill, NC

Marcia Van Riper, PhD, RN
Associate Professor
School of Nursing and the
   Carolina Center for Genome
   Sciences
The University of North Carolina
   at Chapel Hill
Chapel Hill, NC

**Judith A. Vessey, PhD, RN,
   FAAN**
Lelia Holden Carroll Endowed
   Professor
William F. Connell School of
   Nursing
Boston College
Chestnut Hill, MA

Chapter 1

Enhancing Nursing Research With Children and Families Using a Developmental Science Perspective

MARGARET SHANDOR MILES AND DIANE HOLDITCH-DAVIS

ABSTRACT

Nursing scholarship on children and their families has increased rapidly over the past decades. This research focuses on infants, children, and adolescents and their families facing acute or chronic illness, as well as on promoting health and preventing disease in children. While the amount and scope of research in pediatric nursing has increased, the methods and theories used are diverse and are often not based on the most recent science in the broader fields of developmental research. Developmental science, which evolved over the past two decades into a new interdisciplinary framework for the study of human development, involves an integrated holistic, developmental, and systems-oriented perspective. According to this view, the individual functions and develops through dynamic and complex processes involving the integration of many systems within the individual, including mental, biological, and behavioral systems. In addition, individuals function and develop in a continuously ongoing, reciprocal process of interaction with their environment and, as such, have an influence on that environment. These nonlinear, dynamic processes demand complex conceptualizations and research designs if one is to truly understand human development, including health and illness. Key aspects of developmental science important in conceptualization, design, measurement, and data analysis are identified. By providing a framework for critiquing research and presenting recommendations for future research based on developmental science, we hope to move nursing research with children forward toward more developmentally sound knowledge of nursing practice.

1

Nursing has a holistic perspective. Nurses focus on broad aspects of individuals, families, and communities, including physical, psychological, and social domains (Barry, 1996). Many types of knowledge from diverse disciplinary perspectives are important for nursing practice. Nowhere is this holistic perspective more important than in the care of children. Nursing care of children involves understanding the complex and interrelated aspects of each child, as well as the ecology of their experiences and those of their families (Broome, Woodring, & O'Connor-Von, 1996; Craft-Rosenberg, Krajicek, & Shin, 2002; Pridham, 1998). Nurses working with children, whether in the community or in a health care setting, are concerned about developmental changes in physiological growth and function; in health, health behaviors, and illness; and in social and cognitive abilities. Furthermore, nurses characteristically try to understand the processes underlying development and know that development is a process that involves changes across the life span. Thus developmentally based research is of fundamental importance to nursing.

Developmental research focuses on the processes and outcomes of development. For example, child psychology has been defined very broadly to encompass diverse aspects of development, including social, behavioral, personality, and cognitive domains from infancy to adolescence (Mussen, 1983). Life span psychology and recent advances in understanding the developmental processes of aging have broadened the scope of developmental research. Mussen in his definition of child psychology included fields such as comparative-developmental psychology and developmental aspects of ethology and evolutionary psychology. Thus developmental research has long been multidisciplinary (Cairns, 1998). Applied fields concerned with developmental research include pediatric psychology, child development, pediatric medicine, maternal and child health, education, social work, and nursing. Applied disciplines have tended to lag behind the more research-focused fields in the application of new and evolving developmental concepts and methods in their research. Moreover, some applied fields derived their research methods and theories from biological and psychopathological models of clinical psychology and medicine rather than from a developmental perspective (Bearison, 1998).

More recently, advances in developmental research have crystallized into the concept of "developmental science." Developmental science goes beyond any individual discipline in synthesizing developmental theories and methods (Cairns, 2000). As such, it recognizes the complexity of development; incorporates a holistic, contextual, ecological, and interactional perspective; and views individual functioning at multiple levels from genes to culture (Carolina Consortium on Human Development, 1996). The authors have been involved for over a decade with the Center for Developmental Science and its training arm, the Carolina Consortium on Human Development, recognized internationally as one of the key centers for the development of this evolving perspective (Cairns, 2000; Cairns, Elder, & Costello, 1996).

Although nurse researchers increasingly are trained in developmental research methods, many nurses studying infants and children still do not conceptualize their studies from a developmental perspective. As a result, nurses are not building a developmentally sound science for practice as rapidly as needed. In a review of the history of pediatric nursing research, Vessey (1998) presented a quote by Isabel Stewart from 1929 that is still apt today: "If nursing is ever to justify its name as an applied science, if it is ever to free itself from these old superficial, haphazard methods, some way must be found to submit all our practice as rapidly as possible to the most searching test which modern science can devise" (p. 3).

It is essential, then, that future nursing research with children and their families be based on current theory and methods. One of the goals of this volume of the *Annual Review of Nursing Research* is to examine select bodies of research focused on children and their parents from the developmental science perspective. Our hope is that by providing a framework for critiquing research from this perspective and by presenting recommendations for future research based on developmental science, we can move nursing research with children forward toward a developmentally sound knowledge base for nursing practice.

NURSING RESEARCH WITH CHILDREN AND FAMILIES

Nursing scholarship focused on children and their families has increased rapidly over the past decades, although the number of studies remains low in comparison to the need (Lipman & Hayman, 2000; Moore, 2000). Topics range from infants, children, and teenagers and their families facing acute and chronic illness to promoting health and preventing disease in children (Barnard, 1983; Broome, Knafl, Pridham, & Feetham, 1998; Denyes, 1983; Lipman & Hayman, 2000; Walker, 1992). While the amount and scope of research in neonatal and pediatric nursing have increased, the methods and theories used are diverse and often not based on the most recent science from the broader fields of developmental research.

A number of historical influences are important in understanding where nursing science related to children and families is today. The early domains of study and their prevailing paradigms constitute one influence. Much of the early research in pediatric nursing focused on the hospitalized child and its family (Faux, 1998). This research evolved from the work of Blake (1954), Bowlby (1958), Erickson (1958), Prugh, Staub, Sands, Kirschbaum, and Lenihan (1953), and Robertson (1958), all of whom were influenced by psychoanalytic theories of development. These theories also were emphasized in the early graduate programs in pediatric nursing (Blake, 1954; Erickson, 1965). Nursing scholarship during this era primarily consisted of clinical papers, case studies, and descriptive research. This literature led to improvements in the care of children and changes in hospital practices, such as those that separated children from their parents or neglected to emotionally prepare children for surgery and painful procedures (Blake, 1964; Faux, 1998; Vessey, 1998). However, few research programs resulted (Barnes, Bandak, & Beardslee, 1990). Thus, with some important exceptions (Fagin, 1966; Visintainer & Wolfer, 1975), nursing research in the 1950s through the 1970s was fragmented, lacked clear conceptual or theoretical frameworks, and used limited and primarily descriptive designs (Barnard, 1983; Denyes, 1983; Vessey, this volume).

On the other hand, research focusing on mothers and infants, both preterm and full term, was more developmentally based, although there was still little focus on processes over time (Barnard, 1983). This developmental focus was likely due to the pioneering nurse researchers in this area, such as Mary Neal and Kathryn Barnard, who were trained in developmental psychology (Barnard & Neal, 1997; Vessey, 1998). Neal, Barnard, and others also led the way in training nurses in developmental research with infants and parents and, as a result, increased the number of developmentally trained nurse scholars with programs of research in perinatal and neonatal nursing (Barnard, Morisset, & Spieker, 1993; Becker, 2001; Holditch-Davis & Miles, 1997; Moore, 2000; Pridham, 1998; Walker, 1992).

Research with children and families was also held back by lack of well-articulated and developmentally sound conceptual models. Reviews conducted by a number of authors indicated that studies done in the 1960s and 1970s were often atheoretical descriptive studies or used frameworks that were not family or developmentally based (Barnard, 1983; Barnard & Neal, 1977; Barnes et al., 1990; Beal & Betz, 1992; Denyes, 1983; Walker,

1992). Later, researchers based their studies on conceptual models and theories developed for adults. Grand conceptual frameworks and theories of nursing were explored for their potential usefulness in designing research with children, but they did not easily fit (Grey, 1998). Nurses also adapted adult-oriented frameworks and theories from psychology, public health, and other disciplines for research with children; many of these, such as stress and coping theory, were not family focused or developmentally based. Health promotion research with school-aged children and adolescents is often based on adult-based cognitive theories of health behavior. These models varied widely in the attention given to developmental issues, such as the influence of multiple contexts on the health behaviors of youth and explorations of the processes and mechanisms of change over time (Grey, 1998; Hayman, 1998).

Professional organizations also were an important influence in improving the quality and amount of research (Vessey, 1998). Neonatal nurses and pediatric oncology nurses were encouraged in their research by professional organizations such as the Association for Pediatric Oncology Nurses; the Association for Women's Health, Obstetric, Gynecologic, and Neonatal Nursing; and the National Association of Neonatal Nurses (Hinds et al., 1990; Moore, 2000; Walker, 1992). These organizations provided seed money for research and encouraged the publication of research in their clinical journals. However, no professional organization focused on general pediatric nursing until the founding of the Society of Pediatric Nursing in 1990 (Miles, 1996). As a result, until recently there were few sources of funding for pilot research in general pediatrics or pediatric health promotion. Additionally, the National Center for Nursing Research, later the National Institute of Nursing Research, actively solicited research focused on high-risk infants, particularly preterm infants, for decades, while only recently have they indicated interest in research on broader aspects of child health or on children with chronic and terminal illness.

Further, nursing has become more and more specialized even within neonatal and pediatric nursing. While this specialization was important in focusing our scholarship (Walker, 1992), it also led to isolation, which prevented our science from moving forward (Craft-Rosenberg et al., 2002). Specialization has resulted in an intense focus on one age group (e.g., preterm infants, adolescence), one aspect of health (e.g., perinatal, neonatal, primary care), specific health problems (e.g., diabetes, cancer), or specific phenomena (e.g., pain) without an understanding of the broader literature in nursing and other disciplines that would place the problem within a more holistic perspective. For example, pediatric oncology researchers may focus on cancer and its treatments and neglect broader ecological and developmental issues. Neonatal researchers may focus on research with preterm infants and their parents but be unfamiliar with developmental and parenting literature focused on normal infants and preschool children, which might inform their research. Conversely, researchers who focus on older children may not keep up with the rich literature on high-risk infants. Indeed, in a recent review of research on children and families in health and illness, the focus seems to be on children after infancy, and the research of the key developmental researchers studying preterm infants is barely referenced (Broome et al., 1998). Specialization, then, may be causing neonatal and pediatric nurse researchers to "lose the forest for the trees." As nursing research has become more focused and narrow, nurses may have lost touch with the broader issues involved in studying children and their families.

Another influence on nursing research with children is the relatively recent maturation of doctoral education in nursing (Brodie, 1986; Vessey, 1998). As recently as two decades ago, most doctorates of pediatric nurse researchers were in the fields of education, psychology, sociology, anthropology, and child development. Although developmental science was evolving in that period, many programs in psychology and child development did not use this perspective. More recently, nurses have begun to pursue doctoral education in nursing. But, since few pediatric nurses have doctoral degrees, and many with doctorates are not trained in developmental programs, there is now a serious shortage of faculty with backgrounds in neonatal and pediatric nursing as well as in developmental science that can train doctoral students. Many doctoral programs have adult-focused nurse researchers to train doctoral students interested in research with children. Thus these students often are not exposed to the unique body of knowledge that is needed to conduct research with children, such as the theories, models, and methods of developmental science. However, beginning in the 1970s and 1980s, many nurses received doctoral degrees in developmentally focused disciplines and are now experienced faculty members and researchers. As a result, some nursing doctoral programs have faculty equipped to prepare doctoral students as developmental researchers, and some offer substantive courses focused on developmental theories and methods that are important in studying children and families. In addition, faculty expertise may be supplemented through elective courses in developmental psychology or child development. Thus the cadre of nurse researchers with strong backgrounds in developmental research is growing, albeit slowly.

In summary, while the amount of research in pediatric nursing has gradually increased over the past decades, many gaps in the understanding of the health needs of children and their families remain. Although the focus of nursing research is broad, it is also reductionistic, concentrating on very narrow aspects of the child's health or development without considering system interactions or ecological influences. There is limited use of the evolving research methods of developmental research. Many studies use cross-sectional designs that do not allow for the study of processes over time. Furthermore, measures used with children are often inadequate to capture phenomena of interest in a developmentally appropriate way. More importantly, much of our research is atheoretical or is built on models that are not relevant for children or on developmental models that are narrow or outdated. Thus the ecological aspects of a child's development and health are often ignored. Moreover, too often nursing research is individualistic, in that many nurse researchers do not build on the studies of other researchers. This practice limits the development of a scientific base. It is time, then, to conceptualize and design research with children and their families from a sound developmental perspective.

ROOTS OF THE DEVELOPMENTAL SCIENCE PERSPECTIVE

The developmental science perspective has evolved over the past two decades into a new interdisciplinary framework for the study of human development. As such, developmental science transcends the constructs, methods, and focus of any one discipline. Rather, it involves a synthesis of conceptualizations and methods that are rooted in developmental principles and that are meant to guide work and thinking on development, including biology and social behaviors and their interactions over ontogeny (Magnusson & Cairns, 1996).

The developmental science perspective has roots in embryology, behavioral biology, developmental psychobiology, and comparative psychology (Kuo, 1967; Gottlieb, 1970; Schneirla, 1966), all of which emphasize the importance of the origins of behavior, processes in behavioral change, and bidirectionality (Cairns & Valsiner, 1984; Cairns, 1998; Gottlieb, 1996). Of particular importance is developmental systems theory, adapted from Bertalanffy (1962). Systems theory focuses attention on the child as a complex system of hierarchically organized and functionally interdependent elements. These elements are themselves systems that are characterized by simultaneous interactions of component parts and ongoing mutual feedback within the system, with the interactions functioning to maintain system equilibrium (Thelen, 1990; Thelen & Smith, 1998; Thoman, Acebo, & Becker, 1983; Shoner & Kelso, 1988). In this framework, developmental changes occur through interactions of system elements.

The ecological theory of development of Bronfenbrenner (1989) challenged developmental researchers to move beyond the superficial "social address" model (e.g., treating socioeconomic status, gender, parental education, and so forth as though they explain findings) toward determining broader ecological influences on children, including parents, family, neighborhoods, schools, culture, and public policy (Brooks-Gunn, 1995). Recently renamed the "bioecological model of development," this framework focuses on the interactions of various levels of environmental influences on development (Bronfenbrenner & Morris, 1998). Another influence on the developmental science perspective was life course theory from sociology, which suggests that individual lives are influenced by their ever-changing historical context and which deals with developmental transitions and the social context of development (Elder, 1998). Furthermore, life course theory considers development as a linear progression from conception to death and includes linkages between generations as well as intergenerational effects. The work of Rutter (1983), Werner (Werner & Smith, 1989; Werner, 1990), and others (Haggerty, Sherrod, Garmezy, & Rutter, 1994) was important in stressing the importance of individual differences in vulnerability and resilience. The holistic perspective of Magnusson (1995; Magnusson & Stattin, 1998) and the new person-oriented perspectives on design and analysis (Bergman & Magnusson, 1997) also emphasized the importance of focusing on the individual.

KEY ASSUMPTIONS OF THE DEVELOPMENTAL SCIENCE PERSPECTIVE

A key assumption of developmental science is that human development is complex and reflects the interaction of biological, social, and ecological factors within and without the person over the life course. As noted by Magnusson and Cairns (1996), "Individual functioning depends upon and influences the reciprocal interaction among subsystems within the individual: namely, the organization of interactional perceptual-cognitive, emotional, physiological, morphological, perceptual, and neurobiological factors over time" (p. 15). The developmental science perspective recognizes this complexity of development as the first step toward understanding its coherence. It calls for a holistic research approach that uses complex designs to study systems over time. These designs link phenomena such as gender, behavior, perception, cognition, biology, and biological adaptation. The full range of research designs, including experimental, naturalistic-ethnological, and comparative, are important. However, longitudinal designs are at the heart of developmental research because they accurately reflect the integration of processes within individuals and sequential changes over time (Cairns, 1998; Magnussen, 1995; Wohlwill, 1973). While cross-sectional research designs are economical and appropriate for describing age-related changes, they do not allow for the study of stability and change, patterns operating within subsystems over time, or mechanisms of change.

Furthermore, measures and constructs must be developmentally appropriate and must take into account the changing abilities of the child. An essential component of a developmental design is attention to timing, including the timing of data collection and the time intervals for data collection as related to developmental transitions (Magnusson & Cairns, 1996; Wohlwill, 1973). Attention to timing also extends to the analysis of longitudinal data. The statistical methods used must be appropriate for repeated measures on individuals and must be able to detect developmental change and stability. Longitudinal statistics should allow for the complexity of data collection at multiple time points in order to examine the processes underlying development.

Another approach to design and analysis used in developmental science involves focusing on individuals (Bergman & Magnussen, 1997; Cairns, Bergman, & Kagan, 1998). In traditional variable-oriented research, the focus is on the relationships among variables and comparisons of group means. Person-oriented analysis emphasizes learning more about outliers rather than focusing only on normative development. Research questions and analysis focus on the individual and allow for the study of participants who are at the extreme ends of the continuum, including an exploration of how they develop over time and in different contexts. Thus a person-oriented analysis examines individuals' diverse pathways and outcomes. It calls for a broad array of designs and analytic techniques, including qualitative, in-depth designs as well as quantitative, longitudinal designs that involve grouping individuals with similar profiles according to variables of interest and exploring factors associated with differing profiles.

Individual functioning is also influenced by complex interactions among sociological, biological, genetic, familial, and intergenerational events that occur in specific ecological contexts (Carolina Consortium on Human Development, 1996). The ecology of development must be considered in design because there is a continuously ongoing, reciprocal interaction between an individual and his or her broader environments (Brooks-Gunn, 1995; Magnusson, 1995). Research designs need to integrate events within the individual with the social context and culture. Of utmost importance is the focus on parents and family, including intergenerational aspects of the family, as a critical part of the child's ecology. Additionally, attention must be paid to how socioeconomic status, ethnicity and culture, and characteristics of community influence developmental processes and outcomes.

In summary, developmental science involves an integrated holistic, developmental, and systems-oriented perspective (Magnusson, 1995; Wapner & Demick, 1998). According to this view, the individual is seen as functioning and developing as a total integrated organism; therefore, a focus on a single aspect of development, taken out of context of the whole person, is inadequate. Individual functioning must be considered a dynamic and complex process involving the integration of many factors within the individual, such as mental, biological, and behavioral factors, as well as environmental factors. According to Magnusson (1995), "The individual functions and develops in a continuously ongoing, reciprocal process of interaction with his or her environment" (p. 26). Thus the individual not only is influenced by his environment but also has an influence on that environment. All of these and many other factors operate in a nonlinear, dynamic process that demands a complex conceptual framework and complex research designs to truly understand human development, including health and illness.

IMPLICATIONS FOR NURSING SCIENCE

Developmental science has many implications for nursing research that is focused on the health and illness of infants, children, youth, and their families. Developmental outcomes encompass many aspects of the individual important to nursing science, including morphology and physiology; neurological and cognitive development; and social, behavioral, personality, sexual, and emotional development. Of utmost importance is the systems view of development in which these complex aspects interact with each other and function on multiple levels. This complex, holistic view of development fits with the holistic view of individuals espoused by nursing and thus is important in studies of health-related developmental issues. In fact, health can be operationalized as the state in which children show optimal physiological, physical, cognitive, and psychological development.

Another important aspect of developmental science is the focus on the broader ecological systems in which the individual operates. Thus, ecological factors influencing a child's health, health behaviors, or adaptation to acute and chronic illness include parents, siblings, extended family, peers, schools, and the wider community. Furthermore, the child and his or her ecological system interact with each other. Characteristics such as child gender interactively influence and are influenced by the child's ecology, which in turn influences the child's social, physical, and emotional development. Likewise, a child's response to the diagnosis of cancer is influenced by the ecology of the health care system and by the ecology of the family, particularly parental responses. At the same time, the child's responses to his or her illness and treatments also influence the health care team and parental responses to the child.

Of particular importance is how culture, ethnicity, and socioeconomic factors influence health and development through beliefs, values, and health care access issues. Equally important is how the child and family's culture, ethnicity, and socioeconomic background influence adaptation to acute and chronic illness. There is an urgent need to study how children at various socioeconomic levels and with different cultural backgrounds adapt to acute or chronic illness. Further, intergenerational aspects of health (e.g., family history of heart disease, parental chronic illness), health behaviors (e.g., teen pregnancy or family smoking patterns), and response to illness (e.g., unresolved feelings about the previous death of a child) are important influences that need to be included in studies.

Developmental science has many implications for the design of nursing research with children. Its focus on exploring phenomena and processes over time fits with nursing's concern with fundamental processes related to health and health outcomes across time and place (Pridham, 1998; Walker, 1992). However, simple cross-sectional designs for one point in time are insufficient for understanding the complex interactions of the child and his ecology. Rather, designs informed by complex ecological models and in-depth longitudinal designs are needed to understand the mechanisms that influence children's health and their adaptation to health problems.

The focus on individuals put forth in person-oriented approaches to design and analysis places the individual, rather than the group, at the center of research (Bergman & Magnusson, 1997; Cairns et al., 1998). This approach fits with nursing's concern with the responses and outcomes of individuals. The emphasis is on learning more about individuals, including those who are outliers or extreme in their responses. Such an approach is especially important in understanding individual differences in response to stressors such as poverty and illness and, ultimately, in understanding how person-environment interactions influence vulnerability or resilience (Rutter, 1983). Thus qualitative methods as well as methods using sophisticated cluster analyses and multilevel analyses to examine high-risk samples are important.

An example of the application of developmental science to health-related studies is research on cardiovascular risk in children. Cardiovascular risk involves behaviors such as exercise, smoking, and eating and health parameters such as obesity, blood pressure, and cholesterol levels. In assessing these aspects in a child, one must consider gender; physical development, including height and weight and pubertal level; social development such as peer relationships; physiological changes that affect cholesterol and weight; and aspects of behavioral development that influence risk behaviors (Harrell, Bangdiwala, Deng, Webb, & Bradley, 1998). Further, the bidirectionality of these risks needs to be explored. To be developmentally sound, studies of cardiovascular risks in children and youth also must use a holistic conceptual model that includes ecological factors in the child's environment such as family and peer health behaviors and values and aspects of the school environment such as exercise availability, smoking rules, and school lunch nutrition (Lee & Cubbin, 2002). Intergenerational biological factors, such as familial history of cardiovascular disease, are also important. Longitudinal studies are essential to understand the processes and mechanisms through which these multiple factors interactively influence cardiovascular risk in children.

Developmental and respiratory outcomes of preterm infants with chronic lung disease are another example. Studies of these developmental and health outcomes must include not only infant medical complications but also the child's ecology. For example, parental responses to the neonatal intensive care unit, such as depression and post-traumatic stress disorder, parental stresses and daily hassles, the family constellation, and marital relationships are an important context for an infant's development. Furthermore, the infant's impact on parents also needs to be explored. Intergenerational effects might include how the parents were parented and what parental health behaviors, such as smoking, they follow. Additional ecological factors could include ethnic group, socioeconomic status, and rural versus urban location, because prematurely born children from minority groups and poor families are known to have poorer outcomes (Berlin, Brooks-Gunn, Spiker, & Zaslow, 1995; Brooks-Gunn, Kelbanov, & Duncan, 1996; Engelke, Engelke, Helm, & Holbert, 1995; Vohr et al., 2000). In addition, community supports, such as public health nurses, early intervention, and the quality of child care, are factors influencing outcomes. Moreover, these factors interact with each other; for example, a 700-gm-birthweight, prematurely born boy going home to a single mother who already has three boys and thus wants a girl and who smokes and lives in a polluted urban area would be at increased risk for health and developmental problems.

CRITERIA FOR REVIEW OF RESEARCH FROM A DEVELOPMENTAL SCIENCE PERSPECTIVE

Developmental science, which evolved over decades, has many important implications for the conceptualization and design of nursing research focused on children and their families. As a step toward increasing the application of developmental science in nursing studies of infants, children, youth, and their families, we focused this issue of the *Annual Review of Nursing Research* on an evaluation of the state of nursing research vis-à-vis developmental science. Chapters in this volume include papers summarizing programs of research focused on the care of preterm infants and parenting children with chronic health problems. Chapters also focus on research related to children's health, including physical symptoms in adolescents, symptom experiences in children with cancer, psychosocial adjustment of children with cystic fibrosis, stressors and coping in children with chronic illness, and children's psychological responses to hospitalization. The additional papers focus on siblings of children with chronic illness and disability and on the maternal mental health of mothers parenting children in poverty. The key aspects of developmental science that were considered in this review are outlined below.

1. Conceptualization

We asked the authors in this volume to examine whether or not the research in their reviews used a conceptual or theoretical model that incorporated a holistic view of development. Authors also explored whether there was a focus on gender and maturational changes, and whether the complex nature of the health and development of children was recognized. The authors also determined the extent to which the conceptualization of the research encompassed the ecological and sociocultural context of the child and family, such as community, school, peer group, culture, and ethnicity. The authors examined whether intergenerational influences were considered. Finally, because of the importance of systems theory to developmental science, the authors examined the extent to which the studies used a systems model that encompassed interaction, process, and bidirectionality.

2. Design

We also asked the authors to examine whether the design of the studies they reviewed focused on stability and change in developmental processes and patterns operating within subsystems. Thus the authors examined whether the design was longitudinal and used appropriate longitudinal approaches to analysis. For cross-sectional designs, they determined whether development and processes within development were examined. A related issue was whether attention was paid to the timing of data collection and the timing of developmental transitions. Another point considered was whether broader ecological and cultural issues such as ethnicity, gender, socioeconomic status, and intergenerational effects were measured and examined.

3. Measurement

The volume's authors determined the extent to which the measures, instruments, and other data collection methods were developmentally appropriate and sensitive for the population under study (e.g., infants, children, and/ or youth). They also examined whether the measures and constructs took into account the changing properties of the individual and the social context of development. Another aspect examined was whether the study integrated multilevel measures (e.g., biological, physiological, behavioral, cognitive, emotional, environmental, and contextual). Finally, the authors examined the extent to which there were links between domains of health and development.

4. Data Analysis

We also asked the authors in this volume to determine whether the statistical methods used were appropriate for the understanding of processes and change over time. The use of individual-focused analysis as compared to variable-oriented analytic methods was identified, since person-oriented methods explore processes within individuals better than methods that explore relationships and differences among variables found in groups of individuals.

5. Discussion

Finally, the authors determined whether each study's discussion section incorporated developmental issues and processes. In addition, they examined whether the study investigators pointed out the limitations of the study vis-à-vis developmental processes and whether the need for further more developmentally related research was discussed.

CONCLUSIONS

In summary, developmental science offers a paradigm and method for the study of health and development in infants, children, and adolescents and their families. Cairns et al. (1996) identified five domains of developmental research that can be considered under the rubric of developmental science. These include "the development of human personality and social action, the ontogeny and evolution of behavioral adaptations in nonhuman animals, the development of perception, movement, and language in infants and young children, the development of psychopathology and emotional disorders, and the development of cognitive processes in children and older adults" (p. 223). To date, there is limited use of developmental science in health-related research with children and their families. Therefore, it is time for nurse scholars to become more aware of these advances in developmental research and incorporate them into nursing science related to children's health.

ACKNOWLEDGMENTS

The authors wish to acknowledge support from Grant NR05263, National Institute of Nursing Research, NIH. The authors also wish to acknowledge the mentoring of the late Robert B. Cairns, PhD, Boshamer Professor, Department of Psychology, and Founding Director of the Center for Developmental Science, University of North Carolina at Chapel Hill. We wish to thank Gilbert Gottlieb, PhD, Emeritus Professor, University of North Carolina at Greensboro, and Research Professor, Center for Developmental Science, University of North Carolina at Chapel Hill; and Jaan Valsiner, PhD, Professor, Department of Psychology, Clark University, for their consultation.

REFERENCES

Barnard, K. E. (1983). Nursing research related to infants and young children. In H. H. Werley & J. J. Fitzpatrick (Eds.), *Annual review of nursing research* (Vol. 1, pp. 3–26). New York: Springer.

Barnard, K. E., Morisset, C. E., & Spieker, S. J. (1993). Preventive interventions: Enhancing parent-infant relationship. In C. Zeanah (Ed.), *Handbook on infant mental health* (pp. 386–401). New York: Guilford Press.

Barnard, K. E., & Neal, M. (1977). Maternal-child nursing research. *Nursing Research, 26,* 193–198.

Barnes, C. M., Bandak, A. G., & Beardslee, C. I. (1990). Content analysis of 186 descriptive case studies of hospitalized children. *Maternal-Child Nursing Journal, 19,* 281–296.

Barry, P. D. (1996). *Psychosocial nursing.* Philadelphia, PA: Lippincott-Raven.

Beal, J., & Betz, C. (1992). Intervention studies in pediatric nursing research: A decade of review. *Pediatric Nursing, 18,* 586–590.

Bearison, D. J. (1998). Pediatric psychology and children's medical problems. In I. E. Sigel, K. A. Renninger, & W. Damon (Eds.), *Handbook of child psychology:*

Vol. 4. Child psychology in practice (5th ed., pp. 635–711). New York: John Wiley.

Becker, P. (2001). Contexts and systems in studies of maternal and child health. *Research in Nursing and Health, 24,* 155–156.

Bergman, L. R., & Magnusson, D. (1997). A person-oriented approach in research on developmental psychopathology. *Development and Psychopathology, 9,* 291–319.

Berlin, L. J., Brooks-Gunn, J., Spiker, D., & Zaslow, M. J. (1995). Examining observational measures of emotional support and cognitive stimulation in black and white mothers of preschoolers. *Journal of Family Issues, 16*(5), 664–686.

Bertalanffy, L. von (1962). *Modern theories of development: An introduction to theoretical biology* (J. H. Woodger, Trans.). New York: Harper. (Originally published in 1933.)

Blake, F. (1954). *The child, his parents and the nurse.* Philadelphia: J. B. Lippincott.

Blake, F. (1964). *Family-centered pediatric nursing care.* Columbus, OH: Ross Laboratories.

Bowlby, J. (1958). The nature of a child's ties to his mother. *International Journal of Psychoanalysis, 39,* 350–373.

Brodie, B. (1986). Impact of doctoral programs on nursing education. *Journal of Professional Nursing, 2,* 350–357.

Bronfenbrenner, U. (1989). Ecological systems theory. *Annals of Child Development, 6,* 185–246.

Bronfenbrenner, U., & Morris, P. A. (1998). The ecology of developmental processes. In R. M. Lerner & W. Damon (Eds.), *Handbook of child psychology: Vol. I. Theoretical models of human development* (5th ed., pp. 993–1028). New York: John Wiley.

Brooks-Gunn, J. (1995). Children in families in communities: Risk and intervention in the Bronfenbrenner tradition. In P. Moen, G. H. Elder, & K. Luscher (Eds.), *Examining lives in context* (pp. 467–522). Washington, DC: American Psychological Association.

Brooks-Gunn, J., Kelbanov, P. K., & Duncan, G. J. (1996). Ethnic differences in children's intelligence test scores: Role of economic deprivation, home environment, and maternal characteristics. *Child Development, 67,* 396–408.

Broome, M., Knafl, K., Pridham, K., & Feetham, S. (Eds.). (1998). *Children and families: State of the science in nursing.* Newbury Park, CA: Sage.

Broome, M. E., Woodring, B., & O'Connor-Von, S. (1996). Research priorities for the nursing of children and their families: A Delphi study. *Journal of Pediatric Nursing, 11,* 281–287.

Cairns, R. B. (1998). The making of developmental psychology. In R. M. Lerner & W. Damon (Eds.), *Handbook of child psychology: Vol. I. Theoretical models of human development* (5th ed., pp. 25–106). New York: John Wiley.

Cairns, R. B. (2000). Developmental science: Three audacious implications. In L. R. Bergman, R. B. Cairns, L. Nilsson, & L. Nystedt (Eds.), *Developmental science and the holistic approach* (pp. 49–72). Mahway, NJ: Lawrence Erlbaum.

Cairns, R. B., Bergman, L. R., & Kagan, J. (1998). *Methods and models for studying the individual.* Thousand Oaks, CA: Sage.

Cairns, R. B., Elder, G. H., & Costello, E. J. (1996). The making of developmental science. In R. B. Cairns, G. H. Elder, & E. J. Costello (Eds.), *Developmental science* (pp. 223–234). New York: Cambridge University Press.

Cairns, R. B., & Valsiner, J. (1984). Child psychology. *Annual Review of Psychology, 35,* 553–577.

Carolina Consortium on Human Development. (1996). Developmental science: A collaborative statement. In R. B. Cairns, G. H. Elder, & E. J. Costello (Eds.), *Developmental science* (pp. 1–6). New York: Cambridge University Press.

Craft-Rosenberg, M., Krajicek, M. J., & Shin, D. (2002). Report of the American Academy of Nursing Child-Family Expert Panel: Identification of quality and outcome indicators for maternal child nursing. *Nursing Outlook, 50,* 57–60.

Denyes, M. (1983). Nursing research related to school age children and adolescents. In H. Werley & J. Fitzpatrick (Eds.), *Annual review of nursing research* (Vol. 1, pp. 27–43). New York: Springer.

Elder, G. H. (1998). The life course as developmental theory. *Child Development, 69,* 1–12.

Engelke, S. C., Engelke, M. K., Helm, J. M., & Holbert, D. (1995). Cognitive failure to thrive in high-risk infants: The importance of the psychosocial environment. *Journal of Perinatology, 15,* 325–329.

Erickson, F. (1965). The nurse in modern pediatrics. *International Journal of Nursing Studies, 2,* 139–144.

Erickson, F. H. (1958). Play interviews for four-year-old hospitalized children. *Monographs of the Society for Research in Child Development, 23,* 1–69.

Fagan, C. M. (1966). *The effects of maternal attendance during hospitalization on the posthospital behavior of young children.* Philadelphia: F. A. Davis.

Faux, S. A. (1998). Historical overview of responses of children and their families to chronic illness. In M. E. Broome, K. Knafl, K. Pridham, & S. Feetham (Eds.), *Children and families in health and illness* (pp. 179–195). Thousand Oaks, CA: Sage.

Gottlieb, G. (1970). Conceptions of prenatal behavior. In L. R. Aronson, E. Tobach, D. S. Lehrman, & J. S. Rosenblatt (Eds.), *Development and evolution of behavior* (pp. 111–137). San Francisco, CA: W. H. Freeman.

Gottlieb, G. (1996). A systems view of psychobiological development. In D. Magnusson (Ed.), *Individual development over the lifespan: Biological and psychosocial perspectives* (pp. 76–103). New York: Cambridge University Press.

Grey, M. (1998). Integrative review of assessment models for health promotion of children and their families. In M. E. Broome, K. Knafl, K. Pridham, & S. Feetham (Eds.), *Children and families in health and illness* (pp. 15–55). Thousand Oaks, CA: Sage.

Haggerty, R. J., Sherrod, L. R., Garmezy, N., & Rutter, M. (1994). *Stress, risk, and resilience in children and adolescents: Processes, mechanisms, and interventions.* New York: Cambridge University Press.

Harrell, J. S., Bangdiwala, S. I., Deng, S., Webb, J. P., & Bradley, C. (1998). Smoking initiation in youth: The roles of gender, race, socioeconomics, and developmental status. *Journal of Adolescent Health, 23,* 271–279.

Hayman, L. L. (1998). Integrative review of intervention models for health promotion for children and families. In M. E. Broome, K. Knafl, K. Pridham, & S. Feetham (Eds.), *Children and families in health and illness* (pp. 56–79). Thousand Oaks, CA: Sage.

Hinds, P., Norville, R., Anthony, L., Briscoe, B., Gattuso, J., Quargnenti, A., et al. (1990). Pediatric cancer nursing research priorities: A Delphi study. *Journal of Pediatric Oncology Nursing, 7,* 51–52.

Holditch-Davis, D., & Miles, M. S. (1997). Parenting the prematurely born child. In J. J. Fitzpatrick & J. Norbeck (Eds.), *Annual review of nursing research* (Vol. 15, pp. 3–34). New York: Springer.

Kuo, Z-Y. (1967). *The dynamics of behavioral development: An epigenetic view.* New York: Random House.

Lee, R. E., & Cubbin, C. (2002). Neighborhood context and youth cardiovascular health behaviors. *American Journal of Public Health, 92,* 428–436.

Lipman, T. H., & Hayman, L. L. (2000). Pediatric nursing research: A 25-year review—1976–2000. *MCN: American Journal of Maternal-Child Nursing, 25,* 331–335.

Magnusson, D. (1995). Individual development: A holistic, integrated model. In P. Moen, G. H. Elder, & K. Luscher (Eds.), *Examining lives in context* (pp. 19–60). Washington, DC: American Psychological Association.

Magnusson, D., & Cairns, R. B. (1996). Developmental science: Toward a unified framework. In R. B. Cairns, G. H. Elder, & E. J. Costello (Eds.), *Developmental science* (pp. 7–30). New York: Cambridge University Press.

Magnusson, D., & Stattin, H. (1998). Person-context interaction theories. In R. M. Lerner & W. Damon (Eds.), *Handbook of child psychology: Vol. I. Theoretical models of human development* (5th ed., pp. 685–760). New York: John Wiley.

Miles, M. S. (1996). A historical perspective on the Society of Pediatric Nurses. *Journal of the Society of Pediatric Nurses, 1,* 46–47.

Moore, M. L. (2000). Perinatal nursing research: A 25-year review—1976–2000. *MCN: American Journal of Maternal-Child Nursing, 25,* 305–310.

Mussen, P. H. (Ed.) (1983). *Handbook of child psychology* (4th ed.). New York: Wiley.

Pridham, K. F. (1998). Implications for practice, education, and research in health promotion of children and their families. In M. E. Broome, K. Knafl, K. Pridham, & S. Feetham (Eds.), *Children and families in health and illness* (pp. 80–96). Thousand Oaks, CA: Sage.

Prugh, D. G., Staub, E. M., Sands, H. H., Kirschbaum, R. M., & Lenihan, E. A. (1953). A study of the emotional reactions of children and families to hospitalization and illness. *American Journal of Orthopsychiatry, 23,* 700–106.

Robertson, J. (1958). *Young children in hospitals.* New York: Basic Books.

Rutter, M. (1983). Stress, coping and development: Some issues and some questions. In N. Garmezy & M. Rutter (Eds.), *Stress, coping, and development in children* (pp. 1–41). New York: McGraw-Hill.

Schneirla, T. C. (1966). Behavioral development and comparative psychology. *Quarterly Review of Biology, 41,* 283–302.

Shoner, G., & Kelso, J. A. S. (1988). Dynamic pattern generation in behavioral and neural systems. *Science, 239,* 1513–1520.

Stewart, I. (1929). The science and art of nursing [editorial]. *Nursing Education Bulletin, 2,* 107–137.

Thelen, E. (1990). Dynamical systems and the generation of individual differences. In J. Colombo & J. Fagen (Eds.), *Individual differences in infancy: Reliability, stability, prediction* (pp. 19–43). Hillsdale, NJ: Erlbaum.

Thelen, E., & Smith, L. B. (1998). Dynamic systems theories. In R. M. Lerner & W. Damon (Eds.), *Handbook of child psychology: Vol. I. Theoretical models of human development* (5th ed., pp. 563–634). New York: John Wiley.

Thoman, E. B., Acebo, C., & Becker, P. T. (1983). Infant crying and stability in the mother-infant relationship: A systems analysis. *Child Development, 54,* 653–659.

Vessey, J. A. (1998). Historical overview of responses of children and their families to acute illness. In M. E. Broome, K. Knafl, K. Pridham, & S. Feetham (Eds.), *Children and families in health and illness* (pp. 99–114). Thousand Oaks, CA: Sage.

Visintainer, M. A., & Wolfer, J. A. (1975). Pediatric surgical patients' and parents' stress responses and adjustment as a function of psychological preparation and stress-point nursing care. *Nursing Research, 24,* 24–255.

Vohr, B. R., Wright, L. L., Dusick, A. M., Mele, L., Verter, J., Steichen, J. J., et al. (2000). Neurodevelopmental and functional outcomes of extremely low birth weight infants in the National Institute of Child Health and Development Neonatal Research Network, 1993–1994. *Pediatrics, 105,* 1216–1226.

Walker, L. (1992). *Parent-infant nursing science.* Philadelphia: F. A. Davis.

Wapner, S., & Demick, J. (1998). Developmental analysis: A holistic, developmental, systems-oriented perspective. In R. M. Lerner & W. Damon (Eds.), *Handbook of child psychology: Vol. I. Theoretical models of human development* (5th ed., pp. 761–800). New York: John Wiley.

Werner, E. E. (1990). Protective factors and individual resilience. In S. J. Meisels & J. P. Shankoff (Eds.), *Handbook of early childhood intervention* (pp. 97–116). Cambridge, England: Cambridge University Press.

Werner, E. E., & Smith, R. S. (1989). *Vulnerable but invincible: A longitudinal study of resilient children and youth.* New York: Adams-Banister-Cox.

Wohlwill, J. F. (1973). *The study of behavioral development.* New York: Academic Press.

PART I

Preterm Infants

Chapter 2

Care of Preterm Infants: Programs of Research and Their Relationship to Developmental Science

DIANE HOLDITCH-DAVIS AND BETH PERRY BLACK

ABSTRACT

The purpose of this review was to examine the topics covered in current programs of nursing research on the care of the preterm infant and to determine the extent to which this research is informed by developmental science. A researcher was considered to have a current program of research if he or she had at least five publications published since 1990 and was the first author on at least three of them. The infants in a study could be any age from birth throughout childhood; studies focusing on parenting, nursing, or other populations of infants were not included.

Seventeen nurse researchers had current programs of research in this area. These programs had four themes. Those of Becker, Evans, Pridham, Shiao, and Zahr focused on infant responses to the neonatal intensive care unit (NICU) environment and treatments. Franck, Johnston, and Stevens focused on pain management. Harrison, Ludington-Hoe, and White-Traut's research focused on infant stimulation. Holditch-Davis, McCain, McGrath, Medoff-Cooper, Schraeder, and Youngblut studied infant behavior and development.

These research programs had many strengths, including strong interdisciplinary focus and clinical relevance. However, additional emphasis is needed on the care of the critically ill infant. Also, despite the fact that the preterm infant's neurological system develops rapidly over the first year, only three of these researchers used a developmental science perspective. Only research on infant behavior and development focused on the developmental changes that the infants were experiencing. Most of the studies were longitudinal, but many did not use statistics appropriate for identifying stability and change over time. The response of individual infants and the broader ecological context as evidenced by factors such as gender, ethnic group, culture, and intergenerational effects were rarely examined. Thus research on the care of preterm infants could be expanded if the developmental science perspective formed the basis of more studies.

Research on the care of preterm infants refutes the frequent criticism that nursing lacks programs of research. Nurses have developed strong research programs in this area that date back to the late 1970s and early 1980s (Anderson & Vidyasagur, 1979; Barnard & Bee, 1983). From the beginning, these programs have involved interdisciplinary collaborations (e.g., Anderson & Vidyasagur, 1979) and have been published in interdisciplinary outlets as well as in nursing journals (e.g., Blackburn & Barnard, 1985). Their number has continued to grow over the years. By the late 1990s, Medoff-Cooper and Holditch-Davis (1999) identified at least 13 programs of research on preterm infants.

At the same time that these programs were being established, a new perspective, that of developmental science, was becoming accepted in the field of child development. According to this perspective (Cairns, Elder, & Costello, 1996; Zeanah, Boris, & Larrieu, 1997), children develop in a continuous, ongoing, reciprocal interaction with their environment (Gottlieb, 1996; Magnusson, 1995). The child and social environment form a complex system consisting of elements that are themselves systems, such as the mother and child. The various elements interact together so that the total system shows less variability than the individual elements (Thoman, Acebo, & Becker, 1983). The child is an active participant, constantly changing the environment while being influenced by it. Subsystems within the child, such as physiological processes, temperament, and medical complications, affect the overall system and in turn are affected by it. Interactions, rather than causation, are the focus of this perspective. Since interactions between elements are simultaneous and bidirectional, no action of one element can be said to cause the action of another. Research using a developmental science perspective also emphasizes identifying developmental patterns; examining stability and change in phenomena over time; identifying processes underlying development; determining the effects of the broader ecological context, including culture, gender, ethnicity, socioeconomic status, and multiple generations; and studying developmental processes within individuals.

This holistic perspective provides a particularly useful framework for nursing research on preterm infants, one that is compatible with most frameworks currently being used in nursing. Its explicit focus on developmental change is important for research conducted in the preterm period, when the infant's neurological system is developing rapidly. In addition, the focus on bidirectional relationships and complex interactions between the child and his or her environment provides an appropriate framework for studies of the long-term developmental outcomes of prematurely born children, a major area of nursing research.

The purpose of this review was to examine the topics covered in current and ongoing programs of nursing research on the care of the preterm infant. In particular, we examined the nurse researchers with programs of research in this area, the topics covered in their studies, and the extent to which these programs have been informed by the developmental science perspective. The focus was on entire programs of research, rather than single papers, since the complex developmental perspective is unlikely to be fully explicated in a single paper.

METHOD

CINAHL and MEDLINE were searched to identify nursing research (database-based) written since 1990 on the care of preterm infants. The initial search was limited to studies published since 1990 so that only current programs would be included. Special attention was paid to authors with two or more first-author citations in the Medoff-Cooper and Holditch-Davis (1999) review. Studies that examined other infants as well as preterms were included if preterms made up more than half the sample or were an identifiable subgroup. The infants in the study could be any age from birth throughout childhood. Clinical case studies, research reviews, abstracts, theoretical articles, and articles focusing on parenting or health care providers (such as studies that used infant characteristics only to relate to parental outcomes or studies of nursing roles) were excluded. Articles on parental-infant interactions were included if infant behaviors were examined.

For a researcher to be considered as having a current program of research, that researcher had to have at least five publications related to the care of preterm infants published since 1990 and had to be the first author on at least three of these articles. If two authors published together extensively, they were considered to have separate programs of research if each had at least five first-authored articles. Papers coauthored by more than one researcher in this area were listed as part of the first author's program of research. Once a program of research was identified, further searches (including searches of author self-citations) were made on the specific author to identify older research studies. These older studies were included in this review. However, studies focusing on other topics, including parenting or other populations of infants, were not included.

These studies were reviewed to determine the extent to which the study conceptualizations incorporated a developmental science perspective, whether complex interactions between the child and the social and physical environment or biology were considered, whether the research designs were longitudinal, whether the analysis strategies focused on stability and change over time, whether rationales were presented for the timing of data collection, whether the measures were appropriate and sensitive for the study of developing preterm infants, whether there was an emphasis on the broader ecological context (as shown by cultural, gender, socioeconomic, and intergenerational effects), and whether there was evidence of interdisciplinary collaboration.

RESULTS

The literature searches identified 17 nurse researchers with current programs of research on the care of preterm infants. The primary focus of each researcher's program was identified, and researchers were then grouped with other researchers with similar foci. Programs on the care of preterms were found to have four themes: the neonatal intensive care unit (NICU) environment and treatments, pain, infant stimulation, and infant behavior and development.

NICU Environment and Treatments

Five nurse researchers—Jane Evans, Lina Zahr, Shyang-Yun Pamela Shiao, Karen Pridham, and Patricia Becker—had programs of research on the NICU environment. This research focused on the responses of preterms to the NICU environment and medical treatments and interventions to modify the NICU to make it more appropriate for infants. Nurse researchers whose studies focused on descriptions of the NICU are presented before researchers who focused on intervention studies.

JANE EVANS

Jane Evans examined the effects of NICU nursing care on preterms in the first three days of life. She found that weighing, tape removal, and repositioning were associated with hypoxemia and bradycardia (Evans, 1991; Evans, McCartney, & Roth-Sautter, 2000). In response to painful procedures, infants showed negative facial expressions, mouth opening, brow furrowing, hand clenching, muscle rigidity, and moving away, and all but the youngest and sickest preterms cried (Vogelpohl, Evans, & Cedargren, 1995). Similar responses were seen in infants receiving procedures, such as repositioning and intravenous medications, not known to be painful (Evans, Vogelpohl, Bourguignon, & Morcott, 1997). Evans (1992) also found that increasing the FiO_2 prior to suctioning and ventilating with 100% O_2 during suctioning eliminated apnea and bradycardia and reduced the incidence of hypoxia but did not increase blood pressure occurring during suctioning.

Evans's studies examined second-to-second changes in behavioral and physiological responses but did not use a developmental science perspective. Her conceptualizations generally assumed linear causation, rather than a systems perspective. Interactions between infants and the physical environment were not considered. No study used a longitudinal design, and the effect of development on behavior and physiological patterns was not explored except in one study comparing the responses of infants of different gestational ages (Evans et al., 2000). All studies used grouped data, although three presented the responses of individuals descriptively (Evans, 1991; Evans et al., 1997; Vogelpohl et al., 1995). Participants were of various socioeconomic, ethnic, and gender groups, but no analyses examined the effects of these groups. Finally, intergenerational effects were not considered, and the studies did not involve interdisciplinary collaboration.

LINA ZAHR

Lina Zahr's recent research has focused on describing the effects of the NICU environment. She found that preterms change sleep-wake states about six times per hour, and most changes were related to nursing interventions or NICU noise (Zahr & Balian, 1995). Noise and nursing interventions resulted in heart rate increases, oxygen saturation decreases, or respiration rate increases in over a third of infants. She compared the NICU environment in the United States and Lebanon and found that infants in Lebanon experienced less noise and fewer nursing interventions and thus had fewer negative changes in physiological parameters and sleep-wake states (Zahr, 1998). However, the U.S. infants were smaller and sicker than the ones in Lebanon.

In earlier reports, Zahr examined a modification of Als's system (Als et al., 1986) to provide developmental care and teach low-income African American mothers about their preterm infants' behaviors (Parker, Zahr, Cole, & Brecht, 1992; Zahr, Parker, & Cole, 1992). Control infants received developmental care without maternal involvement. The experimental infants scored higher on the Bayley mental scale at 4 and 8 months and on the Bayley motor scale at 4 months (Parker et al., 1992; Zahr et al., 1992). Infant temperament was the most important predictor of mother-infant interaction quality at 4 and 8 months (Zahr, 1991). At 4 months, mothers interacted more favorably with infants who were less dull, were more adaptable, and had higher birthweights. At 8 months, mothers interacted more favorably with difficult infants than with infants with easier temperaments.

The conceptualizations of these studies were primarily empirically based, although one study used Als's (1986) synactive theory (Zahr & Balian, 1995). Zahr did not use a developmental science perspective, but her studies considered interactions between the child and the social environment. Two studies considered interactions between child and the physical environment, specifically noise (Zahr, 1998; Zahr & Balian, 1995), and one examined interactions between behaviors and the biological variable of birthweight (Zahr et al., 1992). Her three maternal intervention studies were longitudinal, but only one of them used repeated measures statistics (Zahr et al., 1992), and no rationale was provided for the timing of data collection. Two studies were interdisciplinary and involved physician and psychologist collaborators (Parker et al., 1992: Zahr et al., 1992). Despite having participants of different ethnic groups and two cross-cultural studies (Zahr, 1998; Zahr & Balian, 1995), cultural and intergenerational effects were not examined in any of her studies.

SHYANG-YUN PAMELA SHIAO

Shyang-Yun Pamela Shiao has investigated the physiological effects of oral feedings with nasogastric tubes in place. Nasogastric tubes were found to interfere with breathing and sucking, resulting in lower tidal volumes (Shiao, 1995; Shiao, Brooker, & DiFiore, 1996; Shiao, Youngblut, Anderson, DiFiore, & Martin, 1995). In addition, infants fed in the morning fed less effectively and showed poorer coordination of sucking and swallowing (Shiao, 1995). Periods of continuous sucking had more negative effects on breathing and sucking, but more formula intake, than periods with intermittent sucking (Shiao, 1997). Infants with desaturation events during feeding took longer to make the transition to full oral feedings (Shiao et al., 1996). In a meta-analysis, Shiao, Chang, Lannon, and Yarandi (1997) found that non-nutritive sucking led to lower heart rates and higher oxygenation during painful procedures and when done without other stimulation. This effect was greater for preterm infants than for fullterms. Shiao (2002) found that arterial oxygen saturation was more accurate in identifying desaturation events than pulse oximetry. Shiao, Andrews, and Ahn (2002) found that Apgar scores, pregnancy-induced hypertension, gestational age, and resuscitation predicted intubation of high-risk infants, but only gestational age and congenital defects predicted the complications of oxygen therapy.

Shiao's studies have contributed to the knowledge of infant physiological responses. These studies were empirically based and lacked a developmental focus or systems conceptualization. In the study comparing morning and afternoon effects on feeding, Shiao did not cite the literature on circadian effects (Shiao, 1995). The studies were not longitudinal, with the exception of Shiao (2002), and cultural, ethnic group, and intergenerational effects were not examined. Gender effects were examined in Shiao et al. (2002). Shiao did have several collaborators, including an engineer and a physician.

KAREN PRIDHAM

Karen Pridham's research has focused primarily on feeding and growth in preterm infants. In a series of studies using medical record reviews, she found that the age when infants with bronchopulmonary dysplasia (BPD) first received nipple feedings was affected by weight, gestational age, and respiratory treatments (Pridham, Sondel, Change, & Green, 1993) and that transition time to nipple feedings was affected by birthweight, the length of tube feeding, and history of apnea and BPD (Pridham et al., 1998). During enteral feedings, very-low-birthweight infants showed stable growth rates, intake of micronutrients, and ratio of carbon dioxide produced to oxygen consumed (Steward & Pridham, 2001). Infants weighing less than 1,000 gm at birth showed decreasing weight percentiles over the period of hospitalization as compared to fetal growth, and infants who took longer to regain their birthweight had a greater loss of percentiles

(Steward & Pridham, 2002). Over the first year, premature infants weighed less than fullterms but grew at the same rate, and girls weighed less and grew more slowly than boys (Pridham, Brown, Sondel, Clark, & Green, 2001). Maternal and infant negative behaviors during feeding related to increased weight growth, whereas illness severity was related to slower growth. Pridham also compared demand nipple feedings with standard nipple feedings. Infants had higher caloric and fluid intake on standard feedings, but the difference decreased over the 5 days of the study (Pridham et al., 1999; Pridham, Kosorok, et al., 2001). On a different topic, Pridham, Becker, and Brown (2000) found that mothers provided more attention-supporting behaviors for 8-month-old premature infants who were exploring toys than they did to fullterms, and that more maternal attention-directing was associated with less infant toy exploration.

Pridham's research was primarily empirically based, although two studies used the transactional model (Pridham et al., 2000; Pridham, Brown, et al., 2001). Her studies included interactions between biology (morbidity and gestational age) and behavior, and two examined interactions between the child and the social environment (Pridham et al., 2000; Pridham, Brown, et al., 2001). However, she did not examine interactions between the child and the physical environment or bidirectional relationships. Her demand feeding studies viewed the infant as affecting the environment. Processes underlying development were studied (Pridham et al., 1998, 2000; Pridham, Brown, et al., 2001; Steward & Pridham, 2001). Her studies were longitudinal, and five used statistical methods appropriate for identifying change over time (Pridham et al., 1998, 1999; Pridham, Brown, et al., 2001; Pridham, Kosorok, et al., 2001; Steward & Pridham, 2001). Yet no study had individual-focused analyses, and no rationales were provided for data collection timing, except in Pridham et al. (2000). The author examined ethnic effects in three studies (Pridham et al., 1998, 1999, 2001) and gender effects in all studies except Steward and Pridham (2001). She did not examine socioeconomic or intergenerational effects. She had interdisciplinary collaborators from medicine, psychology, statistics, and nutrition.

Patricia Becker

Patricia Becker has studied modifying the NICU environment using a version of Als's intervention system for preterm infants (Als et al., 1986). She found improvements in morbidity, higher oxygen saturations, fewer disorganized movements, and more alertness during nursing care in infants receiving the intervention than in controls, but she did not find differences in sleep-wake behaviors at hospital discharge (Becker, 1995; Becker, Grunwald, Moorman, & Stuhr, 1991, 1993). Becker also found that infants receiving developmental handling slept more and had smaller decreases in respiration rate and oxygenation, smaller increases in heart rate, fewer movements, and fewer disorganized movements than infants receiving traditional handling (Becker, 1995; Becker, Brazy, & Grunwald, 1997; Becker, Grunwald, & Brazy, 1997).

Becker's studies used a developmental science perspective (Becker et al., 1997), especially in the conceptualizations of brain-environment interactions by Black and Greenough (1986) and Als (1986). Her studies all included interactions between the social environment and the child, and most examined interactions between the child and the physical environment (Becker, 1995; Becker et al., 1991, 1993) and between biology (morbidity and gestational age) and behavior (Becker et al., 1991, 1993, 1997). Processes underlying development were conceptualized though not studied (Becker, 1995; Becker et al., 1991, 1993, 1997). All studies were longitudinal and, with the exception of Becker et al. (1991), used statistical methods appropriate for identifying change over time, but none had individual-focused analyses. No rationales were provided for the timing of data collection. Her samples were primarily white, and she did not examine ethnic, cultural, gender-based, or intergenerational effects. She had interdisciplinary collaborators from medicine, occupational therapy, and statistics.

Pain Management

Three nurse researchers—C. Celeste Johnston, Bonnie Stevens, and Linda Franck—have studied pain management in preterm infants. These researchers have collaborated extensively, but each has enough first-authored studies to qualify as having a separate program of research.

C. CELESTE JOHNSTON

C. Celeste Johnston's research has focused on pain in preterms. She found that preterms' heart rates and behaviors differed when preterms were reacting to real and sham painful procedures (Johnston, Stevens, Yang, & Horton, 1995). Sucrose-flavored pacifiers were more effective than plain pacifiers in reducing crying by fullterms and preterms during blood drawing, heelsticks, and circumcision, and repeated doses of sucrose were more effective than a single dose (Johnston, Stevens, et al., 1999; Johnston, Stremler, Horton, & Friedman, 1999; Johnston, Stremler, Stevens, & Horton, 1997). The number of cries of preterms differed in those receiving heelsticks without and with pacifiers, but cry duration and frequency did not differ (Johnston, Sherraud, et al., 1999). Rocking did not reduce the frequency of negative facial expressions in response to heelsticks, but it increased the amount of quiet sleep (Johnston et al., 1997). Responses to pain tended to become more obvious as infants matured, but infants who were born at younger gestational ages and thus had more time in the NICU had less mature responses to pain than infants of similar postconceptional ages born at later gestational ages (Johnston & Stevens, 1996). Young preterm infants who were asleep at the beginning of a painful procedure and had recently undergone a painful procedure were the most likely to show only minimal behavioral responses to painful procedures (Johnston, Stevens, et al., 1999; Johnston, Stevens, Yang, & Horton, 1996). A survey of Canadian NICUs indicated that pain management was done primarily for surgical pain, with little done for procedural pain (Johnston, Collinge, Henderson, & Anand, 1997). Opioids were the most frequently given pain medication.

Johnston's research was primarily empirically based, although one study used Als's (1986) synactive theory (Johnston, Stevens, et al., 1999). Her studies included interactions between infants and the social environment and multifactorial causation. Four examined interactions between biology (gestational age, medical complications) and behaviors (Johnston et al., 1995, 1996; Johnston, Stremler, et al., 1997; Johnson & Stevens, 1996), but none included interactions with the physical environment. Only one had a developmental focus, longitudinal design, and repeated measures statistics (Johnston et al., 1996). No rationale for the timing of data collection was presented in any study. Johnston's studies did not give the ethnic background of participants or test for ethnic group, socioeconomic, or intergenerational effects. One examined gender effects (Johnston et al., 1996). All analyses were group-oriented. The author had collaborators from public health, statistics, and medicine (Johnston et al., 1996; Johnston, Collinge, et al., 1997; Johnston, Stevens, et al., 1999).

BONNIE STEVENS

Bonnie Stevens's research has focused on measuring pain responses of preterm infants. In response to painful procedures, such as heelsticks, she found that preterm infants showed mouth opening, brow furrowing, grimacing, muscle rigidity, and moving away (Stevens, Johnston, & Horton, 1993) and that heart rates and intracranial pressure increased and oxygenation decreased (Stevens & Johnston, 1994; Stevens et al., 1993). All but the youngest and sickest infants were likely to cry (Stevens et al., 1993). Older preterms who had not recently experienced another painful procedure and were awake were the most likely to show behavioral responses to pain (Stevens, Johnston, & Horton, 1994). Based on these results, Stevens developed a pain assessment tool, the Premature Infant Pain Profile (PIPP) (Ballantyne, Stevens, McAllister, Dionne, & Jack, 1999; Stevens, Johnston, Petryshen, & Taddio, 1996). This assessment has only been validated for procedural pain. Using the PIPP, Walden et al. (2001) found that infants as young as 27 weeks showed behavioral responses, increases in heart rate, and decreases in respiration rate and oxygen saturation to heelsticks. No developmental changes in these responses occurred between 27 and 32 weeks post conceptional age (PCA). Pacifiers with and without sucrose were more effective in reducing responses to heelsticks than prone positioning (Stevens, Johnston, Franck, et al., 1999). EMLA cream was safe for preterms, but it did not affect responses to heelsticks (Stevens, Johnston, Taddio, et al., 1999). On a different topic, Stevens, Petryshen, Hawkins, Smith, and Taylor (1996) found that developmental care using a version of Als's (1986) protocol did not change the outcomes of preterms but did increase immediate physiological stability.

Stevens used a variety of conceptualizations, including those that were empirically based (Stevens et al., 1993; Stevens & Johnston, 1994; Stevens, Johnston, et al., 1996; Stevens, Johnston, Taddio, et al., 1999), the gate control theory (Stevens et al., 1994), and the synactive theory (Ballantyne et al., 1999; Stevens, Petryshen, et al., 1996; Stevens, Johnston, Franck, et al., 1999; Walden et al., 2001). Only two studies used a systems conceptualization that included multifactorial causation (Stevens, Johnston, et al., 1999; Stevens, Petryshen, et al., 1996). All studies considered interactions between infants and the social environment, although only two considered interactions between the infant and the physical environment (Stevens, Petryshen, et al., 1996; Walden et al., 2001) or between biology (illness severity) and behaviors (Stevens & Johnston, 1994; Stevens, Johnston, Franck, et al., 1999). Two examined development and were longitudinal (Stevens, Petryshen, et al., 1996; Walden et al., 2001), but only Stevens, Petryshen, et al. (1996) used longitudinal statistics. The PIPP was designed to minimize developmental differences. This design feature may be appropriate for clinical use but has limited use in research. Otherwise, the author's measures were appropriate for developing preterms, but no study presented a rationale for the timing of data collection. Her studies did not give the ethnic background of the participants nor test for ethnic group, socioeconomic, gender, or intergenerational effects. No individual-focused analyses were done. Stevens had collaborators from statistics, medicine, and pharmacy (Stevens, Johnston, et al., 1996; Stevens, Johnston, Franck, et al., 1999; Stevens, Johnston, Taddio, et al., 1999; Stevens, Petryshen, et al., 1996).

LINDA FRANCK

Linda Franck has examined infant responses to pain and other NICU experiences. She found that the first dose of morphine after patent ductus ligation had minimal effects on plasma norepinephrine levels, vagal tone, or flexor reflex threshold, possibly because of residual anesthesia (Franck, Boyce, et al., 2000). In a survey of NICUs, Franck (1987) found that nurses used changes in infant behaviors to identify pain and to decide when to administer analgesia and that they used nine different comfort measures to soothe infants. Bathing preterm infants as infrequently as every fourth day was not associated with an increase in pathogen colonization (Franck, Quinn, & Zahr, 2000). Removal of hydrophilic gel caused less damage to preterm infants' skin than did plastic tape or a pectin barrier (Lund et al., 1997). Intubated preterms weighing less than 1,200 gm or less than 30 weeks old tolerated only 20 to 30 minutes of skin-to-skin holding by their mothers (Gale, Franck, & Lund, 1993). In a survey of NICUs, Franck, Bernal, and Gale (2002) found that virtually all allow conventional holding and almost 75% permit skin-to-skin holding.

Franck's studies were empirically based and did not use a developmental science perspective. Only one study examined interactions, those between biology and behaviors (Franck, Boyce, et al., 2000). Two used short-term longitudinal designs (Franck, Quinn, et al., 2000; Lund et al., 1997), but only descriptive analyses were presented. No study presented individually focused analyses. The participants were of various ethnic, socioeconomic, and gender groups, but no analyses examined the effects of these groups or multigenerations. The author had interdisciplinary collaborators from medicine and statistics (Franck, Boyce, et al., 2000; Lund et al., 1997).

Infant Stimulation

Three researchers—Lynda Law Harrison, Susan Ludington-Hoe, and Rosemary White-Traut—have programs of research focusing on infant stimulation, specifically, testing interventions that provide social stimulation that is missing in the technological NICU environment.

Lynda Law Harrison

Lynda Law Harrison's research focuses on describing the effects of touch on preterm infants. In a series of reports, Harrison videotaped mothers, fathers, and grandmothers touching their preterm infants during the first 2 weeks of life. Family members used 14 types of touches; holding, stroking, and contact were the most common (Harrison & Woods, 1991). Mothers spent the most time touching the infant, and fathers the least. The touch addressed to boys and girls showed few differences, but boys were held more. Infants younger than 28 weeks experienced less touch than older infants. Oxygen saturation was lower during parental touching, but only rarely was the decrease clinically significant (Harrison, Leeper, & Yoon, 1990). Heart rate was not affected. Infant gestational age had the greatest effect on oxygen saturation; birthweight and prior handling had the greatest effect on heart rate (Harrison, Leeper, & Yoon, 1991).

Harrison, Olivet, Cunningham, Bodin, and Hicks (1996) provided 15 minutes of daily gentle human touch to preterms in the first 2 weeks of life. Infants had less active sleep and motor activity during the periods of gentle touching. When the frequency of this intervention was increased to three times a day, preterm infants had less active sleep, motor activity, and distress during gentle touching periods but did not differ from controls on any outcome, including vagal tone (Harrison, Williams, Berbaum, Stem, & Leeper, 2000; Harrison, Williams, Leeper, Stern, & Wang, 2000). However, vagal tone did increase with gestational age (Harrison, Williams, Leeper, et al., 2000).

Harrison used a variety of conceptual frameworks, including Weiss's framework of human touch (Harrison et al., 1991), Roy's adaptation model (Harrison et al., 1990), and Porges's polyvagal theory (Harrison, Williams, Leeper, et al., 2000). Only the last-mentioned model is consistent with a developmental science perspective. All of Harrison's studies considered interactions between the child and the social environment, and several examined interactions between biology (vagal tone, medical complications, and gestational age) and behaviors (Harrison et al., 1990, 1991; Harrison,

Williams, Leeper, et al., 2000). However, Harrison did not examine interactions between the child and the physical environment. One study viewed the infant as affecting the environment through behavioral state patterns (Harrison et al., 1991). The author's studies used short-term (less than a month) longitudinal designs, but only three used repeated measures statistics (Harrison et al., 1990, 1996; Harrison, Williams, Berbaum, et al., 2000). Most of her articles include a coauthor from behavioral and community medicine (Harrison et al., 1990, 1991, 1996; Harrison, Williams, Berbaum, et al., 2000; Harrison, Williams, Leeper, et al., 2000). Her measures were appropriate for the study of developing preterms, but no rationale was provided for the timing of measures. Although her participants came from diverse ethnic and socioeconomic groups, ethnic group, gender, and socioeconomic effects were not considered. Harrison did examine intergenerational effects in her comparison of grandmother touch with maternal and paternal touch (Harrison & Woods, 1991).

SUSAN LUDINGTON-HOE

Susan Ludington-Hoe's research has focused on examining the effects of kangaroo care, or skin-to-skin holding, on preterm infants. In studies in Colombia and the United States, she demonstrated that kangaroo care was safe for preterms, even when they had mild grunting, and did not result in hypothermia (Ludington-Hoe, Hadeed, & Anderson, 1991; Ludington-Hoe, Hashemi, Argote, Medeliln, & Rey, 1992; Ludington-Hoe, Nguyen, Swinth, & Satyshur, 2000; Ludington-Hoe et al., 1993). Kangaroo care increased the amount of sleeping, especially quiet sleep, promoted early breastfeeding, and improved respiratory patterns as compared with periods when the infant was alone in the incubator (Ludington, 1990; Ludington-Hoe, Thompson, Swinth, Hadeed, & Anderson, 1994; Ludington-Hoe et al., 1999). Kangaroo care was also safe for ventilated infants (Ludington-Hoe, Ferreira, & Goldstein, 1998) and could be used along with fiber-optic phototherapy for infants with hyperbilirubinemia (Ludington-Hoe & Swinth, 2001). A survey of NICUs in the United States showed that over 80% were practicing kangaroo care (Engler et al., 2002).

Ludington-Hoe's research was based on empirical knowledge of the extrauterine transition and the needs of preterm parents. In one study, her conceptualization included multifactorial causation (Ludington-Hoe et al., 1999). Her studies lacked a developmental focus, and none was longitudinal. All considered interactions between the infant and the social environment, and several included interactions between the infant and the physical environment in the form of temperature (Ludington-Hoe et al., 1991, 1992, 1993, 1999, 2000). Most studies either did not give the ethnic background of the subjects or were conducted in Colombia; thus ethnic group, socioeconomic, gender, or intergenerational effects were not examined. Although the author's studies were group-oriented, she described individual responses in two studies (Ludington-Hoe et al., 1993, 1999). Several studies had physician collaborators (Ludington-Hoe et al., 1991, 1992, 1993, 1994, 1999, 2000).

ROSEMARY WHITE-TRAUT

In a series of studies, Rosemary White-Traut tested a modification of Rice Infant Sensorimotor Stimulation, a 10-minute structured massage, along with verbal stimulation. White-Traut and Pate (1987) found that during the intervention preterms were more alert, but this effect may have been due to temperature changes rather than to the massage. Infants were taken out of the incubator for the massage. As a result, infant temperature decreased slightly, and heart and respiratory rate increased but stabilized before the conclusion of the intervention (White-Traut & Goldman, 1988). The groups did not differ significantly in weight gain or length of hospitalization, but the experimental infants tended to show more rapid weight gain and shorter hospitalizations (White-Traut, Nelson, & Silvestri, 1990; White-Traut & Tubezewski, 1986). In another study, the intervention protocol was altered to be more contingent on infant cues (White-Traut, Nelson, Silvestri, Patel, & Kilgallon, 1993). Again, the experimental infants showed increased alertness during the intervention and continued to be alert for 30 minutes afterwards. In another study, mothers provided the massage stimulation (White-Traut et al., 1990; White-Traut & Nelson, 1988). These mothers showed more positive behaviors on a standardized assessment than mothers receiving control interventions, but infant behaviors did not differ between groups.

In another study, the massage intervention was compared with auditory stimulation, auditory stimulation combined with massage, and auditory, massage, and rocking combined (White-Traut, Nelson, Silvestri, Cunningham, & Patel, 1997). Infants were alert more during the intervention in the massage and massage-plus-auditory groups, whereas the auditory-only group showed more quiet sleep. The massage-, auditory-, and rocking-group infants showed minimal changes during the intervention but were alert for 30 minutes afterwards. The massage-only group had the most episodes of elevated heart rates. Preterm infants with periventricular leukomalacia (PVL) who received the combined auditory, massage, and rocking intervention showed an increase in alertness over the intervention period and were hospitalized for 9 fewer days than other infants with PVL (White-Traut et al., 1999). Heart rate variability after the intervention was related to the type of brain injury, the length of hospital stay, and developmental outcome at 1 year (Hanna et al., 2000).

Although White-Traut's early work was based primarily on empirical evidence, her more recent studies have used complex conceptualizations within the developmental science perspective, including the ecological theory (White-Traut et al., 1999) and Porges's polyvagal theory (Hanna et al., 2000). However, the only interactions considered in her research were those between the infant and the social environment; bidirectional relationships were not mentioned. About half of her studies were longitudinal (Hanna et al., 2000; White-Traut et al., 1993, 1997, 1999; White-Traut & Pate, 1987), but only two used statistical analyses to detect change over time (White-Traut et al., 1993, 1997). The author did not examine ethnic group, gender, cultural, or intergenerational effects, probably because most of her samples were predominately African American. White-Traut had a number of interdisciplinary collaborators. Michael Nelson, a psychologist, was coauthor on most papers. White-Traut also collaborated with several physicians, a statistician, and an engineer.

Infant Behavior and Development

Six nurse researchers have research programs on infant behavior and development: Barbara Medoff-Cooper, Gail McCain, Diane Holditch-Davis, Barbara Schraeder, Margaret McGrath, and JoAnne Youngblut. Studies in this area focus on infant behaviors that are indicators of neurological status and on the long-term outcomes of preterm infants.

BARBARA MEDOFF-COOPER

Barbara Medoff-Cooper has studied the neurobehavioral assessment of preterm infants. Most recently she has focused on nutritive sucking behaviors. Fullterms had higher sucking pressures and consumed more formula than preterms (Medoff-Cooper, Weininger, & Zukowsky, 1989). The average number of sucks and sucking pressure increased, and the time between sucks and time per sucking burst decreased from 32 weeks PCA to term (Medoff-Cooper, McGrath, & Bilker, 2000; Medoff-Cooper, Verklan, &

Carlson, 1993). Infants closer to term age were more likely to be alert during feeding than younger infants (Medoff-Cooper et al., 2000). The author has shown that mean sucking pressure and length of sucking bursts were correlated with the motor development at 6 months (Medoff-Cooper & Gennaro, 1996). Also, sucking patterns could be modeled using a Markov regression (Zhang & Medoff-Cooper, 1996).

In other studies, Medoff-Cooper and Brooten (1987) showed that the time of neurobehavioral assessment within a feeding cycle had minimal effects on its results in preterms. During handling for a neurobehavioral assessment, preterms with chronic lung disease (CLD) showed more stress behaviors than other preterms only 5 of the 24 times tested despite the fact that infants with CLD had more tachycardia, tachypnea, and bradycardia (Medoff-Cooper, 1988). Preterm infants with intraventricular hemorrhages (IVH) had more abnormal findings on a neurobehavioral assessment than other preterms (Medoff-Cooper, Delivora-Papadopoulos, & Brooten, 1991). Magnetic resonance imaging (MRI) differentiated between preterms with and without IVH, and the results of neurobehavioral assessments were correlated with MRI findings (Medoff-Cooper et al., 1991; Younkin et al., 1988). Medoff-Cooper and Schraeder (1982) found that 25% of prematures between 4 and 14 months were at developmental risk, but developmental status and quality of parenting, as measured by the Home Observation for Measurement of the Environment (HOME), were not related. However, the HOME score and infant distractibility and mood were correlated. Prematures had more difficult temperaments than fullterms, and temperament was related to both the HOME score and illness severity (Medoff-Cooper, 1986).

Finally, in studies on unrelated topics, a replication of Brooten and colleagues's (1988) early discharge protocol showed that preterms could be safely discharged home when they were as small as 1,800 gm (Gibson et al., 1998). Lybrand, Medoff-Cooper, and Munro (1990) showed that urine-specific gravity could be reliably obtained from a diaper sample up to 4 hours after voiding.

Most of Medoff-Cooper's studies were empirically based on findings about physiology or neurological development, but a few used Als's (1986) synactive theory (Medoff-Cooper, 1988; Medoff-Cooper et al., 1989; Medoff-Cooper & Gennaro, 1996). Her studies considered interactions between the child and the social environment, but none examined interactions between the child and the physical environment. Most examined interactions between biology (gestational age, chronic lung disease, intraventricular hemorrhage, and medical complications) and behavior (e.g., Medoff-Cooper, 1986, 1988; Medoff-Cooper et al., 1989, 1991; Medoff-Cooper & Brooten, 1987). All but four were longitudinal (Lybrand et al., 1990; Medoff-Cooper & Brooten, 1987; Medoff-Cooper et al., 1989; Zhang & Medoff-Cooper, 1989). However, most only descriptively dealt with the data; only one used appropriate longitudinal statistics (Medoff-Cooper et al., 2000). One study used Markov regression to model individual patterns (Zhang & Medoff-Cooper, 1996), and two others just described individual responses (Medoff-Cooper et al., 1993; Medoff-Cooper & Brooten, 1987). Medoff-Cooper did not provide rationales for the timing of data collection. She did not give the ethnic background of her samples, and ethnic, cultural, gender, and intergenerational effects were not examined. She had interdisciplinary collaborators—physicians, an engineer, and statisticians—and was coauthor on papers in other disciplines (Gibson et al., 1998; Younkin et al., 1988).

GAIL McCAIN

Gail McCain's research has focused on how sleep-wake states are modified by nursing care. She compared the ability of stroking, non-nutritive sucking, and non-nutritive sucking plus rocking to arouse preterms for feedings. Non-nutritive sucking with or without rocking was the most effective in bringing infants to a quiet, waking state and maintaining this state, in which infants are most likely to feed effectively (McCain, 1992, 1995). Infants who did not complete oral feedings were asleep more of the feeding time than were successful feeders (McCain, 1997). McCain also tested using non-nutritive sucking to bring preterms to a waking state prior to feeding (McCain, Gartside, Greenberg, & Lott, 2001). As compared to control infants, intervention infants took 5 fewer days to achieve full oral feedings. In the first 3 days of life, preterms receiving antenatal phenobarbital did not differ in heart rate or sleep-wake states from infants not receiving the medication, suggesting that the antenatal dosage was not sedating (McCain, Donovan, & Gartside, 1999). Finally, upper arm and calf blood pressure measurements in preterms were compared without finding any differences (Kunk & McCain, 1996). Sleep-wake states were not outcomes in this study, but infants were studied only when they were in a quiet, inactive state.

McCain's research did not use a developmental science perspective, but she did consider bidirectional relations (McCain, 1995), multifactorial causation (McCain et al., 1999), and interactions between biology (medications and medical complications) and behaviors (McCain, 1997; McCain et al., 1999, 2001). Three studies were short-term longitudinal designs, but only two used appropriate longitudinal statistics (Kunk & McCain, 1996; McCain et al., 1999). In one study, McCain provided descriptive information about individual responses (McCain, 1995). Like most of the nurse researchers, she did not provide a rationale for the timing of her measures or examine cultural or intergenerational effects. Race and gender effects were examined in one study (McCain et al., 2001). She had interdisciplinary collaborators in two studies (McCain et al., 1999, 2001).

DIANE HOLDITCH-DAVIS

Diane Holditch-Davis's research focuses on the development of sleep-wake states in preterms and infant interactive behaviors. In a series of studies, she found changes over the preterm period in the amount of sleep-wake states, length and frequency of apneic pauses, and organization of sleep states (Holditch-Davis, 1990a; Holditch-Davis & Edwards, 1998a, 1998b; Holditch-Davis, Edwards, & Wigger, 1994). During the first month after term, prematures showed more alertness, nonalert waking activity, and sleep-wake transition and less drowsiness and sleep than fullterm infants (Holditch Davis & Thoman, 1987).

Sleep-wake patterns of preterm infants were affected by illness and treatments. Changes in sleep-wake states were associated with acute medical complications, including hydrocephalus, sepsis, and cold stress (Holditch-Davis & Hudson, 1995). Yet preterm infants with chronic lung disease only differed from other preterms by having more irregular respiration in quiet sleep, more jitters, and fewer smiles (Holditch-Davis & Lee, 1993; Holditch-Davis, 1995) and did not differ from medically fragile infants on developmental outcomes or interactive behaviors (Holditch-Davis, Docherty, Miles, & Burchinal, 2001). Theophylline, used to treat apnea, resulted in more waking and less active sleep in the first month after term (Thoman et al., 1985). Routine nursing care, such as checking vital signs, resulted in less quiet sleep as compared with times when the infant was undisturbed (Brandon, Holditch-Davis & Belyea, 1999; Holditch-Davis, 1990b). The amount of waking was increased and sleep was decreased during uncomfortable procedures (Holditch Davis & Calhoun, 1989). Preterm infants given four naps a day for 1½ hours each showed less quiet waking, longer sleep bouts, a more rapid decline in apnea, and more rapid weight gain than other preterms (Holditch-Davis, Barham, O'Hale, & Tucker, 1995; Torres, Holditch-Davis, O'Hale, &

D'Auria, 1997). Preterms were also found to gain weight faster in cycled light as compared to near darkness (Brandon, Holditch-Davis, & Belyea, 2002).

Infants also affect and were affected by interactions with adults. Hospitalized preterms spent more time in active sleep and sleep-wake transition when they were with nurses, rather than parents (Miller & Holditch-Davis, 1992). As medically fragile infants grew older over the first 6 months, they were alert more and vocalized more; their mothers spent less time feeding, holding, rocking, and touching but talked and played more (Holditch-Davis, Tesh, Burchinal, & Miles, 1999). At 6 months, prematures were more likely to be drowsy or asleep during feeding and alert during nonfeeding periods, and maternal behaviors differed during feeding and nonfeeding periods (Holditch-Davis, Miles, & Belyea, 2000). The behaviors of medically fragile infants at 6 and 12 months were correlated with HOME scores, and the HOME scores were related to mental development (Holditch-Davis, Tesh, Goldman, Miles, & D'Auria, 2000). Three-year-old premature children with normal developmental status had more optimal interactive behaviors and received more optimal parenting than children with developmental concerns (Holditch-Davis, Bartlett, & Belyea, 2000).

Holditch-Davis's research used a developmental science perspective, although this is more obvious in recent studies. All studies assumed multifactorial causation, and most included systems conceptualizations, assumed bidirectional relationships, and viewed the infant as actively changing the environment (e.g., Holditch-Davis et al., 1999, 2001; Holditch-Davis et al., 2000; Holditch-Davis, Miles, et al., 2000). All but three considered interactions between the infant and the social environment (Brandon et al., 2002; Holditch-Davis et al., 1994; Holditch-Davis & Edwards, 1998a). Interactions between infants and the physical environment were occasionally studied (Brandon et al., 1999, 2002; Holditch-Davis et al., 1995; Holditch-Davis & Edwards, 1998a; Torres et al., 1997), and interactions between biology (e.g., theophylline treatment, mechanical ventilation, neurological problems, chronic lung disease) and behaviors were examined (e.g., Holditch-Davis, 1990a, 1995; Holditch-Davis et al., 1999, 2001; Holditch-Davis & Lee, 1993). With four exceptions (Holditch-Davis, Bartlett, et al., 2000; Holditch Davis & Calhoun, 1989; Holditch-Davis, Miles, et al., 2000; Miller & Holditch-Davis, 1992), her studies were longitudinal. Most used longitudinal statistics and examined stability and change over time (e.g., Holditch-Davis et al., 1999, 2001; Holditch-Davis & Edwards,

1998a, 1998b). The statistic she used, the mixed general linear model, includes group and individual development in a single equation, but only two studies presented the individual patterns from the mixed model (Holditch-Davis et al., 1994; Holditch-Davis & Edwards, 1998a). The author did not provide rationales for the timing of data collection. Except for her two earliest papers (Holditch Davis & Thoman, 1987; Thoman et al., 1985), her studies had ethnically diverse samples and often examined ethnic group, socioeconomic, and gender effects (Brandon et al., 1999; Holditch-Davis et al., 1994, 1999; Holditch-Davis & Edwards, 1998a, 1998b). However, she did not examine intergenerational effects. She had collaborators from psychology and statistics.

BARBARA SCHRAEDER

Barbara Schraeder studied factors related to the developmental outcomes of preterm infants. In an early study, Schraeder and Medoff-Cooper (1983) found that HOME scores were unrelated to developmental outcome in toddlers but were related to child temperament. In a series of reports from one longitudinal study, Schraeder further examined the relation between development and home environment. The home environment had a greater effect on the child's development than did biological variables (Schraeder, 1986; Schraeder, Rappaport, & Courtwright, 1987), with language stimulation and stimulation of academic behavior most directly related to development. The quality of the home environment at 6 months was more strongly related to development at 48 months than were demographic and medical variables (Schraeder, Heverly, & Rappaport, 1990b). Children whose temperaments were rhythmic, active, and persistent, but not intense, and who had a high threshold had fewer behavior problems but had poorer learning skills than children with other temperament characteristics (Schraeder, Heverly, & Rappaport, 1990a). At 5 years, children who were more immature and hyperactive had caretakers who had more daily stress and less positive home environments (Tobey & Schraeder, 1990).

At school age, the sample was compared to a matched group of fullterm children (Schraeder, Heverly, O'Brien, & McEvoy-Shields, 1992a, 1996b). Environmental variables—age of mother at first birth and quality of the home environment—had the largest impact on cognitive abilities and academic achievement. Birthweight did not affect academic achievement and had minor effects on cognitive abilities. Prematurely born children were retained in grade more than fullterms, required more special education, and had lower mathematics scores (Schraeder, Heverly,

O'Brien, & Goodman, 1997). Prematures also had slightly poorer lung function (Schraeder, Czajka, Kalman, & McGeady, 1998) and were more likely to fail tests of binocular vision and ocular motor muscle balance (Shraeder & McEvoy-Shields, 1991). Classroom behavior problems were related to goodness of fit with mothers' and teachers' expectations (Schraeder, Heverly, & O'Brien, 1996a). Mothers did not perceive premature children as being more vulnerable, but vulnerability was related to temperament (Schraeder, Heverly, O'Brien, & McEvoy-Shields, 1992b).

Most of Schraeder's studies used an empirical framework. Two (Schraeder, 1986; Schraeder et al., 1996b) used the transactional model, a theory consistent with developmental science except that the child is seen as a passive recipient of environmental risks (Sameroff & Chandler, 1975). Her studies generally considered bidirectional feedback and interactions between the child and the social environment and between biology (gestational age and medical complications) and behaviors. Although her studies were longitudinal, she usually did not use repeated measures statistics, but rather multiple regression and correlations over ages. The exception was Schraeder et al. (1997), which used the repeated measures analysis of variance. Thus, despite having an 11-year longitudinal study, Schraeder examined stability and changes in child developmental status in only a few studies (Schraeder, 1986; Schraeder et al., 1987, 1996b, 1997; Schraeder & Medoff-Cooper, 1983). Her measures were appropriate for rapidly developing preterm infants, but she did not provide rationales for the timing of these measures, and she relied heavily on maternal report measures, especially in her early studies. She did not examine ethnic group, cultural, or intergenerational effects but did correlate socioeconomic status and medical risk with outcomes in one study (Schraeder et al., 1996b) and examined gender difference in behavioral problems in another (Schraeder et al., 1996a). Only one study had interdisciplinary collaborators (Schrader et al., 1998).

MARGARET MCGRATH

Margaret McGrath's research focuses on the effects of environmental and medical risks on premature infants' developmental outcomes. Infants were divided into five medical risk groups: healthy fullterms, healthy preterms, sick preterms, small-for-gestational-age infants, and preterms with neonatal neurological complications. At 4 years, the prematurely born children had poorer motor outcomes, and motor skills were related to medical complications and maternal depression and responsiveness (McGrath &

Sullivan, 1999). Also, mastery motivation (exploration, persistence, positive affect, and attention) was related to better cognitive outcomes, and infants at higher medical risk had lower mastery motivation (McGrath, Sullivan, Brem, & Rocherolle, 1995). Fullterms and healthy preterms showed good development through age 8, whereas the other groups showed increasing percentages of infants with developmental problems; infants with neurological problems had the highest percentage of developmental problems (McGrath, Sullivan, Lester, & Oh, 2000). Interaction patterns also differed by medical risk, with mothers showing higher involvement with preterms at medical risk, and child developmental outcomes were related to maternal interaction patterns (McGrath, Sullivan, & Seifer, 1998). In other reports, prematures whose mothers' perceptions of their cries were similar to the acoustic analysis of the infants' cries had better language and cognitive development at 18 month than prematures whose mothers' perceptions differed from the acoustic analysis (Lester et al., 1995). Preterm and fullterm infants showed different pattern of changes in heart rate variability during visual orientation at 1 month, and this heart rate variability was related to development at 8 months (Lester et al., 1990).

McGrath's research used a developmental science perspective. She used the transactional model modified by concepts of neural plasticity and goodness of fit so that the child was seen as actively affecting the environment (Lester et al., 1995; McGrath et al., 1995, 1998; McGrath & Sullivan, 1999). Her studies all considered interactions between the child and social environment and between biology (medical risk group) and behaviors. Her studies were primarily longitudinal but did not use repeated measures statistics (Lester et al., 1990, 1995; McGrath et al., 2000; McGrath & Sullivan, 1999). Thus stability and change over time were seldom examined and then only using correlations or Chi Square tests (McGrath et al., 2000). Her measures were appropriate for growing prematures, but no rationale for the timing of data collection was presented. Her sample was primarily white and middle class; she did not examine socioeconomic, gender, cultural, ethnic group, or intergenerational effects. Her studies were conducted as part of a multidisciplinary team effort. Not only did she have interdisciplinary coauthors from psychology and medicine on her first-authored papers, but she was also a coauthor on papers published in other disciplines.

JOANNE YOUNGBLUT

JoAnne Youngblut's research program has focused on the effects of maternal employment. Studies with mothers of premature infants showed that the more the mother worked and the more choice she felt she had about employment, the better the cognitive and motor outcomes of her infant (Youngblut, Loveland-Cherry, & Horan, 1991, 1993, 1994). Similar findings occurred when mothers of premature and fullterm infants were compared, and the developmental outcomes of the premature and fullterm infants did not differ (Youngblut et al., 2001). A history of child care protected preschool children born prematurely and at term from developing aggressive behaviors after hospitalization (Youngblut & Brooten, 1999). In another study, metal and nonmetal incubators were found to exhibit similar amounts of vibration, but the metal incubators transmitted less vibration to the mattress (Youngblut, Lewandowski, Casper, & Youngblut, 1994).

Youngblut did not use a developmental science perspective, although two studies used theories compatible with developmental science: ecological theory (Youngblut et al., 2001) and attachment theory (Youngblut & Brooten, 1999). Multifactorial causation and interactions between the child and the social environment were examined, but bidirectional relationships or interactions between the child and the physical environment were not considered. Several studies examined interactions between biology (prematurity) and behavior (Youngblut et al., 1993, 2001; Youngblut & Brooten, 1999). Two were longitudinal and used appropriate statistics to identify change over time (Youngblut et al., 1993; Youngblut, Loveland-Cherry, et al., 1994). She did not conduct individual-focused analyses, provide rationales for the timing of measures, or examine ethnic group, gender, or intergenerational effects, in some cases because of the homogeneity of her sample (Youngblut et al., 1991, 1993; Youngblut, Loveland-Cherry, et al., 1994). A psychologist and an engineer were coauthors on two studies (Youngblut et al., 2001; Youngblut, Lewandowski, et al., 1994).

DISCUSSION

The 17 current programs of nursing research on the care of preterm infants are both strong and extensive, particularly considering that several of the nurse researchers identified by Medoff-Cooper and Holditch-Davis (1999), such as Gene Anderson and Kathryn Barnard, no longer have a current program of research in this area. Most of the identified nurse researchers have significant research depth, and 11 of them would still have qualified as having a research program had a more restrictive definition of having six first-authored papers been used. Yet few of these investigators conduct research solely on the care of preterms; rather, most also study parenting or other groups of infants. These researchers also cross-collaborate extensively with each other. Twelve have coauthored papers with another researcher with a research program on this topic.

The topics covered by these nurses were notable for their clinical relevance. Their studies examined everything from the NICU environment in the first few days of life to outcomes at 11 years of age. Care of the critically ill infant was the sole exception. Only studies on sleep-wake states, suctioning, and the NICU environment examined critical care infants (Brandon et al., 2002; Evans, 1991, 1992; Evans et al., 1997, 2000; McCain et al., 1999; Shiao, 2002; Shiao et al., 2002; Vogelpohl et al., 1995). Even the extensive literature on pain management has focused primarily on procedural pain, rather than pain due to mechanical ventilation or surgery, common problems in critically ill infants. Two factors probably account for this lack. First, the vulnerability of critically ill infants makes them difficult to study. Second, all nurses with research programs on this topic are nursing faculty members. Thus they may lack direct clinical involvement in the intensive care unit.

Another strength of these research programs was their interdisciplinary foci. All of these researchers, except Evans, had collaborators from other disciplines such as medicine, psychology, statistics, and engineering. Most, except Harrison, Pridham, and Shiao, have published in interdisciplinary journals as well as nursing ones, as shown in the reference list. Several also were coauthors in papers by collaborators from other disciplines (Gibson et al., 1998; Hanna et al., 2000; Lester et al., 1990, 1995; Parker et al., 1992; Thoman et al., 1985; Younkin et al., 1988).

On the other hand, the developmental science perspective was not widely used by these researchers despite its consistency with nursing's conceptual frameworks. Only four—Becker, Holditch-Davis, McGrath, and Pridham—clearly used this perspective. Several researchers used theories compatible with developmental science, such as the ecological framework (White-Traut et al., 1999; Youngblut et al., 2001), the transactional model (e.g., Schraeder et al., 1996b), the synactive theory (e.g., Johnston, Stevens, et al., 1999; Medoff-Cooper & Gennaro, 1996; Stevens, Johnston, Franck, et al., 1999; Zahr & Balian, 1995), and the polyvagal theory (Hanna et al., 2000; Harrison, Williams, Leeper, et al., 2000). Empirically based conceptualizations, however, were the most common bases for studies. Despite the limited use of developmental science, these researchers used components of this perspective, such as interactions between the child and the social environment and multifactorial causation. Yet only a few discussed bidirectional relationships (Holditch-Davis and McCain) or examined interactions between the physical environment and the child (Becker, Harrison, Holditch-Davis, Ludington-Hoe, Stevens, and Zahr). Most, except Holditch-Davis, McGrath, Pridham, and Schraeder, viewed the infant as a passive recipient of environmental stimulation. Thus a widespread adoption of the developmental science perspective could expand the conceptualizations in research on the care of preterm infants.

A surprising finding was the limited focus on change and timing in these programs of research even though preterms are known to be developing rapidly. These nurse researchers, except Ludington-Hoe, used longitudinal designs in their research, but only research in the area of infant behavior and development included infant developmental patterns as a major focus. Researchers in other areas often ignored the longitudinal nature of their data when it came to analysis (e.g., Evans, 1992; Medoff-Cooper, 1988), and many studies examining development did not use longitudinal statistics. Either data from only two time points were compared (e.g., Harrison & Woods, 1991; Schraeder et al., 1996b; Walden et al., 2001) or developmental patterns were identified only descriptively (Medoff-Cooper, 1991). These strategies were understandable in the 1980s, but since then longitudinal statistics have been developed that can deal with mistimed and missing data (e.g., Holditch-Davis et al., 1994; Pridham, Brown, et al., 2001). Also, only one study (Pridham et al., 2000) provided a rationale for the timing of data collection.

These researchers used a wide variety of physiological and behavioral measures in their studies, all of which were appropriate for developing preterms. The physiological measures used were primarily vital sign measures, such as heart rate and oxygenation. However, more complex measures, such as intracranial pressure (Stevens et al., 1993), MRI (Medoff-Cooper et al., 1991), and norepinephrine levels (Franck, Boyce, et al., 2000), have also been used. Research on preterms could be expanded by the use of other physiological measures, such as biochemical or genetic measures. Physiological measures were primarily used as outcomes. When interactions between biology and behaviors were examined, the biological measures were usually limited to medical complications or gestational age. The only exceptions were Holditch-Davis and McCain, who studied medication effects, and Harrison and White-Traut, who examined heart rate variability (Hanna et al., 2000; Harrison et al., 2000; Holditch-Davis &

Edwards, 1998a, 1998b; Holditch-Davis et al., 1994; McCain et al., 1999). Thus, research is needed on the interactions between biology and the behaviors of preterms that uses biological measures beyond medical complications.

Another limitation of the research programs on the care of preterm infants was the lack of studies on individuals. Although nursing emphasizes meeting the needs of individuals, most studies only used group analyses. A few studies presented individual data descriptively (Evans, 1991; Evans et al., 1997; Ludington-Hoe et al., 1993, 1999; McCain, 1995; Medoff-Cooper et al., 1993; Medoff-Cooper & Brooten, 1987; Vogelpohl et al., 1995), but only two researchers conducted individual-focused statistical analyses (Holditch-Davis et al., 1994; Holditch-Davis & Edwards, 1998a; Zhang & Medoff-Cooper, 1996). Clearly, more individual-focused analyses of preterm infants' responses are needed, since the responses of individuals cannot be extrapolated from group patterns. Currently, most nursing research emphasizes group analyses, and the importance of individual-focused analyses is not always recognized. For example, most of the individual data were removed from the Holditch et al. (1994) article during the final copyediting by a production editor.

Finally, these programs of research had a limited focus on the broader ecological context, as shown by cultural, gender, socioeconomic, or intergenerational effects. Only two researchers studied the effects of ethnic group (e.g., Holditch-Davis et al., 1999; Pridham et al., 1999), five studied gender effects (e.g., Holditch-Davis & Edwards, 1998a; Johnston et al., 1996; Pridham et al., 2000; Schraeder et al., 1996a; Shiao et al., 2002), two studied socioeconomic effects (Holditch-Davis et al., 1999; Schraeder et al., 1996b), and one examined intergenerational effects (Harrison & Woods, 1991). Although two researchers conducted studies in developing countries, neither examined cultural effects (Ludington-Hoe et al., 1992, 1993; Zahr, 1998; Zahr & Balian, 1995).

Three reasons may explain this limited attention to the broader ecological context. Many studies had samples that were too small to permit statistical examination of group differences. Others had samples that were homogeneous in ethnic or socioeconomic status (Becker, McGrath, White-Traut, Youngblut, Zahr). This homogeneity prevented the researchers from examining group differences. Also, many researchers believe that these variables have effects solely through socialization that occurs after the preterm period. However, these variables also have biological effects. Gender differences are due to prenatal hormone exposure as well as socialization, and minority status and poverty are associated with higher rates of perinatal complications. Thus both gender and ethnic differences have been found in the preterm period (Holditch-Davis et al., 1994; Holditch-Davis & Edwards, 1998a). These variables are even more important in outcome studies, since older children are subject to socialization effects. Yet no studies after the first year examined the effects of these contextual variables, except Schraeder et al. (1996a), who found gender effects on behavioral problems.

In conclusion, there are a number of strong programs of nursing research on the care of the preterm infants. However, research on this topic needs more emphasis on the intensive care period, developmental changes especially during the preterm period, individual differences, and the broader ecological context. A more widespread adoption of the developmental science perspective could lead to these expansions in nursing research that is focused on these vulnerable infants.

ACKNOWLEDGMENTS

The preparation of this paper was partially supported by Grant NR01894 from the National Institute for Nursing Research, National Institutes of Health, to the first author.

REFERENCES

Als, H. (1986). A synactive model of neonatal behavioral organization: Framework for the assessment of neurobehavioral development in the premature infant and for support of infants and parents in the neonatal intensive care environment: Part 1. Theoretical framework. *Physical and Occupational Therapy in Pediatrics, 6,* 1–53.

Als, H., Lawhon, G., Brown, E., Gibes, R., Duffy, F. H., McAnulty, G., et al. (1986). Individualized behavioral and environmental care for the very low birth weight preterm infant at high risk for bronchopulmonary dysplasia: Neonatal intensive care unit and developmental outcome. *Pediatrics, 78,* 1123–1132.

Anderson, G. C., & Vidyasagur, D. (1979). Development of sucking in premature infants from 1 to 7 days post birth. *Birth Defects: Original Article Series, 15*(7), 145–171.

Ballantyne, M., Stevens, B., McAllister, M., Dionne, K., & Jack, A. (1999). Validation of the premature infant pain profile in the clinical setting. *Clinical Journal of Pain, 15,* 297–303.

Barnard, K. E., & Bee, H. L. (1983). The impact of temporally patterned stimulation on the development of preterm infants. *Child Development, 54,* 1156–1167.

Becker, P. T. (1995). Studies of developmental nursing care for very low birth weight infants. In S. G. Funk, E. M. Tornquist, M. T. Champagne, & R. A. Wiese (Eds.), *Key aspects of caring for the acutely ill: Technological aspects, patient education, and quality of life* (pp. 79–94). New York: Springer.

Becker, P. T., Brazy, J. E., & Grunwald, P. C. (1997). Behavioral state organization of very low birth weight infants: Effects of developmental handling during caregiving. *Infant Behavior and Development, 20,* 503–514.

Becker, P. T., Grunwald, P. C., & Brazy, J. E. (1997). Motor organization in very low birth weight infants during caregiving: Effects of a developmental intervention. *Journal of Developmental and Behavioral Pediatrics, 20,* 344–354.

Becker, P. T., Grunwald, P. C., Moorman, J., & Stuhr, S. (1991). Outcomes of developmentally supportive nursing care for very low birth weight infants. *Nursing Research, 40,* 150–155.

Becker, P. T., Grunwald, P. C., Moorman, J., & Stuhr, S. (1993). Effects of developmental care on behavioral organization in very-low-birth-weight infants. *Nursing Research, 42,* 214–220.

Black, J. E., & Greenough, W. T. (1986). Induction of pattern in neural structure by experience: Implications for cognitive development. In M. E. Lamb, A. L. Brown, & B. Rogoff (Eds.), *Advances in developmental psychology* (Vol. 4, pp. 1–50). Hillsdale, NJ: Erlbaum.

Blackburn, S. T., & Barnard, K. E. (1985). Analysis of caregiving events relating to preterm infants in the special care unit. In A. W. Gottfried & J. L. Gaiter (Eds.), *Infant stress under intensive care: Environmental neonatology* (pp. 113–129). Baltimore: University Park Press.

Brandon, D. H., Holditch-Davis, D., & Belyea, M. (1999). Nursing care and the development of sleeping and waking behaviors in preterm infants. *Research in Nursing and Health, 22,* 217–229.

Brandon, D. H., Holditch-Davis, D., & Belyea, M. (2002). Preterm infants born at less than 31 weeks' gestation have improved growth in cycled light compared with continuous near darkness. *Journal of Pediatrics, 140,* 192–199.

Brooten, D., Gennaro, S., Brown, L. P., Butts, P., Givons, A. L., Bakewell-Sachs, S., et al. (1988). Anxiety, depression, and hostility in mothers of preterm infants. *Nursing Research, 37,* 213–216.

Cairns, R. B., Elder, G. H., & Costello, E. J. (1996). *Developmental science.* Cambridge, England: Cambridge University Press.

Engler, A. J., Ludington-Hoe, S. M., Cusson, R. M., Adams, R., Bahnsen, M., Brumbaugh, E., et al. (2002). Kangaroo care: National survey of practice, knowledge, barriers, and perceptions. *MCN: American Journal of Maternal-Child Nursing, 27,* 146–161.

Evans, J. C. (1991). Incidence of hypoxemia associated with caregiving in premature infants. *Neonatal Network, 10*(2), 17–24.

Evans, J. (1992). Reducing the hypoxemia, bradycardia, and apnea associated with suctioning in low birthweight infants. *Journal of Perinatology, 12*(2), 137–142.

Evans, J. C., McCartney, E. S., & Roth-Sautter, C. M. (2000). Desaturation and/or bradycardic events following caregiving in the newborn intensive care unit. *Neonatal Intensive Care, 13*(4), 20–25.

Evans, J. C., Vogelpohl, D. G., Bourguignon, C. M., & Morcott, C. S. (1997). Pain behaviors in LBW infants accompany some "nonpainful" caregiving procedures. *Neonatal Network, 16*(3), 33–40.

Franck, L. S. (1987). A national survey of the assessment and treatment of pain and agitation in the neonatal intensive care unit. *Journal of Obstetric, Gynecologic and Neonatal Nursing, 16,* 387–393.

Franck, L., Bernal, H., & Gale, G. (2002). Infant holding policies and practices in neonatal units. *Neonatal Network, 21*(2), 13–20.

Franck, L., Boyce, T., Gregory, G. A., Jemerin, J., Levine, J., & Miaskowski, C. (2000). Plasma norepinephrine levels, vagal tone index, and flexor reflex threshold in premature neonates receiving intravenous morphine during the postoperative period: A pilot study. *Clinical Journal of Pain, 16,* 95–104.

Franck, L. S., Quinn, D., & Zahr, L. (2000). Effect of less frequent bathing of preterm infants on skin flora and pathogen colonization. *Journal of Obstetric, Gynecologic and Neonatal Nursing, 29,* 584–589.

Gale, G., Franck, L., & Lund, C. (1993). Skin-to-skin (kangaroo) holding of the intubated premature infant. *Neonatal Network, 12*(6), 49–57.

Gibson, E., Medoff-Cooper, B., Nuamah, I. F., Gerdes, J., Kirkby, S., & Greenspan, J. (1998). Accelerated discharge of low birth weight infants from neonatal intensive care: A randomized, controlled trial. *Journal of Perinatology, 18,* 517–523.

Gottlieb, G. (1996). A systems view of psychobiological development. In D. Magnusson (Ed.), *The lifespan development of individuals: Behavioral, neurobiological and psychosocial perspectives* (pp. 76–103). Cambridge, England: Cambridge University Press.

Hanna, B. D., Nelson, M. N., White-Traut, R. C., Silvestri, J. M., Vasan, U., Rey, P. M., et al. (2000). Heart rate variability in preterm brain-injured and very-low-birth-weight infants. *Biology of the Neonate, 77,* 147–155.

Harrison, L. L., Leeper, J. D., & Yoon, M. (1990). Effects of early parental touch on preterm infants' heart rates and arterial oxygen saturation levels. *Journal of Advanced Nursing, 15,* 877–885.

Harrison, L. L., Leeper, J., & Yoon, M. (1991). Preterm infants' physiologic responses to early parent touch. *Western Journal of Nursing Research, 13,* 698–713.

Harrison, L., Olivet, L., Cunningham, K., Bodin, M. B., & Hicks, C. (1996). Effects of gentle human touch on preterm infants: Pilot study results. *Neonatal Network, 15*(2), 35–42.

Harrison, L. L., Williams, A. K., Berbaum, M. L., Stem, J. T., & Leeper, J. (2000). Physiologic and behavioral effects of gentle human touch on preterm infants. *Research in Nursing and Health, 23,* 435–446.

Harrison, L. L., Williams, A. K., Leeper, J., Stern, J. T., & Wang, L. (2000). Factors associated with vagal tone responses in preterm infants. *Western Journal of Nursing Research, 22,* 776–795.

Harrison, L. L., & Woods, S. (1991). Early parental touch and preterm infants. *Journal of Obstetric, Gynecologic and Neonatal Nursing, 20,* 299–306.

Holditch-Davis, D. (1990a). The development of sleeping and waking states in high-risk preterm infants. *Infant Behavior and Development, 13,* 513–531.

Holditch-Davis, D. (1990b). The effect of hospital caregiving on preterm infants' sleeping and waking states. In S. G. Funk, E. M. Tornquist, M. T. Champagne, L. A. Copp, & R. A. Wiese (Eds.), *Key aspects of recovery: Improving nutrition, rest, and mobility* (pp. 110–122). New York: Springer.

Holditch-Davis, D. (1995). Behaviors of preterm infants with and without chronic lung disease when alone and when with nurses. *Neonatal Network, 14*(7), 51–57.

Holditch-Davis, D., Barham, L., O'Hale, A., & Tucker, E. (1995). The effect of standardized rest periods on convalescent preterm infants. *Journal of Obstetric, Gynecologic and Neonatal Nursing, 24,* 424–432.

Holditch-Davis, D., Bartlett, T. R., & Belyea, M. (2000). Developmental problems and the interactions between mothers and their three-year-old prematurely born children. *Journal of Pediatric Nursing, 15,* 157–167.

Holditch Davis, D., & Calhoun, M. (1989). Do preterm infants show behavioral responses to painful procedures? In S. G. Funk, E. M. Tornquist, M. T. Champagne, L. A. Copp, & R. A. Wiese (Eds.), *Key aspects of comfort: Management of pain, fatigue, and nausea* (pp. 35–43). New York: Springer.

Holditch-Davis, D., Docherty, S., Miles, M. S., & Burchinal, M. (2001). Developmental outcomes of infants with bronchopulmonary dysplasia: Comparison with other medically fragile infants. *Research in Nursing and Health, 24,* 181–193.

Holditch-Davis, D., & Edwards, L. (1998a). Modeling development of sleep-wake behaviors: II. Results of 2 cohorts of preterms. *Physiology and Behavior, 63,* 319–328.

Holditch-Davis, D., & Edwards, L. (1998b). Temporal organization of sleep-wake states in preterm infants. *Developmental Psychobiology, 33,* 257–269.

Holditch-Davis, D., Edwards, L. J., & Wigger, M. C. (1994). Pathologic apnea and brief respiratory pauses in preterm infants: Relation to sleep state. *Nursing Research, 43,* 293–300.

Holditch-Davis, D., & Hudson, D. C. (1995). Using preterm infant behaviors to identify acute medical complications. In S. G. Funk, E. M. Tornquist, M. T. Champagne, & R. A. Wiese (Eds.), *Key aspects of caring for the acutely ill: Technological aspects, patient education, and quality of life* (pp. 95–120). New York: Springer.

Holditch-Davis, D., & Lee, D. A. (1993). The behaviors and nursing care of preterm infants with chronic lung disease. In S. G. Funk, E. M. Tornquist, M. T. Champagne, & R. A. Wiese (Eds.), *Key aspects of caring for the chronically ill: Hospital and home* (pp. 250–270). New York: Springer.

Holditch-Davis, D., Miles, M., & Belyea, M. (2000). Feeding and non-feeding interactions of mothers and prematures. *Western Journal of Nursing Research, 22,* 320–334.

Holditch-Davis, D., Tesh, E. M., Burchinal, M., & Miles, M. S. (1999). Early interactions between mothers and their medically fragile infants. *Applied Developmental Science, 3,* 155–167.

Holditch-Davis, D., Tesh, E. M., Goldman, B. D., Miles, M. S., & D'Auria, J. (2000). Use of the HOME Inventory with medically fragile infants. *Children's Health Care, 29,* 257–277.

Holditch Davis, D., & Thoman, E. B. (1987). Behavioral states of premature infants: Implications for neural and behavioral development. *Developmental Psychobiology, 20,* 25–38.

Johnston, C. C., Collinge, J. M., Henderson, S. J., & Anand, K. J. S. (1997). A cross-sectional survey of pain and pharmacological analgesia in Canadian neonatal intensive care units. *Clinical Journal of Pain, 13,* 308–312.

Johnston, C. C., Sherraud, A., Stevens, B., Franck, L., Stremler, R., & Jack, A. (1999). Do cry features reflect pain intensity in preterm neonates? *Biology of the Neonate, 76,* 120–124.

Johnston, C. C., & Stevens, B. J. (1996). Experience in a neonatal intensive care unit affects pain response. *Pediatrics, 98,* 925–930.

Johnston, C. C., Stevens, B. J., Franck, L. S., Jack, A., Stremler, R., & Platt, R. (1999). Factors explaining lack of response to heelstick in preterm newborns. *Journal of Obstetric, Gynecologic and Neonatal Nursing, 28,* 587–594.

Johnston, C. C., Stevens, B., Yang, F., & Horton, L. (1995). Differential response to pain by very premature neonates. *Pain, 61,* 471–479.

Johnston, C. C., Stevens, B., Yang, F., & Horton, L. (1996). Developmental changes in response to heelstick in preterm infants: A prospective cohort study. *Developmental Medicine and Child Neurology, 38,* 438–445.

Johnston, C. C., Stremler, R., Horton, L., & Friedman, A. (1999). Effect of repeated doses of sucrose during heel stick procedure in preterm neonates. *Biology of the Neonate, 75,* 160–166.

Johnston, C. C., Stremler, R., Stevens, B., & Horton, L. (1997). Effectiveness of oral sucrose and simulated rocking on pain response in preterm neonates. *Pain, 72,* 193–199.

Kunk, R., & McCain, G. (1996). Comparison of upper arm and calf oscilometric blood pressure measurement in preterm infants. *Journal of Perinatology, 16*(2 Pt. 1), 89–92.

Lester, B. M., Boukydis, Z., Garcia-Coll, C. T., Peucker, M., McGrath, M. M., Vohr, B. R., et al. (1995). Developmental outcome as a function of the goodness of fit between the infant's cry characteristics and the mother's perception of her infant's cry. *Pediatrics, 95,* 516–521.

Lester, B. M., Boukydis, Z., McGrath, M., Censullo, M., Zahr, L., & Brazelton, T. B. (1990). Behavioral and physiologic assessment of the preterm infant. *Clinics in Perinatology, 17*(1), 155–171.

Ludington, S. M. (1990). Energy conservation during skin-to-skin contact between premature infants and their mothers. *Heart and Lung, 19,* 445–451.

Ludington-Hoe, S. M., Anderson, G. C., Simpson, S., Hollingshead, A., Argopte, L. A., Medellin, G., et al. (1993). Skin-to-skin contact beginning in the delivery room for Colombian mothers and their preterm infants. *Journal of Human Lactation, 9,* 241–242.

Ludington-Hoe, S. M., Anderson, G. C., Simpson, S., Hollingsead, A., Argote, L. A., & Rey, H. (1999). Birth-related fatigue in 34–36-week preterm neonates: Rapid recovery with very early kangaroo (skin-to-skin) care. *Journal of Obstetric, Gynecologic and Neonatal Nursing, 28,* 94–103.

Ludington-Hoe, S. M., Ferreira, C. N., & Goldstein, M. R. (1998). Kangaroo care with a ventilated preterm infant. *Acta Paediatrica, 87,* 711–713.

Ludington-Hoe, S. M., Hadeed, A. J., & Anderson, G. C. (1991). Physiological responses to skin-to-skin contact in hospitalized premature infants. *Journal of Perinatology, 11,* 19–24.

Ludington-Hoe, S. M., Hashemi, M. S., Argote, L. A., Medellin, G., & Rey, H. (1992). Selected physiologic measures and behavior during paternal skin contact with Colombian preterm infants. *Journal of Developmental Physiology, 18,* 223–232.

Ludington-Hoe, S. M., Nguyen, N., Swinth, J. Y., & Satyshur, R. D. (2000). Kangaroo care compared to incubators in maintaining body warmth in preterm infants. *Biological Research for Nursing, 2,* 60–73.

Ludington-Hoe, S. M., & Swinth, J. Y. (2001). Kangaroo care during phototherapy: Effect on bilirubin profile. *Neonatal Network, 20*(5), 41–48.

Ludington-Hoe, S. M., Thompson, C., Swinth, J., Hadeed, A. J., & Anderson, G. C. (1994). Kangaroo care: Research results, and practice implications and guidelines. *Neonatal Network, 13*(1), 19–27.

Lund, C. H., Nonata, L. B., Kuller, J. M., Franck, L. S., Cullander, C., & Durand, D. J. (1997). Disruption of barrier function in neonatal skin associated with adhesive removal. *Journal of Pediatrics, 131,* 367–372.

Lybrand, M., Medoff-Cooper, B., & Munro, B. H. (1990). Periodic comparisons of specific gravity using urine from a diaper and collecting bag. *MCN: American Journal of Maternal-Child Nursing, 15,* 238–239.

Magnusson, D. (1995). Individual development: A holistic, integrated model. In P. Moen, G. H. Elder, & K. Luscher (Eds.), *Examining lives in context: Perspectives on the ecology of human development* (pp. 19–60). Washington, DC: American Psychological Association.

McCain, G. C. (1992). Facilitating inactive awake states in preterm infants: A study of three interventions. *Nursing Research, 41,* 157–160.

McCain, G. C. (1995). Promotion of preterm infant nipple feeding with nonnutritive sucking. *Journal of Pediatric Nursing, 10,* 3–8.

McCain, G. C. (1997). Behavioral state activity during nipple feedings for preterm infants. *Neonatal Network, 16*(5), 43–47.

McCain, G. C., Donovan, E. F., & Gartside, P. (1999). Preterm infant behavioral and heart rate responses to antenatal phenobarbital. *Research in Nursing and Health, 22,* 461–470.

McCain, G. C., Gartside, P. S., Greenberg, J. M., & Lott, J. W. (2001). A feeding protocol for healthy preterm infants that shortens time to oral feeding. *Journal of Pediatrics, 139,* 374–379.

McGrath, M. M., & Sullivan, M. C. (1999). Medical and ecological factors in estimating motor outcomes of preschool children. *Research in Nursing and Health, 22,* 155–167.

McGrath, M. M., Sullivan, M. C., Brem, F., & Rocherolle, K. C. (1995). Mastery motivation and cognitive development in 4-year-old children born at various degrees of medical risk. *Journal of Pediatric Nursing, 10,* 287–294.

McGrath, M. M., Sullivan, M. C., Lester, B. M., & Oh, W. (2000). Longitudinal neurologic follow-up in neonatal intensive care unit survivors with various neonatal morbidities. *Pediatrics, 106,* 1397–1405.

McGrath, M. M., Sullivan, M. C., & Seifer, R. (1998). Maternal interaction patterns and preschool competence in high-risk children. *Nursing Research, 47,* 309–317.

Medoff-Cooper, B. (1986). Temperament in very low birth weight infants. *Nursing Research, 35,* 139–143.

Medoff-Cooper, B. (1988). The effects of handling on preterm infants with bronchopulmonary dysplasia. *Image: Journal of Nursing Scholarship, 20,* 132–134.

Medoff-Cooper, B. (1991). Changes in nutritive sucking patterns with increasing gestational age. *Nursing Research, 40,* 245–247.

Medoff-Cooper, B., & Brooten, D. (1987). Relation of the feeding cycle to neurobehavioral assessment in preterm infants: A pilot study. *Nursing Research, 36,* 315–317.

Medoff-Cooper, B., Delivora-Papadoupoulos, M., & Brooten, D. (1991). Serial neurobehavioral assessments in preterm infants. *Nursing Research, 40,* 94–97.

Medoff-Cooper, B., & Gennaro, S. (1996). The correlation of sucking behaviors and bayley scales of infant development at six months of age in VLBW infants. *Nursing Research, 45,* 291–296.

Medoff-Cooper, B., & Holditch-Davis, D. (1999). Therapeutic actions and outcomes for preterm (low birth weight) infants. In A. S. Hinshaw, S. Feetham, & J. Shaver (Eds.), *Handbook of clinical nursing research* (pp. 161–183). Newbury Park, CA: Sage.

Medoff-Cooper, B., McGrath, J., & Bilker, W. (2000). Nutritive sucking and neurobehavioral development in preterm infants from 34 weeks PCA to term. *MCN: American Journal of Maternal-Child Nursing, 25,* 64–70.

Medoff-Cooper, B., & Schraeder, B. D. (1982). Developmental trends and behavioral styles in very low birth weight infants. *Nursing Research, 31,* 68–72.

Medoff-Cooper, B., Verklan, T., & Carlson, S. (1993). The development of sucking patterns and physiologic correlates in very-low-birth-weight infants. *Nursing Research, 42,* 100–105.

Medoff-Cooper, B., Weininger, S., & Zukowsky, K. (1989). Neonatal sucking as a clinical assessment tool: Preliminary findings. *Nursing Research, 38,* 162–165.

Miller, D. B., & Holditch-Davis, D. (1992). Interactions of parents and nurses with high-risk preterm infants. *Research in Nursing and Health, 15,* 187–197.

Parker, S. J., Zahr, L. K., Cole, J. G., & Brecht, M.-L. (1992). Outcome after developmental intervention in the neonatal intensive care unit for mothers of preterm infants with low socioeconomic status. *Journal of Pediatrics, 120,* 780–785.

Pridham, K., Becker, P., & Brown, R. (2000). Effects of infant and caregiver conditions on an infant's focused exploration of toys. *Journal of Advanced Nursing, 31,* 1439–1448.

Pridham, K. F., Brown, R., Sondel, S., Clark, R., & Green, C. (2001). Effects of biologic and experiential conditions on the pattern of growth in weight of premature and full-term infants. *Research in Nursing and Health, 24,* 283–297.

Pridham, K., Brown, R., Sondel, S., Green, C., Wedel, N. Y., & Lai, H.-C. (1998). Transition time to full nipple feeding for premature infants with a history of lung disease. *Journal of Obstetric, Gynecologic and Neonatal Nursing, 27,* 533–545.

Pridham, K., Kosorok, M. R., Greer, F., Carey, P., Kayata, S., & Sondel, S. (1999). The effects of prescribed versus ad libitum feedings and formula caloric density on premature infant dietary intake and weight gain. *Nursing Research, 48,* 86–93.

Pridham, K., Kosorok, M. R., Greer, F., Kayata, S., Bhattacharya, A., & Grunwald, P. (2001). Comparison of caloric intake and weight outcomes of an *ad lib* feeding regimen for preterm infants in two nurseries. *Journal of Advanced Nursing, 35,* 751–759.

Pridham, K. F., Sondel, S., Chang, A., & Green, C. (1993). Nipple feeding for preterm infants with bronchopulmonary dysplasia. *Journal of Obstetric, Gynecologic and Neonatal Nursing, 22,* 147–155.

Sameroff, A. J., & Chandler, M. J. (1975). Reproductive risk and the continuum of caretaking casualty. In F. D. Horowitz (Ed.), *Review of child development research* (Vol. 4, pp. 187–244). Chicago: University of Chicago Press.

Schraeder, B. D. (1986). Developmental progress in very low birth weight infants during the first year of life. *Nursing Research, 35,* 237–242.

Schraeder, B. D., Czajka, C., Kalman, D. D., & McGeady, S. J. (1998). Respiratory health, lung function, and airway responsiveness in school-age survivors of very-low-birth-weight. *Clinical Pediatrics, 37,* 237–246.

Schraeder, B. D., Heverly, M. A., & O'Brien, C. M. (1996a). Home and classroom behavioral adjustment in very low birthweight children: The influences of caregiver stress and goodness of fit. *Children's Health Care, 25,* 117–131.

Schraeder, B. D., Heverly, M. A., & O'Brien, C. (1996b). The influence of early biological risk and the home environment on nine-year outcome of very low birth weight. *Canadian Journal of Nursing Research, 28,* 79–95.

Schraeder, B. D., Heverly, M. A., O'Brien, C., & Goodman, R. (1997). Academic achievement and educational resource use of very low birth weight (VLBW) survivors. *Pediatric Nursing, 23,* 21–25, 44.

Schraeder, B. D., Heverly, M. A., O'Brien, C., & McEvoy-Shields, K. (1992a). Finishing first grade: A study of school achievement in very-low-birth-weight children. *Nursing Research, 41,* 354–361.

Schraeder, B. D., Heverly, M. A., O'Brien, C., & McEvoy-Shields, K. (1992b). Vulnerability and temperament in very low birth weight school-aged children. *Nursing Research, 41,* 101–105.

Schraeder, B. D., Heverly, M. A., & Rappaport, J. (1990a). Temperament, behavior problems, and learning skills in very low birth weight preschoolers. *Research in Nursing and Health, 13,* 17–34.

Schraeder, B. D., Heverly, M. A., & Rappaport, J. (1990b). The value of early home assessment in identifying risk in children who were very low birthweight. *Pediatric Nursing, 16,* 268–272.

Schraeder, B. D., & McEvoy-Shields, K. (1991). Visual acuity, binocular vision, and ocular muscle balance in VLBW children. *Pediatric Nursing, 17,* 30–33.

Schraeder, B. D., & Medoff-Cooper, B. (1983). Development and temperament in very low birth weight infants—The second year. *Nursing Research, 32,* 331–335.

Schraeder, B. D., Rappaport, J., & Courtwright, L. (1987). Preschool development of very low birthweight infants. *Image: Journal of Nursing Scholarship, 19,* 174–178.

Shiao, S.-Y. P. K. (1995). Comparison of morning and afternoon feedings in very low birth weight infants. *Issues in Comprehensive Pediatric Nursing, 18,* 43–53.

Shiao, S.-Y. P. K. (1997). Comparison of continuous versus intermittent sucking in very-low-birth-weight infants. *Journal of Obstetric, Gynecologic and Neonatal Nursing, 26,* 313–319.

Shiao, S.-Y. P. K. (2002). Desaturation events in neonates during mechanical ventilation. *Critical Care Quarterly, 24*(4), 14–29.

Shiao, S.-Y. P. K., Andrews, C. M., & Ahn, C. (2002). Predictors of intubation and oxygenation complications in neonates. *Newborn and Infant Nursing Reviews, 2,* 128–137.

Shiao, S.-Y. P. K., Brooker, J., & DiFiore, T. (1996). Desaturation events during oral feedings with and without a nasogastric tube in very low birth weight infants. *Heart and Lung, 25,* 236–245.

Shiao, S.-Y. P. K., Chang, Y.-J., Lannon, H., & Yarandi, H. (1997). Meta-analysis of the effects of nonnutritive sucking on heart rate and peripheral oxygenation: Research from the past 30 years. *Issues in Comprehensive Pediatric Nursing, 20,* 11–24.

Shiao, S.-Y. P. K., Youngblut, J. M., Anderson, G. C., DiFiore, J. M., & Martin, R. J. (1995). Nasogastric tube placement: Effects on breathing and sucking in very-low-birth-weight infants. *Nursing Research, 44,* 82–88.

Stevens, B. J., & Johnston, C. C. (1994). Physiological responses of premature infants to painful stimuli. *Nursing Research, 43,* 226–231.

Stevens, B. J., Johnston, C. C., Franck, L., Petryshen, P., Jack, A., & Foster, G. (1999). The efficacy of developmentally sensitive interventions and sucrose for relieving procedural pain in very low birth weight neonates. *Nursing Research, 48,* 35–42.

Stevens, B. J., Johnston, C. C., & Horton, L. (1993). Multidimensional pain assessment in premature neonates: A pilot study. *Journal of Obstetric, Gynecologic and Neonatal Nursing, 22,* 531–541.

Stevens, B. J., Johnston, C. C., & Horton, L. (1994). Factors that influence the behavioral pain responses of premature infants. *Pain, 59,* 101–109.

Stevens, B., Johnston, C., Petryshen, P., & Taddio, A. (1996). Premature infant pain profile: Development and validation. *Clinical Journal of Pain, 12,* 13–22.

Stevens, B. J., Johnston, C. C., Taddio, A., Jack, A., Narciso, J., Stremler, R., et al. (1999). Management of pain from heel lance with lidocaine-prilocaine (EMLA) cream: Is it safe and efficacious in preterm infants? *Journal of Developmental and Behavioral Pediatrics, 20,* 216–221.

Stevens, B. J., Petryshen, P., Hawkins, J., Smith, B., & Taylor, P. (1996). Developmental versus conventional care: A comparison of clinical outcomes for very low birth weight infants. *Canadian Journal of Nursing Research, 28,* 97–113.

Steward, D. K., & Pridham, K. F. (2001). Stability of respiratory quotient and growth outcomes of very low birth weight infants. *Biological Research for Nursing, 2,* 198–205.

Steward, D. K., & Pridham, K. F. (2002). Growth patterns of extremely low-birth-weight hospitalized preterm infants. *Journal of Obstetric, Gynecologic and Neo-natal Nursing, 31,* 57–64.

Thoman, E. B., Acebo, C., & Becker, P. T. (1983). Infant crying and stability in the mother-infant relationship: A systems analysis. *Child Development, 54,* 653–659.

Thoman, E. B., Holditch Davis, D., Raye, J. R., Philipps, A. F., Rowe, J. C., & Denenberg, V. H. (1985). Theophylline affects sleep-wake state development in premature infants. *Neuropediatrics, 16,* 13–18.

Tobey, G. Y., & Schraeder, B. D. (1990). Impact of caretaker stress on behavioral adjustment of very low birthweight infants. *Nursing Research, 39,* 84–89.

Torres, C., Holditch-Davis, D., O'Hale, A., & D'Auria, J. (1997). Effect of standardized rest periods on apnea and weight gain of preterm infants. *Neonatal Network, 16*(8), 35–43.

Vogelpohl, D. G., Evans, J. C., & Cedargren, D. H. (1995). Behavioral pain response of the low birth weight premature neonate in the NICU. *Neonatal Intensive Care, 8*(5), 28–33.

Walden, M., Penticuff, J. H., Stevens, B., Lotas, M. J., Kozinetz, C. A., Clark, A., et al. (2001). Maturational changes in physiologic and behavioral responses of preterm neonates to pain. *Advances in Neonatal Care, 1*(2), 94–106.

White-Traut, R. C., & Goldman, M. B. C. (1988). Premature infant massage: Is it safe? *Pediatric Nursing, 14,* 285–289.

White-Traut, R. C., & Nelson, M. N. (1988). Maternally administered tactile, auditory, visual, and vestibular stimulation: Relationship to later interactions between mothers and premature infants. *Research in Nursing and Health, 11,* 31–39.

White-Traut, R. C., Nelson, M. N., & Silvestri, J. M. (1990). The effectiveness of multisensory stimulation in enhancing recovery among preterm infants. In S. G. Funk, E. M. Tornquist, M. T. Champagne, L. A. Copp, & R. A. Wiese (Eds.), *Key aspects of recovery: Improving nutrition, rest, and mobility* (pp. 130–149). New York: Springer.

White-Traut, R. C., Nelson, M. N., Silvestri, J. M., Cunningham, N., & Patel, M. (1997). Response of preterm infants to unimodal and multimodal sensory intervention. *Pediatric Nursing, 23,* 169–175, 193.

White-Traut, R. C., Nelson, M. N., Silvestri, J. M., Patel, M. K., & Kilgallon, D. (1993). Patterns of physiologic and behavioral response of intermediate or preterm infants to intervention. *Pediatric Nursing, 19,* 625–629.

White-Traut, R. C., Nelson, M. N., Silvestri, J. M., Patel, M., Vasan, U., Han, B. K., et al. (1999). Developmental intervention for preterm infants diagnosed with periventricular leukomalcia. *Research in Nursing and Health, 22,* 131–143.

White-Traut, R. C., & Pate, C. M. H. (1987). Modulating infant state in premature infants. *Journal of Pediatric Nursing, 2,* 96–101.

White-Traut, R. C., & Tubezewski, K. A. (1986). Multimodal stimulation of the premature infant. *Journal of Pediatric Nursing, 1,* 90–95.

Youngblut, J. M., & Brooten, D. (1999). Alternate child care, history of hospitalization, and preschool child behavior. *Nursing Research, 48,* 29–34.

Youngblut, J. M., Brooten, D., Singer, L. T., Standing, T., Lee, H., & Rodgers, W. L. (2001). Effects of maternal employment and prematurity on child outcomes in single parent families. *Nursing Research, 50,* 346–355.

Youngblut, J. M., Lewandoswki, W., Casper, G. R., & Youngblut, W. R. (1994). Vibration in metal and non-metal incubators. *Biomedical Instrumentation and Technology, 28,* 476–480.

Youngblut, J. M., Loveland-Cherry, C. J., & Horan, M. (1991). Maternal employment effects on family and preterm infants at three months. *Nursing Research, 40,* 272–275.

Youngblut, J. M., Loveland-Cherry, C. J., & Horan, M. (1993). Maternal employment, family functioning, and preterm infant development at 9 and 12 months. *Research in Nursing and Health, 16,* 33–43.

Youngblut, J. M., Loveland-Cherry, C. J., & Horan, M. (1994). Maternal employment effects on families and preterm infants at 18 months. *Nursing Research, 43,* 331–337.

Younkin, D., Medoff-Cooper, B., Guillet, R., Sinwell, T., Chance, B., & Delivora-Papadopoulos, M. (1988). In vivo ^{31}P nuclear magnetic resonance measurement of chronic changes in cerebral metabolites following neonatal intraventricular hemorrhage. *Pediatrics, 82,* 331–336.

Zahr, L. (1991). Correlates of mother-infant interaction in premature infants from low socioeconomic backgrounds. *Pediatric Nursing, 17,* 259–264.

Zahr, L. K. (1998). Two contrasting NICU environments. *MCN: American Journal of Maternal-Child Nursing, 23,* 28–36.

Zahr, L. K., & Balian, S. (1995). Responses of premature infants to routine nursing interventions and noise in the NICU. *Nursing Research, 44,* 179–185.

Zahr, L. K., Parker, S., & Cole, J. (1992). Comparing the effects of neonatal intensive care unit intervention on premature infants at different weights. *Journal of Developmental and Behavioral Pediatrics, 13,* 165–172.

Zeanah, C. H., Boris, N. W., & Larrieu, J. A. (1997). Infant development and developmental risk: A review of the past 10 years. *Journal of the American Academy of Child and Adolescent Psychiatry, 36,* 165–178.

Zhang, P., & Medoff-Cooper, B. (1996). A Markov regression model for nutritive sucking data. *Biometrics, 52,* 112–124.

Chapter 3

Developmental Transition From Gavage to Oral Feeding in the Preterm Infant

SUZANNE M. THOYRE

ABSTRACT

The development of early oral feeding skills in the preterm infant is an active and complex area of nursing research. This integrative review summarizes the accumulated nursing research since 1990 that describes feeding the preterm infant during the transition from gavage to full oral feeding. Literature was identified through searches of databases covering the fields of nursing and medicine and of journals and nurse researchers who publish in this area of study. Four main areas of research were identified: development of infant feeding skills, descriptive studies on the transition period, studies that focus on identifying infant readiness to begin oral feeding, and studies that explore optimal ways to advance oral feeding as the infant moves toward full oral feeding. Research studies were critiqued from a developmental science perspective, which conceptualizes feeding skill as an emergent property of multiple systems, both within and outside the infant, that are interacting and working together to promote optimal functioning. Through this analysis, areas for future research are identified.

For the preterm infant the task of transitioning from gavage to oral feeding is complex, involving the integration, maturation, and coordination of multiple systems, including the caregiver system. The transition period occurs during the final weeks of the infant's hospitalization and for breastfed infants is likely to extend into the early discharge period. Oral feeding is often the final competency that an infant needs to attain before being discharged home. Supporting the development of oral feeding skills

61

is an important area of nursing practice, and consequently a great deal of attention has focused on understanding preterm infant feeding behaviors and on strategies to support the preterm infant during this transition period. This integrative review summarizes nursing research related to feeding the preterm infant during the transition to full oral feeding, critiques the research in relation to developmental science theory, and identifies areas for future research (Cooper, 1989).

BACKGROUND

To study any aspect of the transition to full oral feeding, a multisystem developmental approach is required (Medoff-Cooper, 2000). Developmental science provides a framework that organizes the multiple foci of feeding research, and it is appropriate for the study of this biological and social process. Rather than taking a purely maturational perspective with the overarching belief that the development of feeding skills is "just a matter of time," or a cognitive-structuralist perspective that views the development of feeding skills as a process that lies within the infant with the environment offering a facilitative role, a developmental science perspective views the process of infant feeding skill development as a reflection of the dynamic interactions between the infant and caregiver and external subsystems. Central to this perspective is the notion that learning to feed orally is a developmental process whereby multiple subsystems "from the subsystems of genetics, neurobiology, and hormones to those of families, social networks, communities, and cultures" (Cairns, Elder, & Costello, 1996, p. 1) interact and cocreate organization of the feeding system. Subsystems within the infant, such as the autonomic system, the state system, hunger, and motor systems serving the infant's posture, oral structures, and upper airway, are in the process of maturing along convergent, but not necessarily synchronous, timelines (Medoff-Cooper, Bilker, & Kaplan, 2001; Thelen, 1989). The social system (typically parents, select family members or significant others, and nurses), the culture of care in the neonatal intensive care unit (NICU), the time period (era of care), and the physical systems, including the type of bottle or nipple used and the activity, sound, and lighting of the room, are all subsystems of feeding that contribute to and cocreate feeding skill.

The transition period spans the time from the introduction of oral feeding through the time when the preterm infant is fully oral feeding.

Both breast and bottle feeding research will be reviewed. Rates of breastfeeding vary in the preterm population by health of the infant, maternal factors, NICU protocols, the larger economic and health care systems, and the definition of breastfeeding used (Bell, Geyer, & Jones, 1995; Furman, Minich, & Hack, 1998; Hill, Ledbetter, & Kavanaugh, 1997; Kliethermes, Cross, Lanese, Johnson, & Simon, 1999; Meier et al., 1993; Stine, 1990; Woldt, 1991). Between 15 and 94% of mothers who intended to breastfeed their preterm infants were at least partially breastfeeding at discharge, with the lowest rates reported for infants with the lowest birthweight (BW) and gestational age at birth (GA) and for infants born in the United States (Furman et al., 1998; Hill et al., 1997; Meier et al., 1993; Nyqvist, Sjoden, & Ewald, 1999; Yip, Lee, & Sheehy, 1996). Since there are now several excellent and thorough reviews available about breastfeeding the preterm infant (e.g., Meier, 2001; Meier & Brown, 1996), emphasis will be on studies that focus on breastfeeding during the transition period.

METHOD

The *Cumulative Index of Nursing and Allied Health Literature, Pubmed,* and *Medline* were searched using several strategies to identify articles for the review. First, the following phrases were used: *preterm and feeding, preterm and bottle, preterm and breast.* In addition, specific journals and authors with research programs on the oral feeding of preterm infants were searched, and, finally, reference lists of all identified articles were searched for additional, potentially missed research articles.

     To be included, (a) research had to be published from 1990 to present, (b) the nurse researcher had to be the first or second author, and (c) there had to be a sample of preterm infants hospitalized in an NICU during the time of the study. Excluded were studies pertaining to the content of the feeding (formula/breast milk quality), non-research-based reports or discussions, abstracts, unpublished manuscripts, and funded studies without published reports. This review is limited to the time period of 1990 to present because of the changes that have occurred in neonatal care. In particular, the advent of surfactant has decreased the number of preterm infants with severe bronchopulmonary dysplasia and allowed younger infants, who are now healthier, to begin oral feeding at a much earlier postconceptional age (PCA). Additionally, the issues and concerns related to oral feeding progression are influenced by current health care goals. NICUs now aim for earlier discharge of infants to reunite families sooner and to contain health care costs. Although preterm infants are now healthier at the time of oral feeding, they are considerably less mature; therefore, the task of transitioning to oral feedings has significantly changed.

Areas of study related to the transition from gavage to full oral feeding have been wide in scope, including when to offer the preterm infant oral feeding, what the overall process of advancement of oral feeding should be, and explorations of specific feeding skills. Units of study have been as short as seconds to as long as the entire transitional period. The bulk of the research has focused on description, understanding relationships, and prediction. However, in the past decade intervention studies have increased, and one meta-analysis on feeding interventions is now in the literature (Daley & Kennedy, 2000). In addition, several "state of the science" papers have been written, one on neonatal sucking behaviors and two on breastfeeding the preterm (Medoff-Cooper & Ray, 1995; Meier, 2001; Meier & Brown, 1996).

The organization of this review and the critique of individual studies were guided by the perspective of developmental science. The development of skills required for oral feeding is discussed first; then follows a description of the transition period and an exploration of research on infant readiness for oral feeding; and finally, a review of research on the advancement of oral feeding is provided. Studies were examined for the extent to which they incorporated a developmental, ecological, and sociocultural approach to the conceptualization, design, measurement, data analysis, and discussion of the research.

Development of Infant Oral Feeding Skills

A significant clinical problem for preterm infants during early feeding is their coordination of suck-swallow-breathe mechanisms. Infant feeding skill is reflected in the infant's ability to coordinate sucking, swallowing, and breathing while obtaining adequate nutritional intake for growth, maintaining physiologic regulation, and remaining engaged in the feeding process. Nursing research aimed at understanding the organization of preterm infant feeding skills has focused on four main skill areas: (a) attaining and maintaining an awake state prior to and during feeding; (b) development of and change in oral-motor behaviors as infants transition to full oral feeding;

(c) coordination of sucking and breathing with regulation of physiologic control during oral feeding; and (d) the role of the caregiver in feeding skill development. While these research foci will be discussed individually, there is a great deal of overlap between them.

ATTAINING AND MAINTAINING AN AWAKE STATE

During the time when preterm infants are learning to oral feed, development of sleep-wake states and state organization is occurring, reflecting the underlying maturation of the central nervous system. In general, between 29 and 39 weeks PCA, infants spend the majority of their time in active sleep. However, over time, active sleep decreases, quiet sleep increases, and behavioral states become more organized (Holditch-Davis, 1990; Holditch-Davis & Edwards, 1998). During the transition to oral feeding most awake states occur during caregiving. Preterm infants have the most bouts of alertness, sleep-wake transitioning, and drowsiness during periods of routine caregiving, such as feeding (Brandon, Holditch-Davis, & Beylea, 1999).

Sleep-wake states have been examined prior to and during oral feedings as an indicator of readiness to feed and as a critical component of feeding behaviors. An awake state prior to feeding is hypothesized to indicate that the infant is behaviorally organized and ready for the task. Infants who begin oral feeding in an awake state are more likely to consume their prescribed feeding volume (Anderson et al., 1990; McCain, 1997; Pickler, Higgins, & Crummette, 1993) and, for those infants with BW less than 1,500 gm, to have improved growth during the transition period (Anderson et al., 1990). Medoff-Cooper, McGrath, and Bilker (2000) longitudinally studied the development of sleep-wake states at 34 weeks PCA and again at 40 weeks PCA. As infants matured, they showed increasing ability to receive stimuli, interact socially, and sustain energy through the feeding. At 34 weeks, infants were more likely to change from drowsiness to sleep after feeding, whereas at 40 weeks, infants were able to stay awake.

Non-nutritive sucking (NNS) has been tested as an intervention to achieve an optimal state prior to feeding (Anderson et al., 1990; Gill, Behnke, Conlon, & Anderson, 1992; McCain, 1992, 1995; Pickler et al., 1993; Pickler, Frankel, Walsh, & Thompson, 1996). In four studies, NNS prior to feeding modulated the state prior to feeding—either bringing the infant up to an awake state from a state of drowsiness or sleep or calming the infant from an active state (Anderson et al., 1990; Gill et al., 1992;

McCain, 1992, 1995; Pickler et al., 1996). In addition, NNS facilitated maintenance of awake states (McCain, 1992, 1995) and higher oxygen saturation (Pickler et al., 1996). Pickler et al. (1993) also tested the effect of NNS on infant state, physiologic regulation, and feeding performance. Infants receiving NNS had higher feeding performance scores (higher intake, shorter feeding) and were more likely to be in a sleep state 5 minutes after the feeding but were not more likely to be in an awake state at the onset of or during feeding.

Several key components of NICU feeding protocols related to infant state are in need of research-based evidence. While maintenance of an awake state is an important component of an infant's ability to oral-feed, no studies tested strategies to arouse an infant who has decreased his or her level of arousal during feeding. Furthermore, despite common recommendations to avoid stimulation of the preterm infant during feeding (such as by arousal strategies like talking to the infant), no studies have evaluated the infant's behavioral responses to external stimulation during feeding.

Another common protocol is the alternation of gavage and oral feeding, which is based on the assumption that younger infants require rest periods between oral feedings to restore energy. Similarly, many nurseries impose a maximum oral feeding time for preterms, with the assumption that longer feedings increase the infant's energy expenditure and potential for fatigue. Yet an ideal feeding length has not been established (Hill, 1992). Infant feeding capacities are likely to vary throughout the day (Shiao, 1995). It may be less tiring for an infant to be orally fed in response to his or her readiness or by incorporating rest periods into the feeding than by using a nonindividualized prescribed plan. Finally, most preterm infants are drowsy or sleeping by the end of the feeding (Medoff-Cooper et al., 2000); however, whether infants are demonstrating satiety or manifesting fatigue is not known. The terms *fatigue, tired,* and *sleep* are used interchangeably to describe problematic and common preterm infant feeding behavior, but no measures other than state have been employed to describe these behaviors. Studies are needed to determine early indicators of fatigue, to understand underlying causes of fatigue, and to examine the effect of feeding pattern and length on infant energy expenditure.

DEVELOPMENT AND ORGANIZATION OF ORAL-MOTOR FEEDING BEHAVIORS

Oral-motor feeding behaviors are the most observable and studied of infant feeding skills. The tasks of breastfeeding and bottle-feeding differ in oral-motor skills. The breastfeeding research provides a broader examination of the relevant components of oral-motor feeding skills: rooting, areolar grasp, latching on, sucking, and swallowing (Meier, 1996; Nyqvist, Rubertsson, Ewald, & Sjoden, 1996; Nyqvist et al., 1999; Nyqvist & Ewald, 1999); the bottle-feeding research has more closely focused on the relevant components of sucking: pressures, rates, burst quality, and pattern (Medoff-Cooper, 1991; Medoff-Cooper et al., 2000, 2001; Medoff-Cooper, Delivoria-Papadopoulos, & Brooten, 1991; Medoff-Cooper & Gennaro, 1996; Medoff-Cooper, Verklan, & Carlson, 1993; Shiao, 1997).

Medoff-Cooper and associates have studied the development of sucking behaviors during bottle-feeding with the aim of assessing developmental changes in sucking parameters in relation to the integrity of the infant's neurological system. Their first study described the differences in sucking behaviors of preterm and fullterm infants and identified six sucking variables (burst length, interburst length, intersuck interval, duration of suck, volume milk consumed per suck, and peak intraoral sucking pressure) (Medoff-Cooper, Weininger, & Zukowsky, 1989). Preterm infants fed for shorter periods of time, exhibited lower sucking pressures, and had shorter sucking bursts. Using these variables, the authors conducted a series of longitudinal, descriptive studies examining the development of sucking behaviors from 32 through 40 weeks PCA. One 5-minute period of sucking was examined at each PCA with samples of 44 to 66 preterm infants. All but one study had a sample of healthy preterm infants; the final study (Medoff-Cooper et al., 2000) included infants with medical complications.

Overall, Medoff-Cooper and colleagues demonstrated that PCA alone is insufficient to predict sucking skill, given that infants have varying levels of health and experiences with oral feeding. There was large variability in findings across studies. For example, sucking pressures were highest at 32 weeks PCA in a preliminary study, at 35 weeks PCA in a second study, and lowest at 40 weeks PCA in a third study (Medoff-Cooper, 1991; Medoff-Cooper et al., 1993, 2000). Since infants entered the study in their first week of oral feeding, the "inexperienced" oral feeder was anywhere from 32 to 35 weeks PCA at the beginning of the study, making findings difficult to interpret. Furthermore, interindividual variability in feeding skill was not described.

A recent study by Medoff-Cooper et al. (2001) examined changes in sucking parameters as a function of GA by studying 186 healthy infants who were able to engage in oral feeding soon after birth. Infants were grouped by GA (33, 34, 35, 36, 37, and term age). Each infant's sucking parameters were measured once during 5 minutes of nutritive sucking in the first week of oral feeding. Sucking skills were found to change across gestational age as well as across the 5-minute feeding period. As gestational age increased, infants engaged in more sucking, organized sucking into longer sucking bursts with shorter interburst intervals, and increased and stabilized sucking pressures. The cross-sectional analysis also demonstrated that individual sucking parameters mature at different rates. For example, between 34 to 35 weeks gestation, infants demonstrate stabilization and organization of sucking: the variability in within-burst intersuck intervals and sucking pressures decreased and sucking was organized into fewer sucking bursts. Later in gestation (36 to 40 weeks), infants built upon these skills, developing the ability to suck more, lengthening sucking bursts, and increasing sucking pressures.

Across the 5-minute feeding period and independent of GA, infants demonstrated a pattern of diminishing sucking skill through minute 4 of the study (sucking decreased, sucking bursts became shorter, and sucking pressures decreased), with partial recovery of feeding skills during the final minute (Medoff-Cooper et al., 2001). Hill, Kurkowski, and Garcia (2000) also found temporal variability in infant sucking parameters within feedings. As a feeding progressed, infants' sucking became less frequent and sucking bursts shortened, while sucking pauses became more frequent and lengthened. More research is needed in this area to better understand how factors such as ventilation, oxygenation, stress, and recovery from distress affect sucking parameters across entire feeding sessions for preterm infants.

Nyqvist and associates and Meier and associates have studied the oral motor feeding skills of breastfeeding preterm infants (Meier, 1996; Nyqvist & Ewald, 1999; Nyqvist, Farnstrand, Eeg-Olofsson, & Ewald, 2001; Nyqvist, Rubertsson, et al., 1996; Nyqvist et al., 1999). Compared to bottle feeding, early sucking patterns during breastfeeding consist of shorter latching-on periods and sucking bursts with less intake but stable physiologic regulation (Meier, 1996). Nyqvist and colleagues provided a longitudinal account of the progression of oral-motor capacity from initiation of breastfeeding through discharge from the NICU of 71 healthy preterm infants (initiated when infants were 27.9 to 35.9 weeks PCA). Mothers were trained to reliably observe and assess their infants' feeding behaviors at breast (rooting, areolar grasp, latching on, sucking, and swallowing) using the Preterm Infant Breastfeeding Behavior Scale (Nyqvist,

Rubertsson, et al., 1996; Nyqvist et al., 1999; Nyqvist & Ewald, 1999). On average, each mother scored 61 breast-feeding sessions. Obvious rooting, grasp of the areola and nipple, and latching on for greater than 15 minutes were observed as early as 28 weeks PCA. By 32 weeks PCA, some infants were capable of repeated sucking bursts of 10 or more sucks, with longest bursts consisting of 30 consecutive sucks or more. Repeated swallowing was noted at 31 weeks, with nutritive sucking occurring as early as 30.6 weeks. By 36 weeks all infants had demonstrated mature rooting and alveolar grasp, and most had attained the ability for repeated long sucking bursts, latching on for at least 15 minutes, and repeated swallowing. The mean PCA when infants were capable of full breastfeeding was 36 weeks, with a wide range of 33.4 to 40 weeks.

COORDINATION OF SUCKING AND BREATHING WITH REGULATION OF PHYSIOLOGIC CONTROL DURING ORAL FEEDING

For both bottle- and breastfeeding, a major criterion for progression of oral feeding skill is the infant's capacity to extend the sucking burst length and develop an organized, rhythmical sucking pattern (Medoff-Cooper et al., 2001; Nyqvist et al., 1999). However, sucking patterns are constrained by the infant's level of physiologic stability. During the transition period from gavage to oral feeding, preterm infants' regulation of breathing is in the process of stabilizing and becoming more organized. The method of feeding (breast- versus bottle-feeding) significantly differs in its impact on the infant's physiologic stability. Bottle-feeding disrupts the preterm infant's breathing pattern to a greater extent and consequently has a greater potential to negatively impact the preterm's oxygen status than does breastfeeding (Dowling, 1999; Marino, O'Brien, & LoRe, 1995; Meier, 1996).

During bottle feeding, sucking has the potential for affecting preterm infants' ventilation. When engaged in a sucking burst, preterm infants either are apneic or demonstrate a range in the quality of interspersed breaths. Shiao and associates examined two common types of sucking: (a) continuous, long sucking bouts (CS) and (b) bouts of intermittent sucking (IS) (Shiao, Youngblut, Anderson, DiFiore, & Martin, 1995; Shiao, 1997). Infants were studied during two feedings that occurred within a 24-hour period. During CS, infants sucked with higher frequency and pressure and consumed a greater amount of milk. Respiratory rate, minute ventilation and tidal volume, and oxygen saturation decreased, while end-tidal carbon dioxide increased. During IS, sucking frequency and pressure decreased and infants had less volume intake while minute ventilation and oxygen saturation increased, although not to the prefeed level.

Very low birthweight infants (VLBW, less than 1,500 gm at birth) have significant numbers of severe oxygen desaturation events during bottle-feeding. Thoyre and Carlson (in press) found that 22 VLBW infants with variation in respiratory health (86% respiratory distress syndrome, RDS; 36% bronchopulmonary dysplasia, BPD) spent 20% of a feeding near discharge with oxygen saturation below 90%. Infants most at risk for oxygen desaturation during feeding were infants with lower PCA, higher BW, less experience feeding, fewer days on supplemental oxygen, no requirement for supplemental oxygen at the time of the study, and lower baseline oxygen saturation prior to feeding. Smaller-BW infants tended to be older PCA near discharge and to continue to require supplemental oxygen. Despite similar baseline oxygen saturation levels, infants who were on supplemental oxygen had 50% fewer oxygen desaturation events and spent 33% less time with suboptimal oxygen saturation.

Shiao, Brooker, and DiFiore (1996) reported data on two complete feeding sessions of 20 VLBW infants at a mean PCA of 35 weeks to describe oxygen desaturation events, compare characteristics of infants prone to desaturate during feeding, and examine the impact of nasogastric tubes in place during oral feeding on infant physiologic stability and sucking. All infants had a history of mechanical ventilation. The 15 infants with desaturation events during feeding had significantly lower oxygen saturation prior to, during and after feeding than infants without desaturation events. Most desaturation events were preceded with a pause in breathing, a decrease in heart rate, and an increase in end-tidal carbon dioxide. Additionally, desaturation events occurred during prolonged sucking bursts. Infants with BPD had more frequent, more prolonged, and more severe desaturation events. The presence of a nasogastric tube, which potentially impacts the preterm's airway, was associated with increased breathing pauses, shallower breathing, and longer and more severe desaturation events. The tube also had a negative effect on sucking frequency, pressure, and volume intake. Further, infants with BPD had nearly twice as many desaturation events when fed with a nasogastric tube in place.

Research is needed to identify effective interventions to minimize the negative ventilatory effects of bottle-feeding for the preterm. While sucking impacts ventilation, lower oxygen during feeding also impacts the infant's ability to remain engaged in feeding. Infants with lower oxygen saturation tend to have shorter sucking bursts and shorter intervals between bursts, potentially signifying that less energy is available for sucking and there is less ability to organize restorative breathing breaks (Shiao et al., 1996; Zhang & Medoff-Cooper, 1996).

ROLE OF THE CAREGIVER IN FEEDING SKILL DEVELOPMENT

Nurse researchers have viewed oral feeding as involving multiple subsystems within the infant. However, inadequate attention has been paid to the role of the caregiver. The environment that the caregiver provides and the interactions between the caregiver and the infant during the feeding both promote and constrain the infant's skill development. The caregiver's feeding skills (how the caregiver feeds and how he or she thinks about feeding) must therefore be incorporated into the study of infant feeding skills. Caregiver behaviors during feeding are likely a reflection of how sensitive and knowledgeable the caregiver is of the needs of the infant. Sensitive caregiving involves attending to an infant's cues to determine when protection and support are needed and to determine when to allow the infant to regulate his or her own behavior (Thoman, 1993). In the context of feeding a preterm infant, sensitive caregiving is likely to involve prompt response to infant behavioral and physiologic cues as well as proactive structuring of the feeding to support infant feeding competencies.

Several studies on behavior-based developmental care with preterms employed a protocol for oral feeding that included no jiggling of the nipple to encourage sucking. These studies demonstrated earlier initiation of oral feeding, higher infant engagement during feeding, shorter transition time to full oral feeding, and improved growth (Becker, Grunwald, Moorman, & Stuhr, 1991, 1993). However, the studies did not explore the direct effect of the caregivers' action (e.g., jiggling) on infant feeding behavior or physiology.

Hill et al. (2000) examined the effect of specific caregiver actions on infant feeding behavior. This study used a randomized crossover design to test the impact of the nurse providing stability to the jaw and pressure on the cheeks (oral support) to assist the organization and efficiency of sucking. Outcomes included sucking parameters and physiologic stability. Infants were selected on the basis of history of poor feeding, 32 to 34 weeks PCA, and absence of medical complications, including respiratory problems or supplemental oxygen requirement. Oral support decreased the length and frequency of sucking pauses without adversely affecting physiologic stability in this healthy sample. No other sucking parameters differed between groups, and effect on intake was not reported. Feedings that included oral support had fewer declines in oxygen saturation post feeding than feedings without oral support, suggesting that oral support may lead to less energy expenditure. This feeding strategy warrants further study, particularly with infants with cardiorespiratory problems that have the greatest feeding difficulty.

Meier et al. (2000) conducted an intervention study in the use of nipple shields to enhance milk transfer during breastfeeding. Mother-infant pairs were selected based on problematic latch-on (61.8%), sleepiness (29.4%), or other factors, such as nipple soreness (8.8%). Theoretically, the nipple shield provides a less pliable surface for the infant to latch on and maintain attachment to, thus providing oral-motor stability. Two consecutive breastfeedings were compared: one without the nipple shield and the next using it. The nipple shield significantly increased the volume of milk transferred during the breastfeeding session and did not negatively influence the duration of breastfeeding for the dyad.

In a study aimed at examining coregulation of feeding by infants and their mothers, Thoyre (1997) examined preterm feeding behaviors and physiologic response to feeding, maternal feeding behaviors, and how mothers were thinking about their role as coregulators of feeding. VLBW infants with a range of respiratory health conditions were fed by their mothers near the time of discharge from the NICU. Jiggling the nipple occurred, on average, 10% of the time. Mothers tended to jiggle the nipple during pauses in sucking when the infant was either awake and catching up on breathing or when the infant appeared to be asleep. When mothers jiggled or moved the nipple during breathing breaks, infants often demonstrated withdrawal behavior and oxygen desaturation events. If the mother jiggled or moved the nipple when the infant appeared asleep, the infant often responded with sucking that was not sustained and tended to return to a long sucking pause. The more mothers jiggled the nipple, the less engaged infants were in feeding. To understand the relationships between maternal behaviors and infant physiologic responses, a wider range of maternal actions under specific infant conditions (such as when the infant is breathing rapidly or distressed) needs to be studied.

How caregivers view feeding, the goals they have for the feeding, the cues they monitor, the meanings they ascribe to infant cues, their expectations regarding infants' feeding abilities, their sense of feeding coregulation, and their beliefs about their own ability to influence the feeding are reflected in caregivers' working models of feeding (Pridham, 1993; Pridham, Knight, & Stephenson, 1989; Pridham, Limbo, Schroeder,

Thoyre, & Van Riper, 1998; Pridham, Schroeder, & Brown, 1999; Pridham, Schroeder, Brown, & Clark, 2001). Working models of feeding have been linked to mothers' feeding behaviors. Mothers of preterm infants at 1 and 4 months post-term age whose working models of feeding were rated highest in responsivity and orientation to the infant as a person also were rated highest in affective involvement and responsiveness in feeding behavior (Pridham, Sondel, Clark, Green, & Brown, 1994). Mothers of both full- and preterm infants whose feeding expectations and intentions were attuned to their infants' needs for support of nutrient intake, developmental advance, and relationship with the mother demonstrated more positive affect and behavior during feeding at 1, 4, 8, and 12 months post-term age (Pridham, Schroeder, et al., 2001).

Very little is known about how mothers or nurses caring for preterm infants think about or experience feeding during the period when the infant is learning to oral-feed in the NICU. Wood (1991) examined the relationship of nurse reciprocity while bottle-feeding the preterm infant. Reciprocity was defined as the ability of both the infant and the caregiver to understand and respond appropriately to each other's cues. Twenty-seven nurses were observed feeding twice (once with a three-patient assignment, and once with a two- or four-patient assignment). An observational empathy scale was used which consisted of 16 items scored 1–5 on behaviors of the feeder, behaviors of the infant, and interaction between feeder and the infant (Harrison, 1982). As the nurses' workload increased, the amount of nurse-infant reciprocity decreased. In addition, feeding during the day shift (as opposed to the night shift) had a negative impact on reciprocity. Reciprocity was not affected by nurse educational level, years of experience, or parental status. Wood points out that, overall, nurses scored lower than mothers who were observed from the same setting (Harrison), calling attention to the unique perspective that mothers bring to feeding their preterm infants.

Near discharge from the NICU, Thoyre (1997) interviewed mothers about feeding using a focused method of video playback from a just-completed feeding. Interviews were scored from 1 to 6 on Pridham's working model dimension of coregulation (Pridham, Schroeder, et al., 1998). Mothers with higher scores on coregulation viewed the infant's participation in the feeding as highly valued and necessary condition for regulation of the feeding. These mothers described being flexible and proactive in the feeding while taking into account their infant's capacities and needs for support. Goals mothers had for the feeding included providing adequate caloric intake, protecting the infant's energy level, promoting a pleasurable infant experience, and developing a positive mother-infant relationship. The higher mothers scored on the coregulation component of the working model measure, the more their infants were engaged in feeding during feeding episodes. Mothers scoring higher on the coregulation measure were significantly older, their infants were younger gestationally at birth, and the infants tended to have been in the NICU and on oxygen longer (Thoyre, 2000).

Research conducted on the caregiver's role in preterm infant feeding demonstrates that infants' feeding skills may be enhanced through appropriate support. That the external environment can affect feeding skill is consistent with developmental science; that is, the feeding skills of infants are not solely within the infant but rather a product of the whole operating together (Thelen & Ulrich, 1991).

In summary, oral feeding can substantially destabilize the preterm infant unless the infant has acquired the ability to safely suck, swallow, and breathe. To accomplish this, infants need to be capable of sustaining attention to the task of feeding for the duration of the feeding; controlling and coordinating their postural, oral, and upper airway motor systems; and protecting their airway from fluid penetration. At the most basic level, this requires maturation of the autonomic system to the point whereby it can respond and adapt to the disruption and alteration in breathing pattern that occurs when the infant pauses to suck and swallow, as well as maturation of the central nervous system so that the infant is capable of orienting to and focusing attention on environmental stimuli. The demands placed on the infant for adaptation during feeding vary by both the method of feeding (breast, bottle, or bottle plus nasogastric tube) and by the caregiver's ability to respond to the infant and proactively promote an optimal feeding session.

Description of the Transition Period

For some preterm infants, the transition from gavage to oral feeding is rocky and prolonged and leads to a delay in discharge. For others, the transition period runs on an expected course and is managed by routine nursing. Understanding the expected length of the transition period and predicting which infants are likely to require more time for the development of feeding skills have been the foci of several studies.

The length of transition has been examined in four different subgroups of preterm infants. Mandich, Ritchie, and Mullett (1996) studied 65 healthy preterm infants who were 28 to 34 weeks gestation at birth. Infants who continued to have apnea during the transition period, regardless of whether they were on aminophylline, had a longer transition to full oral feeding (11 compared to 6.2 days). Infants who began oral feedings at an earlier PCA and those with a lower BW also had longer transition times.

Pickler, Mauck, and Geldmaker (1997) studied 40 bottle-feeding preterm infants. Infants with the most severe medical complications (such as patent ductus arteriosus, grade III or IV intraventricular hemorrhage, seizures, need for resuscitation) began oral feeding up to 2 weeks later and achieved full oral feeding 2 to 5 weeks later than healthier infants. Transition time was longer for infants weighing less than 1,000 gm at birth, for infants of younger GA, and for those who received longer assisted ventilation. Pickler et al. concluded that combining morbidity rating with GA provided a good prediction of an infant's ability to initiate and progress through learning to oral-feed.

Pridham, Sondel, Chang, and Green (1993) studied the progression to full oral feeding of 55 infants with BPD (defined by radiography and supplemental oxygen requirement greater than 28 days). All infants were less than 32 weeks GA and had a mean BW of 1,000 gm. Infants with BPD began oral feeding at an earlier PCA if they had fewer days of ventilation or required fewer days of supplemental oxygen. Therefore, infants who likely had more severe lung disease had a more prolonged transition to full oral feeding.

In 1998, Pridham, Brown, and colleagues examined the transition period with preterm infants who had a history of lung disease. They compared two levels of respiratory health—21 infants with BPD and 15 with RDS. The theoretical model used for this study was based on an ecological framework including infant (BW, gender, type and severity of lung disease, days tube-fed, breastfeeding in addition to bottle, history of apnea, weight and PCA at initiation of oral feeding), environmental (hospital setting), and historical factors (era: 1983–1989, 1990–1995). Ninety percent of the group with RDS reached full oral feeding in 13 days, compared to 19 days for infants with BPD. A longer transition was predicted by the presence of apnea during the transition period, beginning oral feedings at an earlier PCA, and history of more days tube-fed. No gender effect or effect of breastfeeding was demonstrated. There was a significant difference between hospitals, indicating an effect of care practices on length of transition.

Transition time for breastfeeding infants has not been adequately studied for any group of preterms. However, breastfeeding would likely lengthen the transition time because infants are capable of initiating breastfeeding at an earlier PCA. Most samples from the United States report incomplete transition to full breastfeeding at discharge, citing immature feeding behaviors as a major factor that prevents infants from being capable of consuming enough milk at breast to be fully breastfeeding (Hill, Aldag, & Chatterton, 1999; Hill et al., 1997; Kavanaugh, Mead, Meier, & Mangurten, 1995; Meier, Engstrom, Fleming, Streeter, & Lawrence, 1996). Success at feeding at breast is also highly linked with maternal milk supply and with mothers' ability to be with their infants during the hospitalization period (Hill et al., 1996, 1999; Nyqvist et al., 1999). In Nyqvist's studies conducted in Sweden, where mothers are less likely to have employment conflict with visitation, most breastfeeding infants (80%) were found to be capable of full breastfeeding by 36 weeks PCA, before discharge from the NICU (Nyqvist et al., 1999; Nyqvist & Ewald, 1999), demonstrating an effect of the ecological system on attainment of feeding skills.

In summary, neurodevelopmental maturation, positive, and contingent feeding experience, and health of the infant are key components of an infant's ability to initiate and progress to full oral feeding. All four transition-time studies were retrospective, and none of the studies examined criteria used to determine when oral feedings were initiated or how oral feedings were advanced other than to state that it was the nursery's "standard protocol." No studies have examined length of transition in relation to variability in infants' feeding behavior and physiology during feeding or to variability in caregiver actions during feedings. Rather than focus on the length of the transition period, which varies by the criteria used to initiate feedings, a more productive question may be at what PCA the infant is capable of full oral feeding given various conditions of health and experience. Prospective longitudinal studies are needed with a person-oriented approach to adequately describe infant and caregiver feeding behaviors and physiologic variables in relation to the ability to initiate and progress in feeding skill.

Readiness to Begin Oral Feeding

There is little research on determining when a preterm infant is ready to begin oral feedings and is ready for an individual feeding session. Two studies have described criteria nurses use in determining infant readiness. Siddell and Froman (1994) surveyed both head nurses and staff nurses regarding their feeding practice with stable preterm infants in 420 level II (30%) and level III (70%) neonatal nurseries across the United States. The majority of respondents indicated that their nursery had no set protocol for initiating oral feedings and that nurses made recommendations for initiating oral feedings based on the following in order of importance: PCA, weight, and observed interest in sucking. Despite evidence during the time of the survey that it is safer and more appropriate to begin breastfeeding before bottle-feeding (Meier, 1988; Meier & Anderson, 1987; Meier & Pugh, 1985), 86% of head nurses and 93% of staff nurses indicated that bottle-feeding was begun first. Level II nurseries tended to use behavioral indicators in determining readiness, while level III nurseries tended to use medical indicators.

Kinneer and Beachy (1994) surveyed 47 nurses from three hospitals in the United States to rank the importance of factors for determining readiness to oral-feed. The highest-ranked indicators were behavioral factors (NNS, strong gag reflex, crying) and physiologic factors (stable heart rate and color during NNS, stable cardiorespiratory measures throughout tube feedings), followed by PCA (34 weeks) and weight (greater than 1,500 gm). Hospital differences reflected variation in the culture of neonatal nursing care across settings. For example, nurses from hospital 1 ranked weight as a stronger criterion for initiating oral feeding than nurses from hospitals 2 or 3. Eighty percent of the respondents ranked nurses as the most influential clinicians in determining when to begin oral feeding (followed by physicians, physical and occupational therapists, and, rarely, family). Ninety-six percent of the respondents indicated that their nursery's policy on feeding the preterm infant was flexible. This highlights the centrality of the nurse in feeding and the need for nursing research to guide this area of practice.

The question of when to begin the transition from gavage feeding to feeding at the breast has also been examined. In the United States, it is recommended that infants begin to practice breastfeeding as soon as they are extubated from mechanical respirators or as early as 30 weeks PCA, if the breast is partially emptied prior to the feeding session; breastfeeding for nutritive purposes is recommended as early as 32 weeks PCA (Meier, 2001). However, Nyqvist and colleagues demonstrated that PCA may be a poor marker for the ability to breastfeed in the preterm (Nyqvist et al., 1999; Nyqvist & Ewald, 1999). Breastfeeding was initiated either at birth or following termination of mechanical ventilation (27.9 to 35.9 weeks PCA); the longest delay after birth was 20 days. Emptying the breast before feeding was not part of their study procedure. Low GA at birth and low birthweight (two highly correlated variables) predicted earlier emergence of the capacity for efficient breastfeeding and earlier establishment of full breastfeeding. Nyqvist and Ewald (1999) hypothesize that early, frequent, positive, and contingent experiences with the mother and breast enhanced the development of oral-motor skill development. These researchers therefore recommend that readiness for breastfeeding be measured by physiologic stability rather than by age, weight, or maturity.

Very little is understood about the predictive validity of behavioral or physiologic indicators of feeding readiness. If our goal in caring for the preterm infant is to be contingently responsive and sensitively attuned to infants' cues, then we must learn more about how they indicate readiness for feeding, regarding both when to start and when to offer and terminate an individual feeding. Our observations and criteria must become more precise and be placed within the context of the individual infant. For example, an infant at 36 weeks PCA with unstable chronic lung disease will likely suck on a pacifier and have an active gag response yet not be ready for oral feeding. We do not know if physiologic stability during NNS predicts stability during oral feeding or even what the parameters of "stable" are for the physiologic measures of heart rate, oxygen saturation, and respiratory pattern during feeding.

Oral Feeding Advancement

The advancement of oral feeding includes two related concepts: (a) how often and at what pattern to offer oral feedings (for example, every 2, 3, or 4 hours; oral feeding once per day, and so on), and (b) how to determine the quantity per feeding (prescribed versus ad lib). Many nurseries follow protocols for both the frequency of oral feeding and the pattern of oral versus gavage feeding. A typical regimen may be to begin with one oral feeding per day and gradually increase to one oral feeding per 8 hours, then two feedings per 8 hours, and finally to full oral feeding. It is also common for nurseries to prescribe the volume of milk intake the infant will be offered; however, again, there is a continuum of flexibility from prescribing the volume of every feeding to prescribing an interval amount, such as an amount the infant is required to ingest every 8 hours.

Several studies have examined whether preterm infants are capable of regulating the timing and amount per feeding during the period immediately following the transition period. In a unique longitudinal design, Pridham, Kosorok, et al. (1999) blinded nurses to the volume of milk in the bottle to examine the intake of 33 infants fed an ad lib feeding amount on demand (with a 6-hour limit) compared to 45 infants fed a prescribed volume every 3–4 hours. All infants were in the first 5 days of full oral feeding, less than 35 weeks gestation at birth, and free of significant medical conditions, with the exception of lung disease, and most were African American (92.3%). Infants in each feeding regimen were further randomized to 20 kcal versus 24 kcal per ounce formula. Readiness to oral-feed was determined by infant behaviors of stirring, rooting, sucking on hands, putting hand to mouth, being awake, and crying. Terminating the feeding was determined by infant behavioral cues of sleep state, fatigue, failure to resume sucking, or loss of interest in feeding with signs of contentment. Infant condition (BPD) negatively affected intake and growth. Infants who were allowed to initiate and terminate feedings had lower intake of both volume and calories and lower weight gain across the 5 study days than infants on the prescribed feeding pattern. However, as infants gained more experience regulating intake, they approached the volume and caloric intake and growth of infants in the prescribed group.

Building on this study, Pridham et al. (2001) examined the effect of ad lib feeding regimens on fully bottle-fed preterm infants from two different hospitals to determine if there is a hospital effect on development of feeding skills ($n = 78$). In this study, the sample added from the second hospital included infants fed breast milk, treated as 20 kcal per ounce, and fewer African American infants (23.7% compared to 92.3%). Similar research questions were explored. Ad lib demand feeding patterns again predicted less intake and no weight gain advantage. The same pattern of increasing intake across the 5-day study period approaching the prescribed feeding volume was found in this expanded sample. Further study is clearly needed to understand when and under what conditions preterm infants can guide feeding practices. Consistent with developmental science theory, self-regulatory skills are likely an emergent property of the feeding system created by infant development and experience.

Offering infants opportunities for oral feeding appropriately, without going beyond their capacities, is very complex. In contrast to the period when the infant is fully oral-feeding, during the transition period the infant is less mature and skilled and the caregiver's task of understanding infant readiness and nonreadiness cues and appropriately selecting the mode of feeding (gavage versus oral) is difficult. Saunders, Friedman, and Stramoski (1991) examined whether bottle-feeding infants could initiate feedings on demand. In this study, 29 stable infants less than 37 weeks GA at birth were randomized to either a semi-self-regulating or a control group. Infants in the self-regulating group were allowed to feed on demand within a 5-hour window. Readiness for oral feeding was based on behavioral cues. Control group infants were bottle-fed every 3 hours. Both groups were tube-fed if the infant was unable to complete a feeding in 30 minutes or failed to take an adequate amount for two consecutive feedings. Infants who were given the opportunity to self-regulate the time and amount of feeding ($n = 15$) fed less frequently (4 to 7 times per day compared to 8 times) and consumed slightly less formula, but they demonstrated no difference in weight gain. Self-regulated feeders also required fewer tube feedings and met discharge criteria 1 day earlier than the control group. Saunders et al. speculated that less frequent feedings allowed the infant to rest longer between feedings and minimized the exertion of feeding, thereby supporting growth on a smaller intake of calories. This study had several limitations. The small sample was inadequately described and intake was measured in ml/day rather than ml/kg/day. In addition, tests of significance were only provided for length of hospitalization and pattern of weight gain per day.

McCain, Gartside, Greenberg, and Lott (2001) tested a protocol that was successful in shortening the transition time to full oral feeding. Healthy preterm infants were randomized into a nursery routine care group ($n = 41$) and an intervention group ($n = 40$). Both groups began oral feeding at mean age of 32.3 weeks. The study had two phases: the oral-gavage phase and the full oral phase (first 48 hours of full oral feeding). The control group was fed a prescribed volume every 3 hours throughout the study. During the oral-gavage phase, the intervention group was prepared for each oral feeding with 10 minutes of NNS followed by an assessment of their state to determine if an oral feeding would be offered. If the infant was in a quiet sleep state, the infant was allowed to rest for 30 minutes and the behavioral state assessment was repeated. If the infant continued to be in quiet sleep, the feeding was given by gavage. Feedings were completed by gavage if the infant was unable to take the full feeding volume; therefore, both groups of infants received the same volume of milk during the oral-gavage phase. Transition time was shorter for the intervention group (5 ± 4.2 days versus 10 ± 3.1 days) and for lower-BW infants and longer for infants of mixed race and of triplet or multiple gestations. During the full oral phase, the intervention group's feeding times were lengthened with state assessment occurring from 3.5 to 5.0 hours and the infants were offered an ad lib quantity of milk at the oral feeding (McCain et al., 2001). Despite the ability of the intervention group to self-regulate volume of intake during the full oral phase, infants in both groups had similar intakes. Weight gain did not differ between groups. Gender, sex, respiratory health, and GA at birth had no effect.

McCain et al.'s study demonstrated that it was not only safe but advantageous to implement an infant-directed feeding protocol. The finding that lower-BW infants accomplished oral feeding in a shorter period of time warrants further study. Nyqvist's breastfeeding studies also found that lower-BW infants achieved full breastfeeding at an earlier age (Nyqvist & Ewald, 1999; Nyqvist et al., 1999). Earlier achievement of feeding skills in lower-BW infants may reflect an outcome of providing contingent feeding, a practice that supports the emergence of feeding skills that would otherwise not be possible.

Nyqvist describes a pattern of establishing breastfeeding that is new for many nurseries, particularly in the United States (Nyqvist & Ewald, 1999; Nyqvist et al., 1999). Nyqvist's study procedure consisted of breastfeedings initiated early when the infant was stable. Infants were supplemented with tube feedings when they were not demonstrating interest in feeding and with cup if they demonstrated readiness cues when the mother was unavailable. Bottle-feedings were introduced if mothers were not producing enough milk and discharge was impending, or upon the mother's request. To determine if supplementation was required, infants were weighed before and after all breastfeeding sessions until they were consuming the prescribed daily volume. Infants were found to progress more quickly to full breastfeeding if they had less separation from their mothers, if the mothers were of lower educational level, and if the infants were of lower GA at birth, did not require supplemental oxygen or aminophylline for apnea, and had less experience bottle-feeding. More research is needed to understand why bottle-feeding was associated with less breastfeeding success. Nyqvist and colleagues offered several hypotheses: (a) bottle-feeding may have hastened discharge at the expense of developing breastfeeding skills, (b) bottle-feeding may have a negative effect on mothers' interpretation of their capacity to breastfeed, or (c) introduction of the bottle may have created nipple confusion (although preterm infants demonstrate the ability to change their sucking in response to different nipples).

Kliethermes et al. (1999) conducted a similar breastfeeding protocol in a randomized controlled clinical trial with 84 preterm infants in the United States. Infants in this sample were 1,000 to 2,500 gm at birth, within 1 week of birth, and without congenital or neurological problems or severe BPD (criteria for diagnosis not specified). Upon written orders for onset of oral feedings, infants were randomized to one of two patterns of transitioning. Infants in group I (n = 46) received oral feedings by bottle when they indicated interest in oral feeding and their mother was unavailable (standard care in most U.S. nurseries). Infants in group II (n = 38) received nasogastric tube feedings when they indicated interest in oral feeding and the mother was unavailable. Adequacy of breastfeeding was assessed with daily infant weights. For both groups, mothers stayed with their infants continuously during 24 to 48 hours prior to discharge. During this predischarge period, if infants required feeding supplementation, group I infants were supplemented with bottles while group II infants were supplemented with cup or syringe feeding. Pattern of transition to breastfeeding did not affect length of hospitalization or weight at discharge; however, group II infants were 4.5 times more likely to be breastfeeding at the time of discharge. Group II infants continued to have higher rates of breastfeeding after discharge (3 days, 3 months, and 6 months). The study had notable limitations. Infant GA varied, yet age at first breastfeeding was reported in days of life rather than PCA. No data were reported on PCA at discharge. Although the maternal sample was described well on some variables, no data were presented on how often mothers were actually able to breastfeed or how often infants displayed interest in oral feeding and were then gavage-fed. To adopt this type of change in feeding practice for breastfed infants will require an understanding of what mothers can expect of their role in the feeding plan and what minimal amounts of breastfeeding will be required for success.

In summary, research on the advancement of oral feedings during the transition period has utilized several critical developmental concepts. More research on developing feeding self-regulation and determining the appropriate provision of feeding guidance and support, as well as on the appropriate type and effect of experience, will enhance our ability to promote preterm feeding skill development.

CRITIQUE AND FUTURE DIRECTIONS

Development of feeding skills is complex, involving the interaction of multiple systems within and without the infant. Developmental science as an orientation to the study of individual functioning guided this review and critique of research. Directions for future research that will extend our understanding and incorporate principles of developmental science about this highly salient time for infants and their families are addressed.

A number of methodological issues can be derived from looking at the entire body of research. Studies need to describe their samples more completely. At the very least, all studies need to report BW, GA, PCA at all study times, PCA at oral feeding initiation and accomplishment of full feeding, and health, including specifics of respiratory functioning (days on oxygen, days ventilated, respiratory diagnoses, baseline oxygen saturation, and whether the infant required supplemental oxygen on the days of study). Gender and race have commonly been reported in the sample description but have rarely been part of the analysis. Larger samples will allow us to explore the effect, if any, of gender and race on feeding skill development. In addition, samples need to move beyond the healthiest and most stable infants, since medically fragile preterm infants in the NICU are having the most feeding problems. While data on healthy preterms has been necessary to understand typical developmental patterns, we must begin to understand the feeding skills of more vulnerable infants. Multisite studies would enhance our knowledge base about those preterm infants with the most feeding problems.

Studies also will need to account for individual differences within subsets of infants. Grouping infants by diagnosis alone will not enable us to understand the variability in feeding data. The study by Pridham et al. (1993) demonstrates the great variability found in feeding data within subsets of preterm infants and illuminates the limitations of grouping the data of preterm infants and taking a variable approach. For example, in this study of preterm infants with BPD, infants began oral feeding as early as 30.4 weeks to as late as 47.7 weeks PCA and were fully oral-fed as early as 33.3 weeks to as late as 48.8 weeks PCA. A person-oriented approach to analysis of feeding data could enhance our understanding by exploring factors that are associated with various infant feeding profiles. By mapping individual developmental trajectories within these profiles, we would learn more about the common as well as the nonpredicted developmental pathways to skilled oral feeding.

The temporality of feeding skills both within and across feedings needs further exploration. Many studies currently analyze subsections of feedings, for example, a 5-minute window or the first and last 3 minutes of the feeding. Yet infant feeding skills can vary a great deal across a given feeding (Hill et al., 2000; Medoff-Cooper et al., 2001) and across feedings within a day or week, particularly in the early transition period. Researchers will need to expand their window of study to include the entire feeding period and to explore the temporal stability of feeding skills both within and across feedings. The advancement of the science of feeding of preterm infants lies in whether we can account for developmental changes in feeding skills and their dynamic variability. The challenge lies in whether we can put together changes we observe in skills with the contextual, biological, and social features that contribute to the variability.

We must understand the demand for adaptation placed upon the infant during oral feeding and clarify the potential for intervention. To accomplish this, we need to continue to develop methods for assessing the maturation and stability of the neurologic and physiologic systems. Chart review of the history of apnea or descriptive statistics of physiologic data such as means and medians lack sensitivity and reliability. Heart rate variability, oxygen saturation regularity, and respiratory regularity may be fruitful directions to explore. Descriptive research has facilitated mapping the biobehavioral components of infant feeding skill, specifically, infants' ability to attain and maintain engagement for feeding, organize and coordinate oral-motor functions, and engage in physical activity that demands energy and attention while preserving physiological functioning. This research has also mapped the caregivers' ability to provide a supportive, positive, and contingent feeding experience. However, comprehensive descriptions of the feeding behavior of preterms over time that incorporate multiple system levels are lacking. In-depth case studies would add to the feeding literature. Several case studies in the breastfeeding literature offer excellent examples of the level of description that is required to move the science forward (see Mead, Chuffo, Lawlor-Klean, & Meier, 1992; Nyqvist, Ewald, & Sjoden, 1996).

Longitudinal studies are needed both for descriptive purposes and for clinical trials of interventions. These studies need to extend into the postdischarge period to explore paths of feeding development as well as their outcomes. Longitudinal methods that capture individual differences in change over time, such as cluster analyses, individual growth modeling, or mixed general linear modeling, are needed (see, for example, Francis, Fletcher, Stuebing, Davidson, & Thompson, 1991; Holditch-Davis, Edwards, & Helms, 1998).

Intervention studies aimed at advancing oral feeding skills in the preterm are scarce and have measured few outcomes. The most prominent outcome utilized thus far is volume of intake, as evidenced by Daley and

Kennedy's (2000) choice of dependent variable for their meta-analysis of the effects of interventions on preterm infant feeding. Outcome measures need to be more sensitive to the skills we are intervening to support in both the caregiver and the infant. For example, assessing the amount of intake is an insensitive measure of the infant's response to the challenge of feeding. Intervention studies will require mixed methods of data collection (observational, self-report, interview approaches) and mixed variables (for the infant: physiologic, behavioral, intake, growth, feeding skill development; for the caregiver: the caregiver's working model of feeding, under-' standing of and response to infant feeding behaviors, caregiver feeding behaviors). A "successful" feeding outcome should include how comfortable and engaged in feeding the infant was; whether the infant maintained an adequate oxygen saturation throughout the feeding; whether the infant demonstrated tolerance to the feeding through lack of fatigue at the end of feeding and maintenance of oxygen saturation, heart rate, and respiratory rate at the prefeeding baseline level; and whether the caregiver perceived himself or herself to be supportive, protective, and responsive during the feeding. Skilled feeding should demonstrate the ability to flexibly adapt to current and future conditions to meet the changing demands of the task and the biological, social, and physical environment. Intervention outcomes need to reflect both these immediate feeding goals (success at feeding) as well as the ability to move toward long-range developmental goals (skilled feeding).

In light of the evidence of optimal physiologic regulation during breastfeeding, further research to test models of breastfeeding support for families who choose breastfeeding gains added importance. Breastfeeding research also demonstrates that contingently structured interventions promote the infant's skill development. This research has taken the lead in many areas. In particular, there is discussion from a longer-term viewpoint about contingency and the learning that occurs during feeding (e.g., Nyqvist et al., 1999). Compared to bottle-feeding studies, the models for breastfeeding research have had a more ecological framework that involves more subsystems. Perhaps because the mother is undeniably part of the feeding system, her impact on feeding outcome has not been ignored. This is not true, for the most part, with bottle-feeding research. Here, feeding skill tends to be viewed as solely lying within the infant, with the parent or nurse having a minor, facilitative role. Hence we find very little research on the caregiver who is bottle-feeding, and when we do, there is no mention of fathers or others.

We also know very little about the ecology of the NICU, particularly how nurses interact with preterms during feeding or how they relate to parents around the issue of feeding. Nurses model and teach feeding skills to parents. However, the skills of the nurse in feeding the preterm and in working with families to learn these skills have largely been ignored. For example, we know very little about how nurses vary in their feeding skills or in their working models of feeding, or how they influence parental feeding behaviors.

For those families who opt for partial to full bottle-feeding, we must test strategies to minimize physiologic dysregulation during feeding and strategies to increase contingency provided to the infant. More studies are emerging to test various alternatives to using bottles for the breast-fed infant (e.g., Dowling, Meier, DiFiore, Blatz, & Martin, 2002). However, studies are needed to understand which infants would benefit from being offered only one method of oral feeding and which infants would be able to integrate breast- and bottle-feeding. For families who choose to combine breast- and bottle-feeding, there are no studies on how to integrate these methods. The assumption is that this line of research would promote bottle-feeding at the expense of breastfeeding; however, this ignores the ability of an infant to develop two methods of feeding, and also ignores what many families express as their intent and capacity. Many families may be able to extend the length of time their preterm infant receives breast milk if we help those who want to combine methods to meet their goals.

In summary, nurse researchers have contributed much to our understanding of oral feeding for preterm infants. Research has been conducted on a broad range of topics during a narrow period of time, highlighting the importance nurse researchers have placed on learning about this salient developmental process. As technology for the study of biobehavioral processes has expanded, nurse researchers have also expanded their methods to study behavior and physiology at levels that will continue to move the science of oral feeding forward. Clearly this work will enhance the well-being of preterm infants and help families better meet their goals in parenting and nurturing their children.

ACKNOWLEDGMENTS

This study was supported by Grant P30 NR03962 from NINR, NIH, to the Center for Research on Chronic Illness at the University of North Carolina at Chapel Hill and by NINR Grant K01NR07668.

REFERENCES

Anderson, G. C., Behnke, M., Gill, N. E., Conlon, M., Measel, C. P., & McDonie, T. E. (1990). Self-regulatory gavage-to-bottle feeding in preterm infants: Effects of behavioral state, energy expenditure, and weight gain. In S. G. Funk, E. M. Tornquist, M. T. Champayne, L. A. Coop, & R. A. Wiese (Eds.), *Key aspects of recovery: Nutrition, rest, and mobility* (pp. 83–97). New York: Springer.

Becker, P. T., Grunwald, P. C., Moorman, J., & Stuhr, S. (1991). Outcomes of developmentally supportive nursing care for very low birth weight infants. *Nursing Research, 40,* 150–155.

Becker, P. T., Grunwald, P. C., Moorman, J., & Stuhr, S. (1993). Effects of developmental care on behavioral organization in very-low-birth-weight infants. *Nursing Research, 42,* 214–220.

Bell, E. H., Geyer, J., & Jones, L. (1995). A structured intervention improves breastfeeding success for ill or preterm infants. *MCN: American Journal of Maternal-Child Nursing, 20,* 309–314.

Brandon, D. H., Holditch-Davis, D., & Beylea, M. (1999). Nursing care and the development of sleeping and waking behaviors in preterm infants. *Research in Nursing and Health, 22,* 217–229.

Cairns, R. B., Elder, G. H., Jr., & Costello, J. (Eds.). (1996). *Developmental science.* New York: Cambridge University Press.

Cooper, H. M. (1989). *Integrating research: A guide for literature reviews* (2nd ed.). Newbury Park, CA: Sage Publications.

Daley, K. K., & Kennedy, C. M. (2000). Meta analysis: Effects of interventions on premature infants' feeding. *Journal of Perinatal and Neonatal Nursing, 14,* 62–77.

Dowling, D. A. (1999). Physiological responses of preterm infants to breast-feeding and bottle-feeding with the orthodontic nipple. *Nursing Research, 48,* 78–85.

Dowling, D. A., Meier, P. P., DiFiore, J. M., Blatz, M., & Martin, R. J. (2002). Cup-feeding for preterm infants: Mechanics and safety. *Journal of Human Lactation, 18,* 13–20.

Francis, D. J., Fletcher, J. M., Stuebing, K. K., Davidson, K. C., & Thompson, N. M. (1991). Analysis of change: Modeling individual growth. *Journal of Consulting and Clinical Psychology, 59,* 27–37.

Furman, L., Minich, N. M., & Hack, M. (1998). Breastfeeding of very low birth weight infants. *Journal of Human Lactation, 14,* 29–34.

Gill, N. E., Behnke, M., Conlon, M., & Anderson, G. C. (1992). Nonnutritive sucking modulates behavioral state for preterm infants before feeding. *Scandanavian Journal of Caring Sciences, 6,* 3–7.

Harrison, L. L. (1982). *Teaching mothers about their premature infants: Effects on perception and attachment.* Unpublished doctoral dissertation, University of Tennessee, Knoxville, Tennessee.

Hill, A. S. (1992). Preliminary findings: A maximum oral feeding time for premature infants, the relationship to physiological indicators. *Maternal Child Nursing Journal, 20,* 81–92.

Hill, A. S., Kurkowski, T. B., & Garcia, J. (2000). Oral support measures used in feeding the preterm infant. *Nursing Research, 49,* 2–10.

Hill, P. D., Aldag, J. C., & Chatterton, R. T. (1996). The effect of sequential and simultaneous breast pumping on milk volume and prolactin levels: A pilot study. *Journal of Human Lactation, 12,* 193–199.

Hill, P. D., Aldag, J. C., & Chatterton, R. T. (1999). Effects of pumping style on milk production in mothers of non-nursing preterm infants. *Journal of Human Lactation, 15,* 209–216.

Hill, P. D., Ledbetter, R. J., & Kavanaugh, K. L. (1997). Breastfeeding patterns of low-birth-weight infants after hospital discharge. *Journal of Obstetric, Gynecologic and Neonatal Nursing, 26,* 189–197.

Holditch-Davis, D. (1990). The effect of hospital caregiving on preterm infants' sleeping and waking states. In S. G. Funk, E. M. Tornquist, M. T. Champayne, L. A. Coop, & R. A. Wiese (Eds.), *Key aspects of recovery: Improving nutrition, rest, and mobility* (pp. 110–122). New York: Springer.

Holditch-Davis, D., & Edwards, L. J. (1998). Temporal organization of sleep-wake states in preterm infants. *Developmental Psychobiology, 33,* 257–269.

Holditch-Davis, D., Edwards, L. J., & Helms, R. W. (1998). Modeling development of sleep-wake behaviors: I. Using the mixed general linear model. *Physiology and Behavior, 63,* 311–318.

Kavanaugh, K., Mead, L., Meier, P., & Mangurten, H. H. (1995). Getting enough: Mothers' concerns about breastfeeding a preterm infant after discharge. *Journal of Obstetric, Gynecologic and Neonatal Nursing, 24,* 23–32.

Kinneer, M. D., & Beachy, P. (1994). Nipple feeding premature infants in the neonatal intensive-care unit: Factors and decisions. *Journal of Obstetric, Gynecologic and Neonatal Nursing, 23,* 105–112.

Kliethermes, P. A., Cross, M. L., Lanese, M. G., Johnson, K. M., & Simon, S. D. (1999). Transitioning preterm infants with nasogastric tube supplementation: Increased likelihood of breastfeeding. *Journal of Obstetric, Gynecologic and Neonatal Nursing, 28,* 264–273.

Mandich, M. B., Ritchie, S. K., & Mullett, M. (1996). Transition times to oral feeding in premature infants with and without apnea. *Journal of Obstetric, Gynecologic and Neonatal Nursing, 25,* 771–776.

Marino, B. L., O'Brien, P., & LoRe, H. (1995). Oxygen saturations during breast and bottle feedings in infants with congenital heart disease. *Journal of Pediatric Nursing, 10,* 360–364.

McCain, G. C. (1992). Facilitating inactive awake states in preterm infants: A study of three interventions. *Nursing Research, 41,* 157–160.

McCain, G. C. (1995). Promotion of preterm infant nipple feeding with nonnutritive sucking. *Journal of Pediatric Nursing, 10,* 3–8.

McCain, G. C. (1997). Behavioral state activity during nipple feedings for preterm infants. *Neonatal Network, 16*(5), 43–47.

McCain, G. C., Gartside, P. S., Greenberg, J. M., & Lott, J. W. (2001). A feeding protocol for healthy preterm infants that shortens time to oral feeding. *Journal of Pediatrics, 139,* 374–379.

Mead, L. J., Chuffo, R., Lawlor-Klean, P., & Meier, P. P. (1992). Breastfeeding success with preterm quadruplets. *Journal of Obstetric, Gynecologic and Neonatal Nursing, 21,* 221–227.

Medoff-Cooper, B. (1991). Changes in nutritive sucking patterns with increasing gestational age. *Nursing Research, 40,* 245–247.

Medoff-Cooper, B. (2000). Multi-system approach to the assessment of successful feeding. *Acta Paediatrica, 89,* 393–394.

Medoff-Cooper, B., Bilker, W., & Kaplan, J. M. (2001). Suckling behavior as a function of gestational age: A cross–sectional study. *Infant Behavior & Development, 24,* 83–94.

Medoff-Cooper, B., Delivoria-Papadopoulos, M., & Brooten, D. (1991). Serial neurobehavioral assessments in preterm infants. *Nursing Research, 40,* 94–97.

Medoff-Cooper, B., & Gennaro, S. (1996). The correlation of sucking behaviors and Bayley Scales of Infant Development at six months of age in VLBW infants. *Nursing Research, 45,* 291–296.

Medoff-Cooper, B., McGrath, J. M., & Bilker, W. (2000). Nutritive sucking and neurobehavioral development in preterm infants from 34 weeks PCA to term. *MCN: American Journal of Maternal Child Nursing, 25,* 64–70.

Medoff-Cooper, B., & Ray, W. (1995). Neonatal sucking behaviors. *Image: Journal of Nursing Scholarship, 27,* 195–200.

Medoff-Cooper, B., Verklan, T., & Carlson, S. (1993). The development of sucking patterns and physiologic correlates in very-low-birth-weight infants. *Nursing Research, 42,* 100–105.

Medoff-Cooper, B., Weininger, S., & Zukowsky, K. (1989). Neonatal sucking as a clinical assessment tool: Preliminary findings. *Nursing Research, 38,* 162–165.

Meier, P. (1988). Bottle- and breast-feeding: Effects on transcutaneous oxygen pressure and temperature in preterm infants. *Nursing Research, 37,* 36–41.

Meier, P. P. (1996). Suck-breathe patterning during bottle and breastfeeding for preterm infants. In T. J. David (Ed.), *Major controversies in infant nutrition. International congress and symposium series 215* (pp. 9–20). London: Royal Society of Medicine Press.

Meier, P. P. (2001). Breastfeeding in the special care nursery. Prematures and infants with medical problems. *Pediatric Clinics of North America, 48,* 425–442.

Meier, P., & Anderson, G. C. (1987). Responses of small preterm infants to bottle- and breast-feeding. *MCN: American Journal of Maternal Child Nursing, 12,* 97–105.

Meier, P. P., & Brown, L. P. (1996). State of the science. Breastfeeding for mothers and low birth weight infants. *Nursing Clinics of North America, 31,* 351–365.

Meier, P. P., Brown, L. P., Hurst, N. M., Spatz, D. L., Engstrom, J. L., Borucki, L. C., et al. (2000). Nipple shields for preterm infants: Effect on milk transfer and duration of breastfeeding. *Journal of Human Lactation, 16,* 106–114; quiz 129–131.

Meier, P. P., Engstrom, J. L., Fleming, B. A., Streeter, P. L., & Lawrence, P. B. (1996). Estimating milk intake of hospitalized preterm infants who breastfeed. *Journal of Human Lactation, 12,* 21–26.

Meier, P. P., Engstrom, J. L., Mangurten, H. H., Estrada, E., Zimmerman, B., & Kopparthi, R. (1993). Breastfeeding support services in the neonatal intensive-care unit. *Journal of Obstetric, Gynecologic and Neonatal Nursing, 22,* 338–347.

Meier, P., & Pugh, E. J. (1985). Breast-feeding behavior of small preterm infants. *MCN: American Journal of Maternal Child Nursing, 10,* 396–401.

Nyqvist, K. H., & Ewald, U. (1999). Infant and maternal factors in the development of breastfeeding behaviour and breastfeeding outcome in preterm infants. *Acta Paediatrica, 88,* 1194–1203.

Nyqvist, K. H., Ewald, U., & Sjoden, P. O. (1996). Supporting a preterm infant's behaviour during breastfeeding: A case report. *Journal of Human Lactation, 12,* 221–228.

Nyqvist, K. H., Farnstrand, C., Eeg-Olofsson, K. E., & Ewald, U. (2001). Early oral behaviour in preterm infants during breastfeeding: An electromyographic study. *Acta Paediatrica, 90,* 658–663.

Nyqvist, K. H., Rubertsson, C., Ewald, U., & Sjoden, P. O. (1996). Development of the Preterm Infant Breastfeeding Behavior Scale (PIBBS): A study of nurse-mother agreement. *Journal of Human Lactation, 12,* 207–219.

Nyqvist, K. H., Sjoden, P. O., & Ewald, U. (1999). The development of preterm infants' breastfeeding behavior. *Early Human Development, 55,* 247–264.

Pickler, R. H., Frankel, H. B., Walsh, K. M., & Thompson, N. M. (1996). Effects of nonnutritive sucking on behavioral organization and feeding performance in preterm infants. *Nursing Research, 45,* 132–135.

Pickler, R. H., Higgins, K. E., & Crummette, B. D. (1993). The effect of nonnutritive sucking on bottle-feeding stress in preterm infants. *Journal of Obstetric, Gynecologic and Neonatal Nursing, 22,* 230–234.

Pickler, R. H., Mauck, A. G., & Geldmaker, B. (1997). Bottle-feeding histories of preterm infants. *Journal of Obstetric, Gynecologic and Neonatal Nursing, 26,* 414–420.

Pridham, K. F. (1993). Anticipatory guidance of parents of new infants: Potential contribution of the internal working model construct. *Image: Journal of Nursing Scholarship, 25,* 49–56.

Pridham, K., Brown, R., Sondel, S., Green, C., Wedel, N. Y., & Lai, H. C. (1998). Transition time to full nipple feeding for premature infants with a history of lung disease. *Journal of Obstetric, Gynecologic and Neonatal Nursing, 27,* 533–545.

Pridham, K. F., Knight, C. B., & Stephenson, G. R. (1989). Mothers' working models of infant feeding: Description and influencing factors. *Journal of Advanced Nursing, 14,* 1051–1061.

Pridham, K., Kosorok, M. R., Greer, F., Carey, P., Kayata, S., & Sondel, S. (1999). The effects of prescribed versus ad libitum feedings and formula caloric density on premature infant dietary intake and weight gain. *Nursing Research, 48,* 86–93.

Pridham, K. F., Kosorok, M. R., Greer, F., Kayata, S., Bhattacharya, A., & Grunwald, P. (2001). Comparison of caloric intake and weight outcomes of an *ad lib* feeding regimen for preterm infants in two nurseries. *Journal of Advanced Nursing, 35,* 751–759.

Pridham, K. F., Limbo, R., Schroeder, M., Thoyre, S., & Van Riper, M. (1998). Guided participation and development of care-giving competencies for families of low birth-weight infants. *Journal of Advanced Nursing, 28,* 948–958.

Pridham, K. F., Schroeder, M., & Brown, R. (1999). The adaptiveness of mothers' working models of caregiving through the first year: Infant and mother contributions. *Research in Nursing and Health, 22,* 471–485.

Pridham, K. F., Schroeder, M., Brown, R., & Clark, R. (2001). The relationship of a mother's working model of feeding to her feeding behavior. *Journal of Advanced Nursing, 35,* 741–750.

Pridham, K. F., Schroeder, M., Van Riper, M., Thoyre, S., Limbo, R., & Mlynarczyk, S. (1998). *Maternal working model of feeding: An interview protocol and coding manual.* Unpublished manuscript, University of Wisconsin-Madison School of Nursing.

Pridham, K. F., Sondel, S., Chang, A., & Green, C. (1993). Nipple feeding for preterm infants with bronchopulmonary dysplasia. *Journal of Obstetric, Gynecologic and Neonatal Nursing, 22,* 147–155.

Pridham, K. F., Sondel, S., Clark, R., Green, C., & Brown, R. (1994). *Correlates of preterm and term infant feeding outcomes.* Final Report to the National Institute of Nursing Research (Grant NR02348, 7/1/90-6/30/94).

Saunders, R. B., Friedman, C. B., & Stramoski, P. R. (1991). Feeding preterm infants. Schedule or demand? *Journal of Obstetric, Gynecologic and Neonatal Nursing, 20,* 212–218.

Shiao, S. Y. P. K. (1995). Comparison of morning and afternoon feedings in very low birth weight infants. *Issues in Comprehensive Pediatric Nursing, 18,* 43–53.

Shiao, S. Y. P. K. (1997). Comparison of continuous versus intermittent sucking in very-low-birth-weight infants. *Journal of Obstetric, Gynecologic and Neonatal Nursing, 26,* 313–319.

Shiao, S. Y. P. K., Brooker, J., & DiFiore, T. (1996). Desaturation events during oral feedings with and without a nasogastric tube in very low birth weight infants. *Heart and Lung, 25,* 236–245.

Shiao, S. Y. P. K., Youngblut, J. M., Anderson, G. C., DiFiore, J. M., & Martin, R. J. (1995). Nasogastric tube placement: Effects on breathing and sucking in very-low-birth-weight infants. *Nursing Research, 44,* 82–88.

Siddell, E. P., & Froman, R. D. (1994). A national survey of neonatal intensive-care units: Criteria used to determine readiness for oral feedings. *Journal of Obstetric, Gynecologic and Neonatal Nursing, 23,* 783–789.

Stine, M. J. (1990). Breastfeeding the premature newborn: A protocol without bottles. *Journal of Human Lactation, 6,* 167–170.

Thelen, E. (1989). Self-organization in developmental processes: Can systems approaches work? In M. Gunnar & E. Thelen (Eds.), *Systems in development. Minnesota symposia in child psychology* (pp. 77–117). Hillsdale, NJ: Erlbaum.

Thelen, E., & Ulrich, B. D. (1991). Hidden skills: A dynamic systems analysis of treadmill stepping during the first year. *Monographs of the Society for Research in Child Development, 56* (1, Serial No. 223).

Thoman, E. B. (1993). Obligation and option in the premature nursery. *Developmental Review, 13,* 1–30.

Thoyre, S. (1997). *Co-regulation in preterm infant feeding.* Unpublished doctoral dissertation, University of Wisconsin-Madison, Madison, Wisconsin.

Thoyre, S. (2000). Mothers' ideas about their role in feeding their high-risk infants. *Journal of Obstetric, Gynecologic and Neonatal Nursing, 29,* 613–624.

Thoyre, S., & Carlson, J. (in press). Occurrence of oxygen desaturation events during preterm infant bottle feeding near discharge. *Early Human Development.*

Woldt, E. H. (1991). Breastfeeding support group in the NICU. *Neonatal Network, 9*(5), 53–56.

Wood, A. F. (1991). Factors affecting reciprocity between nurses and preterm infants during feeding. *Journal of Perinatal and Neonatal Nursing, 4,* 62–70.

Yip, E., Lee, J., & Sheehy, Y. (1996). Breast-feeding in neonatal intensive care. *Journal of Paediatrics and Child Health, 32,* 296–298.

Zhang, P., & Medoff-Cooper, B. (1996). A Markov regression model for nutritive sucking data. *Biometrics, 52,* 112–124.

PART II

Children With Health Problems

Chapter 4

Physical Symptoms
in Children and Adolescents

HYEKYUN RHEE

ABSTRACT

This chapter summarizes and critiques research on physical symptoms in children
and adolescents from a developmental science perspective. Studies conducted
by researchers from various disciplines, primarily after 1990, were identified
through searches of MEDLINE, CINAHL, and Psyc INFO. This review focuses
on two areas: the prevalence of common physical symptoms—headache, abdominal pain or discomfort, musculoskeletal pain and fatigue—in pediatric populations and the developmental issues associated with these symptom experiences.
Developmental factors were organized into two overarching categories, individual and environmental factors. Findings indicate that demographic factors, including age, pubertal development, gender, and race or ethnicity; psychological
factors, particularly self-esteem, depression, and anxiety; and behavioral factors
have varying relationships to the report of physical symptoms in children and
youth. In addition, family and parents, peers, and the broader school and community ecology of children have an influence on physical symptom complaints.
There is a need for further studies that are strengthened by the use of developmentally sensitive theoretical frameworks and methodologies that address complicated developmental issues.

Physical complaints of various types of symptoms are fairly common in
otherwise healthy youngsters. From a clinical point of view, these symptoms rarely show a clear link to diagnosable disorders. Children with
frequent complaints of physical symptoms constitute a high-risk group in
pediatric primary care because they often exhibit emotional and behavioral

maladjustment (Campo, Jansen-McWilliams, Comer, & Kelleher, 1999). Some youth develop chronic recurrent symptoms that can interfere with everyday functioning and thus further disrupt physical and psychosocial development. Thus considerable interest has been generated to explain these symptoms in pediatric populations and to understand their psychosocial aspects. Like other health conditions, a variety of "nonphysical" aspects, such as demographic, psychological, and social factors, may be triggers of these symptoms. Nonetheless, it is surprising that, given the growing number of nurses working in pediatric primary care practices, nursing research on pediatric symptom problems is so meager.

In order to generate scientific interest among nurse scholars, systematic examination of existing studies on symptom problems in light of various developmental concepts is needed and should ultimately assist nurses in pursuing further developmentally sensitive research. This chapter, then, summarizes and critiques research on physical symptoms in children and adolescents that has been conducted in both clinical and population-based studies over the past two decades. Studies in this review included those dealing with either a single symptom (e.g., headache, abdominal pain, musculoskeletal pain, fatigue) or a combination of several symptoms. This review also assessed the use and applicability of developmental science in this body of research.

The uniformity of findings across the studies on physical symptoms greatly depends on the use of a common definition. To date the term predominantly used in studies of physical symptoms has been *somatic symptom*, which simply refers to bodily discomforts. Many health professionals and researchers have added a psychosocial component to the definition, viewing somatic symptoms as a response to life events or other forms of psychosocial stress in combination with genetic predisposition and learned behavior at both conscious and unconscious levels, in the absence of demonstrable organic bases (Lipowski, 1988). Researchers using these clinical definitions tend to view somatic symptoms at the border between psychiatry and medicine. Although organic origins of somatic symptoms are relatively rare (Kroenke & Mangelsdorff, 1989), there is always the chance that symptoms result from organic pathology. Therefore, labeling physical symptoms as "somatic symptoms" without ruling out organic origins can at best be inconclusive and at worst misleading. Given the uncertain nature of physical symptoms in pediatric populations, using the term *somatic symptoms* may not be justified. Thus the term *physical symptoms* was used throughout the present review.

METHOD

A computer search of literature listed in several databases, including MED-LINE, the Cumulative Index of Nursing and Allied Health Literature (CINAHL), and PsycINFO, was conducted. References were located by combining the keywords *children or adolescents* with one of the following: *physical symptoms, somatic symptoms, headaches, (recurrent) abdominal pain or discomfort, stomachache, musculoskeletal pain, limb pain, back pain,* or *fatigue or tiredness.* Studies reviewed in this chapter involved samples up to the age of 18 in both clinical and community settings. Primary literature published after 1990 was included to ensure currency of this report. However, the inclusion of a few studies from the 1980s was inevitable for issues that have not been investigated in the past decade. The limited literature in nursing necessitated a broadening of the scope to encompass research conducted in other disciplines.

Evaluation of the research focused on whether (a) the study used a developmentally appropriate theory or model and the extent to which the conceptualization reflected developmental perspectives by incorporating the changing nature or multidimensionality of physical symptoms in youngsters; (b) whether the type of research design was appropriate and the extent to which longitudinal designs were used; (c) whether data collection and measurement methods were appropriate to the developmental ages of subjects; (d) whether the samples were diverse and were analyzed looking at race, ethnic background, and socioeconomic status (SES); and (e) whether the data analysis methods were based on the principles of developmental science that include multidimensionality and interactions among multiple factors. This paper also addressed the extent to which nurses contributed to this literature.

Findings of the review focus on two areas: the prevalence of common physical symptoms—headache, abdominal pain or discomfort, musculoskeletal pain and fatigue—in pediatric populations and the developmental issues associated with these symptoms. Developmental factors were organized into two overarching categories: individual and environmental factors.

Common Types of Physical Symptoms and Their Prevalence

Population-based studies have consistently documented headaches, abdominal pain or discomfort, musculoskeletal pain, and fatigue or tiredness as the symptoms most commonly reported by children and adolescents (Eminson, Benjamin, Shortall, Woods, & Faragher, 1996; Garber, Walker, & Zeman, 1991; Larsson, 1991; Rhee, Miles, Halpern, & Holditch-Davis, 2002).

HEADACHES

Headache is experienced by 50% to 90% of youngsters in various countries (Barea, Tannhauser, & Rotta, 1996; Beiter, Ingersoll, Ganser, & Orr, 1991; Carlsson, 1996; Kristjansdottir & Wahlberg, 1993; Mortimer, Kay, & Jaron, 1992; Perquin et al., 2000; Rhee, 2000; Stewart, Lipton, & Liberman, 1996). Ten to thirty percent of children and adolescents in community settings report weekly or more frequent headaches that vary in type and severity. Tension-type headaches and migraines represent the major categories of childhood and adolescence headaches. However, the differentiation between migraine and tension headaches is often not clear-cut, and both may coexist in the same individual. Thus some researchers proposed a headache continuum in which migraine and tension headaches are not discrete entities but are located at each end of a continuum (Holden, Levy, Deichmann, & Galdstein, 1998; Viswanathan, Bridges, Whitehouse, & Newton, 1998).

RECURRENT ABDOMINAL PAIN AND DISCOMFORT

The most characteristic feature of recurrent abdominal pain is repeated episodes of paroxysmal pain before and after which the child is well. Several painful episodes may occur within a short span of time. They may also last for a few minutes or a few hours. Often the definitions of abdominal pain used in epidemiological survey studies have not been as stringent as the above criteria. Researchers tend to use a generic definition of abdominal pain or discomfort and have reported a varying prevalence of recurrent stomachaches; the numbers range from 2% to 60% in community-based studies of children and adolescents (Alfven, 1993; Beiter et al., 1991; Egger, Costello, Erkanli, & Angold, 1999; Garber et al., 1991; Hyams, Burke, Davis, Rzepski, & Andrulonis, 1996; Larsson, 1991; Perquin et al., 2000; Rhee et al., 2002; Sharrer & Ryan-Wenger, 1991). Hyams et al. (1996) reported that 10% to 20% of school-age children experience abdominal pain frequently and severely enough to affect daily activities.

MUSCULOSKELETAL (LIMB) PAIN

Limb pain is another common recurrent pain. *Growing pain* is a colloquial term often used to describe limb pain, but no causal relationship between growth and limb pain has been established. While some researchers have limited its definition to the four extremities (Abu-Arafeh & Russell, 1996; Larsson, 1991; Perquin et al., 2000), others have used the broader term *musculoskeletal pain* (Egger et al., 1999; Mikkelsson, Salminen, & Kautiainen, 1997). To date no distinction has been suggested between the two terms, and they are used interchangeably in survey studies. According to recent survey studies, 10% to 30% of children and adolescents, depending on the definitions used, report at least weekly musculoskeletal pain (Abu-Arafeh & Russell, 1996; Garber et al., 1991; Larsson, 1991; Mikkelsson et al., 1997; Perquin et al., 2000; Rhee et al., 2002). The lifetime prevalence of joint pain, as a specific type of musculoskeletal pain, occurs in up to 39% of adolescents (Eminson et al., 1996).

FATIGUE

The symptom of fatigue has not received major attention in the pediatric population; no single study has focused exclusively on it. Hence, no concentrated attempt has been made to define fatigue. In survey studies of children and adolescents, the operational definition of fatigue varies from study to study and includes low energy (Garber et al., 1991), tiredness (Larsson, 1991), and weakness (Eminson et al., 1996). In several studies, fatigue emerged as one of the most common physical symptoms, with about 23% of children reporting daily fatigue and one-third to one-half of adolescents complaining of fatigue on at least a weekly basis (Belmaker, Espinoza, & Pogrund, 1985; Garber et al., 1991; Larsson, 1991; Rhee et al., 2002). Poikolainen, Kanerva, and Lonnquist (1995) found that the frequent occurrence of fatigue or weakness was the most common physical symptom and was experienced by 30%.

MULTIPLE SYMPTOM COMPLAINTS

Clusters of coexisting physical symptoms are frequently reported by children and adolescents (Alfven, 1993; Aromaa, Sillanpaa, Rautava, & Helenius, 1998; Borge, Nordhagen, Moe, Botten, & Bakketeig, 1994; Egger et al., 1999; Eminson et al., 1996; Garber et al., 1991; Knishkowy, Palti, Tima, Adler, & Gofin, 1995; Kristjansdottir, 1997a; Mikkelsson et al., 1997; Perquin et al., 2000; Rhee et al., 2002). Eminson et al. (1996) reported that more than 8% of adolescents 11 to 16 years in the community ($N = 805$) had reported 13 or more symptoms simultaneously, which is the DSM-III threshold for the diagnosis of somatization disorder.[1] Simi-

---

[1]The number of symptoms required for somatization disorder diagnoses in the more recent classification has been reduced to eight in DSM-IV and six in ICD-10 (Garralda, 1996).

larly, the Ontario Child Health Study (Offord et al., 1987) of children aged 12 to 16 years in community settings revealed that 7.6% were diagnosable with somatization disorder. In the United States, combinations of four or more symptoms were reported in 9% to 15% of community samples of children and adolescents (Garber et al., 1991; Rhee et al., 2002). Poikolainen et al. (1995) documented two or more recurrent symptoms occurring among 36% of an adolescent sample. Combinations of recurrent abdominal pain and headaches are the most common (Alfven, 1993; Borge et al., 1994; Kristjansdottir, 1997a; Perquin et al., 2000; Zuckerman, Stevenson, & Baily, 1987), and they are frequently present in conjunction with other types of symptoms, such as fatigue and limb pain (Knishkowy et al., 1995).

Individual-Level Factors Associated With Physical Symptoms

Studies have shown that prevalence varies depending on the demographic characteristics of the samples. Symptoms are also associated with various psychological factors and behavioral conditions.

DEMOGRAPHIC CHARACTERISTICS

Age.   In general, physical symptoms increase across childhood into adolescence (Aro, Paronen, & Aro, 1987; McGrath et al., 2000; Garber et al., 1991; Offord et al., 1987; Perquin et al., 2000; Rhee et al., 2002), but despite the increasing trend, the peak age for physical symptoms is not late adolescence. Studies have consistently indicated that physical complaints peak in late childhood or early adolescence (Belmaker, 1984; Garber et al., 1991; Larsson, 1991; Perquin et al., 2000; Rauste-von Wright & von Wright, 1981). Given the wide variation in the speed and sequence of physical maturation even in the same age group, specific consideration of pubertal development is of particular value in studies of adolescence.

Pubertal Development.   Puberty is a period of transition in physical development. Belmaker (1984) found the increasing prevalence of physical symptoms in the early adolescent period and attributed this phenomenon to negative or ambivalent feelings associated with the rapid physical changes of early puberty. A few later studies have shown that the reports of physical symptoms were indeed significantly associated with pubertal development (Aro & Taipale, 1987; Rhee, 2002). In a longitudinal design, Aro and Taipale (1987) examined the effect of puberty on physical symptoms of 14- to 16-year-old girls. Using menarche as a benchmark, they found that physical symptoms increased with pubertal development and were more common in earlier-maturing girls than in on-time or late-maturing girls. However, subjects entered this study when they were already in midadolescence. Therefore, the findings may have been biased by recollection errors. In addition, the literature has shown that menarche as a single parameter of puberty may not be sufficient to detect pubertal development in girls because it is only one aspect of a complex process (Moffitt, Caspi, Belsky, & Silva, 1992). Moreover, if physical changes of puberty are viewed as a major source of distress in adolescent girls, the onset of menarche is not the best indicator, since most growth and secondary sex characteristics occur in girls before menarche (Angold & Worthman, 1993). The exclusive focus on menarche has resulted in another limitation, ignorance about boys and their responses to physical maturation with the reports of physical symptoms.

In acknowledging these limitations, Rhee (2002) incorporated multiple indices of pubertal changes specific to each gender and examined the extent to which pubertal status was associated with symptom reports. Symptom reports were significantly associated with overall pubertal status in both girls and boys; the rates of headache and musculoskeletal pain particularly increased with maturation in both genders. Stomachache and feeling hot decreased as boys became physically mature, and overall symptom reports in girls consistently increased with physical maturation.

Gender.   Studies have also consistently shown that the prevalence of most physical symptoms is higher in girls (Egger et al., 1999; Eminson et al., 1996; Garber et al., 1991; Kujala, Taimela, & Viljanen, 1999; Perquin et al., 2000; Rhee et al., 2002). Gender differences seem to emerge in adolescence (Eminson et al., 1996; Garber et al., 1991; Tamminen et al., 1991; Zuckerman et al., 1987) as girls show an increase in physical symptoms (Aro et al., 1987; Eminson et al., 1996; Garber et al., 1991; Knishkowy et al., 1995; Larsson, 1991; Poikolainen et al., 1995; Tamminen et al., 1991; Taylor, Szatmari, Boyle, & Offord, 1996).

Three possible explanations of these gender effects have been proposed. First, hormonal changes associated with pubertal events may directly contribute to the increased physical symptoms in adolescent girls

(Aro & Taipale, 1987; Belmaker, 1984; Eminson et al., 1996; Perquin et al., 2000). Second, rather indirectly, the expected or perceived social role changes in girls after childhood may either produce distress or reinforce a symptom propensity (Silverstein, McKoy, Clauson, Perdue, & Raben, 1995). Reaction to pain may be intertwined with sociocultural backgrounds in which females' pain complaints and emotional difficulties are more acceptable than males' (Poikolainen et al., 1995; Rauste-von Wright & von Wright, 1992; Walker & Zeman, 1992). Finally, differences in pain response have also been proposed as a possible explanation (Unruh, Ritchie, & Merskey, 1999). That is, females are either more sensitive to bodily changes or more reactive to self-report measures, regardless of actual pain, than males.

The issues related to age, gender, and pubertal status are very important in this area of research. Magnusson and Cairns (1996) defined physical maturation in terms of the developmental integration of time (age) and space (context) and contended that physical maturation operates in conjunction with social environments that are influenced greatly by gender. As such, they emphasized the importance of age, pubertal maturation, and gender in developmental science research. Since the changes in pubertal development over time are dynamic and differ for males and females, longitudinal designs that explore the differing trajectories of boys and girls are mandatory to understand the relationships between symptoms and maturation in the two genders. Most findings, however, rely on cross-sectional designs that are not as effective as a longitudinal design in determining changes in the developmental trajectory of physical symptoms. In lieu of a longitudinal design, studies have used heterogeneous samples undergoing different developmental stages and have examined how each age group behaves differently in a cross-sectional design. Although this type of study can generate information on differences among ages, this situation inevitably invokes critical questions about changes in the individual over time and about the uniformity of data collection methods (e.g., informers and measurements) for subjects of differing developmental stages. While relatively consistent research findings have been obtained regarding variations in symptom experiences according to age, pubertal status, and gender, prospective longitudinal designs are needed to confirm these findings and to identify processes that affect report of physical symptoms.

Race and Ethnicity.   Using clinical samples of school-age children, some researchers found that physical symptoms were greater among minority groups than among whites (Campo et al., 1999; Starfield et al., 1980). In contrast, Jolly et al. (1994) showed that somatic symptoms were more prevalent among Caucasian adolescents than among African Americans. In an attempt to reconcile these contradictory findings, it has been speculated that both white and minority children are afflicted with physical symptom complaints at similar rates but report different symptoms. A recent study found that whites were more prone to headaches, musculoskeletal pain, and dizziness, whereas urinary symptoms, cold sweat, feeling hot, and chest pain were more prevalent among blacks (Rhee, 2002).

Explanations for racial differences include differences in biological traits among the groups (Stewart et al., 1996) and sociocultural contexts (Gureje, Simon, Ustun, & Goldberg, 1997). Although none of these speculations have been tested, sociocultural mechanisms have more often been discussed. Cultures differ in the ways their members express physical symptoms and pain; therefore, they influence not only views of illness but also attitudes toward physical and psychological problems. In addition, race is often confounded with SES in the United States; thus, racial differences in symptom reports might actually represent SES differences. A recent study (Reynolds, O'Koon, Papademetriou, Szczygiel, & Grant, 2001) reported strikingly high rates of physical complaints in a low-income sample in which minority adolescents constituted 96% of the total sample. Despite the study's intriguing results, this report did not provide any information regarding whether such prevalence was significantly higher than in whites. On the other hand, Rhee (2002) found that blacks were more prone to certain symptoms such as chest pain, feeling hot, urinary problems, and cold sweat than whites and that these racial differences either disappeared or became minute after taking into account SES.

In conclusion, the literature on pediatric physical symptoms has by and large ignored race and ethnic issues. Most prior reports were primarily based on clinical samples that were not representative of general pediatric populations. In addition, race and ethnic issues in physical symptoms have rarely been approached from an ecological perspective that incorporates multiple factors beyond apparent differences in skin color (e.g., biological factors, sociocultural components) and that focuses on interactions among these factors.

PSYCHOLOGICAL FACTORS

Self-Esteem.   Youngsters' negative perceptions of themselves are associated with physical symptom experiences (Garber et al., 1991; Garrick,

Ostrov, & Offer, 1988; Kronenberger, Laite, & Laclave, 1995; Marlowe, 1998; Poikolainen et al., 1995; Rauste-von Wright & von Wright, 1992; Rhee, 2000; Silverstein et al., 1995; Walker, Garber, & Smith, 2001). Garrick et al. (1988) found that high scores on a self-report measure of somatization were related to negative self-concept in a community sample of adolescents. Garber et al. (1991) used a scale measuring children's global perceptions of their worth and esteem as one way of establishing construct validity for the Children's Somatization Inventory (CSI). In comparison with healthy control subjects, adolescents with functional physical complaints had significantly lower scores on measures of self-esteem or global self-worth (Walker et al., 2001). Preadolescents who had been referred to a psychiatry consultation service and diagnosed with somatoform disorders using DSM-III-R criteria also expressed lower self-esteem than those who did not present with these diagnoses (Kronenberger et al., 1995). Poikolainen et al. (2000) tested the extent to which self-esteem contributed to the development or maintenance of somatizing symptom patterns and reported self-esteem as an important factor predicting recurrent physical symptoms within 5 years. Likewise, Rhee (2000) showed that the likelihood that low self-esteem predicted headaches within a year was three times as high as the likelihood that headache predicted low self-esteem.

Self-esteem is a basis of personal satisfaction and effective functioning in every aspect of life. Despite its developmental importance, in most studies of physical symptoms self-esteem has been treated as a "piggyback" concept, rather than one deserving major consideration. Even when studies examined self-esteem as a primary research focus, their findings have been limited by the methodology they used. For instance, Kronenberger et al.'s study (1995) lacked a representative study sample, and Garrick et al.'s (1988) study was limited by a cross-sectional design. Rhee's study (2000) avoided these two shortcomings, but may also have fallen short in areas by focusing on a single symptom (headache) and developmental stage (adolescence) and by failing to examine many levels of human functioning within an ecological framework.

Depression.   Depression is a psychological condition most frequently studied in association with physical symptoms. Physical complaints have stronger associations with severity of depression than with any other factors (Egger et al., 1999; McCauley, Carlson, & Calderon, 1991; Tamminen et al., 1991). Children who had been clinically referred because of physical symptoms reported higher levels of depressive symptoms than healthy controls or clinical groups of children without symptom complaints (Andrasik et al., 1988; Cunningham et al., 1987; McCauley et al., 1991). Strong associations between physical symptoms and depression are also found in community samples of children and adolescents (Beidel, Christ, & Long, 1991; Carlsson, Larsson, & Mark, 1995; Egger et al., 1999; Eminson et al., 1996; Garber et al., 1991; Larsson, 1991; Poikolainen et al., 1995; Rauste-von Wright & von Wright, 1992; Rhee, 2000; Tamminen et al., 1991; Taylor et al., 1996; Zwaigenbaum, Szatmari, Boyle, & Offord, 1999). The likelihood of depression increases as the number and intensity of symptoms increase (Garber et al., 1991; Rhee, 2002).

The frequent concurrence of physical symptoms and depression leaves open the question of the direction of causation. Two equally plausible possibilities have been raised: depression as a consequence and depression as an antecedent of physical symptoms. The supposition that physical symptoms lead to depression is based on the assumption that increased social withdrawal and isolation and perceived life interference as a result of chronic symptoms may contribute to the development or continuance of depression (Rudy, Kerns, & Turk, 1988). Kristjansdottir (1997b) concluded that physical symptoms are strong determinants of emotional distress. A recent prospective longitudinal study (Zwaigenbaum et al., 1999) involving a community sample of 500 adolescents showed that high levels of physical symptoms emerged as a significant risk factor for major depression 4 years later, whereas emotional disorders at baseline or gender differences did not. Longitudinal birth cohort studies following children over 3 decades revealed that headache (Fearon & Hotopf, 2001) and abdominal pain (Hotopf, Siobhan, Mayou, Wadsworth, & Wessely, 1998) in childhood in the absence of defined organic diseases were the precursors of psychiatric disorders in adulthood.

On the other hand, depression could be an antecedent of physical symptoms. The physical symptoms in youngsters may be an avenue for expressing negative emotional conditions (McCauley et al., 1991), a position supported by several longitudinal epidemiologic studies (Egger et al., 1999; Pine, Cohen, & Brook, 1996; Rhee, 2000). Egger et al. (1999) noted that musculoskeletal pains were associated with depression in adolescents, whereas restricted activity because of the pains was not. Pine et al.'s (1996) prospective longitudinal study using a sample of children aged 9 to 18 ($N = 776$) found that headache was about twice as common in depressed as in nondepressed adolescents and that depression without current or past headache history prospectively predicted a new onset of headaches in young adulthood. Among adolescents with no history of chronic headaches, those with current depression faced a nearly tenfold increased risk of developing functionally impairing headaches at some time during the following 7 years. Similarly, Rhee (2000, 2002) demonstrated the sequential path from depression to a single symptom, headache, and to multiple symptoms in a 1-year longitudinal study.

Anxiety.   Physical symptoms also are associated with anxiety in children in clinical settings (Bernstein, Garfinkel, & Hoberman, 1989; Jolly et al, 1994; Last, 1991; McCauley et al., 1991) and community settings (Beidel et al., 1991; Carlsson et al., 1995; Egger et al., 1998, 1999; Eminson et al., 1996; Garber et al., 1991; Larsson, 1991; Poikolainen et al., 1995; Rauste-von Wright & von Wright, 1992; Tamminen et al., 1991; Taylor et al., 1996). Children with comorbid anxiety and depression symptoms appear more likely to experience physical symptoms than those with depressive symptoms alone (Jolly et al., 1994; McCauley et al., 1991).

Anxiety disorders also bear an independent relationship with physical symptoms (Jolley et al., 1994). In a clinical sample, anxiety emerged as a better predictor of the persistence of headache over time than depression (Guidetti et al., 1998). Egger et al. (1999) found that girls with an anxiety disorder had nearly 100 times greater prevalence of headaches and stomachaches than those without the disorder. Separation anxiety disorder (SAD) and panic disorder were also related to increased somatic complaints in children (Last, 1991; Livingston, Taylor, & Grawford, 1988). SAD and avoidant disorder are specifically associated with stomach complaints (Bernstein et al., 1997). Children with social phobia reported the most pervasive somatic responses (Beidel et al., 1991).

In short, extensive research has documented an association between physical symptoms of youngsters and such emotional states as depression and anxiety, regardless of temporal sequences or causality. However, most studies, if not all, suffer from a lack of theoretical frameworks and have methodological shortcomings, such as cross-sectional designs, small sample sizes, unrepresentative samples, and a lack of sensitivity about development.

BEHAVIORAL FACTORS

Faull and Nicol (1986) reported higher antisocial scores measured by tantrums and irritability, disobedience, destructiveness, and restlessness among preschool children with abdominal pains. Andrasik et al.'s (1988) study found that a clinical sample of school-age headache sufferers scored higher than matched controls on externalizing behavior problems such as hyperactivity, delinquency, and aggression. More specific behavioral problems (e.g., truancy, drinking problems) were also reported among adolescents suffering from recurrent headaches and abdominal pains from the general population (Beiter et al., 1991; Larsson, 1988). Although this trend seems true for both genders, the increased behavioral risk is greater for boys (Beiter et al., 1991). Likewise, adolescents with physical symptoms are likely to engage in unhealthy habits, such as smoking, drinking, and sexual activity, and they present an aggressive mode of coping, an immature defense style, and the absence of active or constructive coping efforts (Aro & Taipale, 1987; Poikolainen et al., 1995; Rauste-von Wright & von Wright, 1992). Furthermore, symptom complaints in adolescents, especially in boys, have been shown to be associated with several disruptive behavior disorders based on DSM criteria, such as Conduct Disorder (CD), Oppositional Deficit Disorder (ODD), and Attention Deficit Hyperactivity Disorder (ADHD) (Egger, Angold, & Costello, 1998; Egger et al., 1999; Taylor et al., 1996).

A speculation that behavioral difficulty may lead to physical symptom problems follows findings of an association between antisocial behavior during adolescence and somatic complaints in young adulthood (Newcomb & Bentler, 1987). Indeed, behavior problems such as substance abuse have been shown to be the precursors of physical symptom complaints in adolescents in a 6-year longitudinal study (Hansell & White, 1991). On the other hand, Zwaigenbaum et al. (1999) showed that a high somatizing tendency in childhood did not predict substance abuse or dependency in adolescence despite significant relationships between symptoms and these behaviors in a cross-sectional analysis.

Certain vulnerable temperamental characteristics manifested in the early developmental stages, such as higher levels of activity, irregularity, and withdrawal in new situations (Davison, Faull, & Nicol, 1986), may determine children's later coping with stress. Yet mechanisms explaining the relationships between behavior problems and physical symptom reports remain to be discovered through an ecological model that captures multiple levels of functioning within and outside the children and their reciprocal interactions over time.

Environmental Factors Associated With Physical Symptoms

FAMILIAL AND PARENTAL FACTORS

Certain features of the family appear to promote physical symptoms in children. Family stressors and a child's dissatisfaction with his or her family situation are related to current physical symptoms (Rauste-von Wright & von Wright, 1981; Sharrer & Ryan-Wenger, 1991). Thus, symptom complaints are common in children from nonintact or dysfunctional families with parental marital discord or other family conflicts (Campo et al., 1999; Fearon & Hotopf, 2001; Poikolainen et al., 1995; Rhee, 2002; Tamminen et al., 1991). Often family stress becomes heightened with a deficit in financial resources. This situation may account for findings that the rates of physical symptoms are high in children from working-class and low-SES families (Fearon & Hotopf, 2001; Poikolainen et al., 1995; Reynolds et al., 2001; Rhee, 2002; Tamminen et al., 1991). Similarly, many have documented the higher prevalence of physical symptoms in socially and economically underprivileged pediatric samples (Aro et al., 1987; Campo et al., 1999; Fearon & Hotopf, 2001; Flato, Aasland, Vandvik, & Forre, 1997; Hotopf et al., 1998; Hansell & White, 1991; Steptoe & Butler, 1996). Family also functions as an important "breeding ground" for physical symptoms via shared genetic information and shared environment. A family history of physical symptoms is extremely common in children with physical symptoms (Garber et al., 1991; Mikail & von Baeyer, 1990; Walker, Garber, & Greene, 1991). Such a strong family tendency has been explained through genetic predisposition (Aromaa, Rautava, Helenius, & Sillanpaa, 1998) and a social-learning process through "modeling" (Osborne, Hatcher, & Richtsmeier, 1989; Walker & Greene, 1989).

Parents' mental health (e.g., depression, anxiety) (Fearon & Hotopf, 2001; Garber, Zeman, & Walker, 1990; Poikolainen et al., 1995; Walker & Greene, 1989) and chronic physical illness or disability (Fearon & Hotopf, 2001; Hotoft et al., 1998; Mikail & von Baeyer, 1990) are also associated with children's report of physical symptoms. Such associations could be due to coping with the parents' illness (Mikail & von Baeyer, 1990; Zuckerman et al., 1987) or to modeling of parents' vulnerability (Garralda, 1999; Osborne et al., 1989).

Parental personalities also affect children's symptom complaints. The parents of symptom-prone children tend to be anxious, critical, insensitive to the needs of the child, punitive, cold, or distant (Hotoft et al., 1998). Grunau, Whitfield, Petrie, and Fryer (1994) identified poor maternal sensitivity and maternal overinvolvement as precursors to somatization in children. In a retrospective longitudinal study, adult patients with physical symptoms were more likely than patients with other psychological problems to report a childhood pattern of lack of parental care and unsatisfactory relationships with their parents (Craig, Boardman, Mills, Daly-Jones, & Drake, 1993). A poor parent-child relationship has been consistently found to be associated with physical symptoms in adolescents in both community settings (Aro, 1987; Tanaka, Tamai, Terashima, Takenaka, & Tanaka, 2000) and clinical settings (Greene, Walker, Hickson, & Thompson, 1985).

Parental responses to physical symptoms in their children also influence the development and persistence of these symptoms. Parents may reinforce the child's symptoms by providing increased attention and special privileges and allowing withdrawal from stressful situations. These secondary gains may contribute to initiating or prolonging the episode of physical symptoms in some children (Osborne et al., 1989; Walker, Lynn, Garber, & Greene, 1993).

The literature on family and parental factors in pediatric physical symptoms has been limited because researchers have not examined the dynamic processes that influence children's symptom reports over time and within the context of evolving and changing family issues. As a result, the importance of incorporating family dynamics into intervention efforts in managing physical symptoms has not been convincingly shown.

Peer Relationships

Despite its importance to children and adolescents, the effect of peer relationship on children's physical symptoms has received little attention in the literature. A few cross-sectional studies suggest that adolescents with physical symptoms tend to experience difficulties such as a lack of friends, poor relationships with peers, and loneliness (Aro, Hanninen, & Paronen, 1989; Kristjansdottir & Rhee, 2002; Natvig, Albrektsen, Anderssen, & Qvarnstrom, 1999; Rauste-von Wright & von Wright, 1992; Taylor et al., 1996). Most studies have lacked clear definitions of peer relationships. Some studies examined this concept from a "social support" standpoint (Kristjansdottir & Rhee, 2002; Natvig et al., 1999), whereas others simply focused on a quantitative aspect such as number of close friends (Aro et al., 1989). Recently, Rhee (2002) showed that an adolescent's somatizing tendency was negatively affected by friendship quality but positively influenced by quantity. That is, adolescents perceiving high levels of care from friends tended to report fewer physical symptoms, while those who reported having a large number of close friends and spending more time with them showed a higher tendency to somatization. This suggests that these two aspects of peer relationships have different associations with physical symptom experiences. Thus, the specification of the concept seems necessary in researching the roles of peer relationship in pediatric symptom complaints. It is also not clear whether functional impairments resulting from frequent experiences of physical symptoms motivate poor peer relationships or whether a particular emotional or behavioral tendency (e.g., depressiveness, delinquent behaviors) found in youngsters with physical symptoms prevents them from maintaining satisfying relationships with their peers. A longitudinal study based on a developmental science framework could provide a developmentally appropriate understanding of the causal relationships between peer relationships and physical symptoms.

SCHOOL AND COMMUNITY FACTORS

A few studies have found associations between children's physical symptoms and problems in social functioning, particularly in the school context. Physical symptoms in children and adolescents have been related to difficulties in adapting to school (Faull & Nicol, 1986), being bullied in school (Williams, Chambers, Logan, & Robinson, 1996), and feelings of alienation at school (Natvig et al., 1999). Children with physical symptoms often have low motivation for further education, diminished school-related self-efficacy, poor school performance, and high rates of absenteeism (Aro et al., 1987; Campo et al., 1999; Garber et al., 1991; Poikolainen et al., 1995; Rauste-von Wright & von Wright, 1992; Tamminen et al., 1991; Tanaka et al., 2000; Walker, Garber, van Slyke, & Greene, 1995). Frequent school absenteeism and its associated loss of peer relationships and an increase in academic difficulties may pose a serious threat to social and cognitive development and place these children at risk for emotional difficulties, further aggravating physical symptoms. Thus, physical symptoms, if they become chronic and severe, can give rise to serious problems in psychosocial development in childhood and adolescence. The connections between physical symptoms and psychosocial functioning and well-being underscore the need for a systematic investigation of how these factors interrelate.

Certain community characteristics are also associated with pediatric symptom problems. Alfven (1993) showed that these symptoms were more common among children living in unstable social environments. Campbell and Schwarz (1996) pointed out that exposure to community violence can have a potential impact on adolescents' symptom experiences. A lack of literature has hampered a comprehensive discussion of the influence of the community on pediatric symptom reports, and an examination of the particular environments in which children and adolescents are at risk for physical symptoms is needed.

SUMMARY AND CRITIQUE

This review has highlighted three major contributions of contemporary research on pediatric physical symptoms conducted by researchers in various disciplines. First, the prevalence of physical symptoms in otherwise healthy youngsters has been identified. The most frequently reported symptoms are headache, abdominal pain or discomfort, musculoskeletal pain, and fatigue. Second, this review clearly indicated that the phenomena of physical symptoms reported by children and youth have complex associations with demographic, psychological, behavioral, and environmental aspects of the child and his life and need to be studied accordingly. Thus, research using an ecological and developmental science framework with an emphasis on multidimensionality and multicausality is necessary to facilitate a holistic understanding of symptom phenomena. Lastly, studies have implied the existence of complicated mechanisms by which physical symptoms maintain either direct or indirect relationships with multiple developmental factors. The identification of mechanisms is necessary in order to reconcile seemingly contradictory findings about the causal relationships between physical symptoms and certain developmental outcomes, such as psychological and behavioral maladjustments. These mechanisms may involve "mediators" or "moderators" that capture particular processes. Developmental perspectives and methods are important in identifying the mechanisms by which different levels of developmental functioning are affected by physical symptoms and also in identifying factors that affect recurrent reports of physical symptoms in children and youth.

Unfortunately, much of the existing literature on physical symptoms is limited because many studies have been atheoretical and confined to a descriptive or exploratory level. Therefore, their findings have not been systemically constructed in a meaningful and coherent way. Accordingly, a theory based on the principles of a developmental science that emphasizes multidimensionality and interactions among factors will facilitate not only the research process but also the transformation and solidification of findings into a theory about physical symptoms in youngsters.

The vast majority of studies of physical symptoms have used cross-sectional designs. Thus, only two-dimensional snapshots in which factors are statistically associated have been obtained. However, in real life, both individuals and environments keep changing, and these changes shape the individual's "being" and "becoming." Thus, the concept of "change" has constituted a core of developmental science (Magnusson & Cairns, 1996). Accurate accounts are not attainable without an appropriate method of capturing those changes and processes. Longitudinal studies will help produce dynamic information that can more readily be applied to the life situations of youngsters with physical symptoms.

An important methodological issue involves sampling. Two types of studies, clinical- and population-based, have resulted even for identical research questions because of the types of a sample used. For instance, compared to population-based samples of children, clinical samples consist of small numbers of subjects who overrepresent the seriously and chronically afflicted population whose parents are financially able to afford medical care. In population-based studies, the representativeness of a sample is critical. In most studies conducted in Europe, the representativeness of samples has been relatively well maintained. On the other hand, population studies in the United States have been limited not only by small sample sizes but also by less vigorous procedures in ensuring the representativeness of their samples, particularly in terms of race/ethnic ratios, SES, and geographic regions. The use of representative study samples is essential when establishing the prevalence of physical symptoms and examining these symptoms within a normal ecological, developmental context.

Another limitation is the broad age ranges used in many studies. Because of the rapid development of children, even a year's difference in age can be enough to produce remarkable differences in responses. Accordingly, researchers should use more homogeneous age samples where possible. However, ensuring homogeneity of samples by recruiting children of the same age group is not always the best solution. Using heterogeneous age groups in a cross-sectional study can produce information about symptom trajectory over age without using longitudinal designs.

However, a researcher needs to analyze findings by developmental age as well as acknowledge the limitations of cross-sectional study.

Furthermore, developmentally appropriate data collection methods that properly assess the physical domain of interest must be selected. Issues such as choosing proper informants (e.g., parents, teachers, or children), types of measurements (e.g., interview, paper-pencil, observation or physiological measures), and the reading level of instruments are important considerations. Objective methods such as physiological measures that help ensure the comparability of data from subjects of different ages are highly desirable. Recently, understanding development as a product of continuous interactions among multiple levels of human functioning including the biological level has sparked an interest in using biological measures in developmental sciences (Gottlieb, Wahlsten, & Lickliter, 1998). Although physiological factors have been speculated to play a determining role triggering symptom experiences, researchers have rarely studied this aspect. Thus, combining a physiological measure with other data collection tools would strengthen study findings and provide an understanding of the dynamic processes at various levels that affect physical symptoms.

Studies of physical symptoms need more appropriate analytic strategies. Many studies employed cross-sectional analytic techniques, predominantly correlational methods. Yet the interpretations of their results surpassed their data and included statements about causality. On the other hand, longitudinal research designs frequently use regression methods without using appropriate diagnostic procedures such as multicolinearity assessment, residual analyses, and influential statistics; therefore, the credibility of the findings may be questioned. In addition, regression methods focus on variables and deal with group means and ignore individual differences. Thus, "the modeling/description of variables over individuals can be very difficult to translate into properties characterizing single individuals because of the variable-oriented, not individual-oriented, nature of the information provided by the statistical method used" (Bergman, 1998, p. 83). As a remedy for this problem, Bergman and Magnusson (1997) proposed a person-oriented approach in which the unit of analysis is "persons." This analysis focuses on identifying patterns by which information from multiple dimensions is grouped and organized in such a way that the clustered information can describe an individual as a totality. Rhee (2002) demonstrated the feasibility and unique contributions of the person-oriented approach in a study of physical symptoms. Adolescents were classified according to the patterns of multiple symptoms, and each group was further described by a variety of psychosocial variables. The importance and utility of person-oriented approaches in developmental research have gradually gained recognition (Magnusson & Cairns, 1996), and the applicability of this method in symptom research is expected to be further tested in future studies.

Overall, nurses' contribution to physical symptom literature is not remarkable. Only a few publications had nurse researchers as first authors. This review identified four nurse researchers in this area of study. Regrettably, not all these nurse researchers have established programs of research in this field, considering that two of them (Natvig and Sharrer) have published no additional work on a similar topic. Only one nurse researcher, Kristjansdottir from Iceland, has a program of research, as evidenced in her multiple publications focused on headache, stomachache, and back pain (Kristjansdottir, 1997a, 1977b; Kristjansdottir & Rhee, 2002; Kristjansdottir & Wahlber, 1993). In addition, Rhee has begun a program of research on various physical symptoms using a large nationally representative sample of adolescents from the National Longitudinal Study of Adolescent Health (Rhee, 2000, 2002; Rhee et al., 2002).

In summary, research on pediatric physical symptoms has begun to evolve from the simplest model depicting a relationship between a single symptom and an associating factor to a highly complicated system model that is considered superior to the former in light of developmental science. More studies of physical symptoms based on developmental science are needed to reflect the intricate relationships among multiple factors associated with the symptom phenomena and to capture dynamic processes over time. The application of developmental perspectives in physical symptom research could not only enhance understanding but also maximize nurses' contribution to the expansion of knowledge by integrating various research traditions from different disciplines, such as medicine, biology, psychology, sociology, and public health. Moreover, information produced from developmentally appropriate research can be of particular value for nurses working in primary pediatric settings and school health systems as they deal with physical symptom complaints from children and youth.

REFERENCES

Abu-Arafeh, I., & Russell, G. (1996). Recurrent limb pain in schoolchildren. *Archives of Diseases in Childhood, 74,* 336–339.

Alfven, G. (1993). The covariation of common psychosomatic symptoms among children from socio-economically differing residential areas: An epidemiological study. *Acta Paediatrica, 82,* 484–487.

Andrasik, F., Kabela, E., Quinn, S., Attanasio, V., Blanchard, E. B., & Rosenblum, E. L. (1988). Psychological functioning of children who have recurrent migraine. *Pain, 34,* 43–52.

Angold, A., & Worthman, C. W. (1993). Puberty onset of gender differences in rates of depression: A developmental, epidemiologic and neuroendocrine perspective. *Journal of Affective Disorders, 29,* 145–158.

Aro, H. (1987). Life stress and psychosomatic symptoms among 14- to 16-year-old Finnish adolescents. *Psychological Medicine, 17,* 191–201.

Aro, H., Hanninen, V., & Paronen, O. (1989). Social support, life events and psychosomatic symptoms among 14–16-year-old adolescents. *Social Science Medicine, 29,* 1051–1056.

Aro, H., Paronen, O., & Aro, S. (1987). Psychosomatic symptoms among 14–16 year old Finnish adolescents. *Social Psychiatry, 22,* 171–176.

Aro, H., & Taipale, V. (1987). The impact of timing of puberty on psychosomatic symptoms among fourteen- to sixteen-year-old Finnish girls. *Child Development, 58,* 261–268.

Aromaa, M., Rautava, P., Helenius, H., & Sillanpaa, M. (1998). Factors of early life as predictors of headache in children at school entry. *Headache, 38,* 23–30.

Aromaa, M., Sillanpaa, M. L., Rautava, P., & Helenius, H. (1998). Childhood headache at school entry: A controlled clinical study. *Neurology, 50,* 1729–1736.

Barea, L. M., Tannhauser, M., & Rotta, N. T. (1996). An epidemiologic study of headache among children and adolescents of southern Brazil. *Cephalalgia, 16,* 545–549.

Beidel, D. C., Christ, M. A., & Long, P. J. (1991). Somatic complaints in anxious children. *Journal of Abnormal Child Psychology, 19,* 659–670.

Beiter, M., Ingersoll, G., Ganser, J., & Orr, D. P. (1991). Relationships of somatic symptoms to behavioral and emotional risk in young adolescents. *Journal of Pediatrics, 118,* 473–478.

Belmaker, E. (1984). Nonspecific somatic symptoms in early adolescent girls. *Journal of Adolescent Health Care, 5,* 30–33.

Belmaker, E., Espinoza, R., & Pogrund, R. (1985). Use of medical services by adolescents with non-specific somatic symptoms. *International Journal of Adolescent Medicine and Health, 1,* 150–156.

Bergman, L. R. (1998). A pattern-oriented approach to studying individual development: Snapshots and processes. In R. B. Cairns, L. Bergman, & J. Kagan (Eds.), *Methods and models for studying the individual* (pp. 83–121). Thousand Oaks, CA: Sage.

Bergman, L. R., & Magnusson, D. (1997). A person-oriented approach in research on developmental psychopathology. *Development and Psychopathology, 9,* 291–319.

Bernstein, G. A., Garfinkel, B. D., & Hoberman, H. M. (1989). Self-reported anxiety in adolescents. *American Journal of Psychiatry, 14,* 384–386.

Bernstein, G. A., Massie, E. D., Thuras, P. D., Perwien, A. R., Borchardt, C. M., & Crosby, R. D. (1997). Somatic symptoms in anxious-depressed school refusers. *Journal of the American Academy of Child and Adolescent Psychiatry, 36,* 661–668.

Borge, A. I., Nordhagen, R., Moe, B., Botten, G., & Bakketeig, L. S. (1994). Prevalence and persistence of stomachache and headache among children. Follow-up of a cohort of Norwegian children from 4 to 10 years of age. *Acta Paediatrica, 83,* 433–437.

Campbell, C., & Schwarz, D. F. (1996). Prevalence and impact of exposure to interpersonal violence among suburban and urban middle school students. *Pediatrics, 98,* 396–402.

Campo, J. V., Jansen-McWilliams, L., Comer, D. M., & Kelleher, K. J. (1999). Somatization in pediatric primary care: Association with psychopathology, functional impairment, and use of services. *Journal of the American Academy of Child and Adolescent Psychiatry, 38,* 1093–1101.

Carlsson, J. (1996). Prevalence of headache in schoolchildren relation to family and school factors. *Acta Paediatrica, 85,* 692–696.

Carlsson, J., Larsson, B., & Mark, A. (1995). Psychosocial functioning in schoolchildren with recurrent headaches. *Headache, 36,* 77–82.

Craig, T. K., Boardman, A. P., Mills, K., Daly-Jones, O., & Drake, H. (1993). The south London somatization study: I. Longitudinal course and the influence of early life experiences. *British Journal of Psychiatry, 163,* 579–588.

Cunningham, S. J., McGrath, P., Ferguson, H., Humphreys, P., D'Astous, J., Latter, J., et al. (1987). Personality and behavioral characteristics in pediatric migraine. *Headache, 27,* 16–20.

Davison, I. S., Faull, C., & Nicol, A. R. (1986). Research note: Temperament and behavior in six-year-olds with recurrent abdominal pain: A follow up. *Journal of Child Psychology and Psychiatry, 27,* 539–544.

Egger, H. L., Angold, A., & Costello, J. (1998). Headaches and psychopathology in children and adolescents. *Journal of the American Academy of Child and Adolescent Psychiatry, 37,* 951–958.

Egger, H. L., Costello, E. J., Erkanli, A., & Angold, A. (1999). Somatic complaints and psychopathology in children and adolescents: Stomach aches, musculoskeletal pains and headaches. *Journal of the American Academy of Child and Adolescent Psychiatry, 38,* 852–860.

Eminson, M., Benjamin, S., Shortall, A., Woods, T., & Faragher, B. (1996). Physical symptoms and illness attitudes in adolescents: An epidemiological study. *Journal of Child Psychology and Psychiatry, 37,* 519–528.

Faull, C., & Nicol, A. R. (1986). Abdominal pain in six-year-olds: An epidemiological study in a new town. *Journal of Child Psychology and Psychiatry and Allied Disciplines, 27,* 251–260.

Fearon, P., & Hotopf, M. (2001). Relation between headache in childhood and physical and psychiatric symptoms in adulthood: National cohort study. *British Medical Journal, 322,* 1–6.

Flato, B., Aasland, A., Vandvik, I. H., & Forre, O. (1997). Outcome and predictive factors in children with chronic idiopathic musculoskeletal pain. *Clinical and Experimental Rheumatology, 15,* 569–577.

Garber, J., Walker, L. S., & Zeman, J. (1991). Somatization symptoms in a community sample of children and adolescents: Further validation of the children's somatization inventory. *Psychological Assessment: A Journal of Consulting and Clinical Psychology, 3,* 588–595.

Garber, J., Zeman, J., & Walker, L. S. (1990). Recurrent abdominal pain in children: Psychiatric diagnoses and parental psychopathology. *Journal of the American Academy of Child and Adolescent Psychiatry, 29,* 648–656.

Garralda, M. E. (1996). Somatization in children. *Journal of Child Psychology and Psychiatry, 37,* 13–33.

Garralda, M. E. (1999). Practitioner review: Assessment and management of somatization in childhood and adolescence; a practical perspective. *Journal of Child Psychology and Psychiatry, 40,* 1159–1167.

Garrick, T., Ostrov, E., & Offer, D. (1988). Physical symptoms and self-image in a group of normal adolescents. *Psychosomatics, 29,* 73–80.

Gottlieb, G., Wahlsten, D., & Lickliter, R. (1998). The significance of biology for human development: A developmental psychobiological systems view. In W. Damon (General Ed.) & R. M. Lerner (Series Ed.), *Handbook of child psychology: Vol. 1. Theoretical models of human development* (5th ed., pp. 233–273). New York: Wiley.

Greene, J. W., Walker, L. S., Hickson, G., & Thompson, J. (1985). Stressful life events and somatic complaints in adolescence. *Pediatrics, 75,* 19–22.

Grunau, R. W., Whitfield, M. F., Petrie, J. H., & Fryer, E. L. (1994). Early pain experience, child and family factors, as precursors of somatization: A prospective study of extremely premature and fullterm children. *Pain, 56,* 353–359.

Guidetti, V., Galli, F., Fabrizi, P., Giannantoni, A. S., Napoli, L., Bruni, O., et al. (1998). Headache and psychiatric comorbidity: Clinical aspects and outcome in an 8-year follow-up study. *Cephalalgia, 18,* 455–462.

Gureje, O., Simon, G. E., Ustun, T. B., & Goldberg, D. P. (1997). Somatization in cross-cultural perspective: A World Health Organization study in primary care. *American Journal of Psychiatry, 154,* 989–995.

Hansell, S., & White, H. R. (1991). Adolescent drug use, psychological distress, and physical symptoms. *Journal of Health and Social Behavior, 32,* 288–301.

Holden, E. W., Levy, J. D., Deichmann, M. M., & Galdstein, J. (1998). Recurrent pediatric headaches: Assessment and intervention. *Developmental and Behavioral Pediatrics, 19,* 109–117.

Hotopf, M., Siobhan, C., Mayou, R., Wadsworth, M., & Wessely, S. (1998). Why do children have chronic abdominal pain, and what happens to them when they grow up? Population based cohort study. *British Medical Journal, 316,* 1196–1200.

Hyams, J. S., Burke, G., Davis, P. M., Rzepski, B., & Andrulonis, P. A. (1996). Abdominal pain and irritable bowel syndrome in adolescents: A community-based study. *Journal of Pediatrics, 129,* 220–226.

Jolly, J. B., Wherry, J. N., Wiesner, D. C., Reed, D. H., Rule, J. C., & Jolly, J. M. (1994). The mediating role of anxiety in self-reported somatic complaints of depressed adolescents. *Journal of Abnormal Child Psychology, 22,* 691–702.

Knishkowy, B., Palti, H., Tima, C., Adler, B., & Gofin, R. (1995). Symptom clusters among young adolescents. *Adolescence, 30,* 351–362.

Kristjansdottir, G. (1997a). Prevalence of pain combinations and overall pain: A study of headache, stomach pain and back pain among school-children. *Scandinavian Journal of Social Medicine, 25,* 58–63.

Kristjansdottir, G. (1997b). The relationship between pains and various discomforts in school children. *Childhood, 4,* 491–504.

Kristjansdottir, G., & Rhee, H. (2002). Risk factors of back pain in schoolchildren: A search for explanations to a public health problem. *Acta Paediatrica, 91,* 849–854.

Kristjansdottir, G., & Wahlberg, V. (1993). Sociodemographic differences in the prevalence of self-reported headaches in Icelandic school-children. *Headache, 33,* 376–380.

Kroenke, K., & Mangelsdorff, A. D. (1989). Common symptoms in ambulatory care: Incidence evaluation, therapy and outcome. *American Journal of Medicine, 86,* 262–266.

Kronenberger, W. G., Laite, G., & Laclave, L. (1995). Self-esteem and depressive symptomatology in children with somatoform disorders. *Psychosomatics, 36,* 564–569.

Kujala, U. M., Taimela, S., & Viljanen, T. (1999). Leisure physical activity and various pain symptoms among adolescents. *British Journal of Sports Medicine, 33,* 325–328.

Larsson, B. (1988). The role of psychological, health-behavior and medical factors in adolescent headache. *Developmental Medicine and Child Neurology, 30,* 616–625.

Larsson, B. S. (1991). Somatic complaints and their relationship to depressive symptoms in Swedish adolescents. *Journal of Child Psychology and Psychiatry, 32,* 821–832.

Last, C. G. (1991). Somatic complaints in anxiety disordered children. *Journal of Anxiety Disorder, 5,* 125–138.

Lipowski, Z. J. (1988). Somatization: The concept and its clinical application. *American Journal of Psychiatry, 145,* 1358–1368.

Livingston, R., Taylor, J. L., & Grawford, S. L. (1988). A study of somatic complaints and psychiatric diagnosis in children. *Journal of the American Academy of Child and Adolescent Psychiatry, 27,* 185–187.

Magnusson, D., & Cairns, R. B. (1996). Developmental science: Toward a unified framework. In R. B. Cairns, G. H. Elder, & E. J. Costello (Eds.), *Developmental science* (pp. 7–30). New York: Cambridge University Press.

Marlowe, N. (1998). Self-efficacy moderates the impact of stressful events on headache. *Headache, 38,* 662–667.

McCauley, E., Carlson, G. A., & Calderon, R. (1991). The role of somatic complaints in the diagnosis of depression in children and adolescents. *Journal of the American Academy of Child and Adolescent Psychiatry, 30,* 631–635.

McGrath, P. A., Speechley, K. N., Seifert, C. E., Biehn, J. T., Cairney, A. E. L., Gorodzinsky, F. P., et al. (2000). A survey of children's acute, recurrent and chronic pain: Validation of the pain experience interview. *Pain, 87,* 59–73.

Mikail, S. F., & von Baeyer, C. L. (1990). Pain, somatic focus, and emotional adjustment in children of chronic headache sufferers and controls. *Social Science and Medicine, 31,* 51–59.

Mikkelsson, M., Salminen, J. J., & Kautiainen, H. (1997). Non-specific musculoskeletal pain in preadolescents: Prevalence and 1-year persistence. *Pain, 73,* 29–135.

Moffitt, T. E., Caspi, A., Belsky, J., & Silva, P. A. (1992). Childhood experience and the onset of menarche: A test of a sociobiological model. *Child Development, 63,* 47–58.

Mortimer, M. J., Kay, J., & Jaron, A. (1992). Childhood migraine in general practice: Clinical features and characteristics. *Cephalalgia, 12,* 238–243.

Natvig, G. K., Albrektsen, G., Anderssen, N., & Qvarnstrom, U. (1999). School-related stress and psychosomatic symptoms among school adolescents. *Journal of School Health, 69,* 362–368.

Newcomb, M. D., & Bentler, P. M. (1987). Changes in drug use from high school to young adulthood: Effects of living arrangement and current life pursuit. *Journal of Applied Developmental Psychology, 8,* 221–246.

Offord, D. R., Boyle, M. H., Szatmari, P., Rae-Grant, N. I., Links, P. S., Cadman, D. T., et al. (1987). Ontario Child Health Study: II. Six-month prevalence of disorder and rates of service utilization. *Archives of General Psychiatry, 44,* 832–836.

Osborne, R. B., Hatcher, J. W., & Richtsmeier, A. J. (1989). The role of social modeling in unexplained pediatric pain. *Journal of Pediatric Psychology, 14,* 43–61.

Perquin, C. W., Hazebroek-Kampschreur, A., Hunfeld, J., Bohnen, A. M., Suijlekom-Smit, L., Passchier, J., et al. (2000). Pain in children and adolescents: A common experience. *Pain, 87,* 51–58.

Pine, D. S., Cohen, P., & Brook, J. (1996). The association between major depression and headache: Results of a longitudinal epidemiologic study in youth. *Journal of Child and Adolescent Psychopharmacology, 6,* 153–164.

Poikolainen, K., Aalto-Setala, T., Marttunen, M., Tuulio-Henriksson, A., & Lonnqvist, J. (2000). Predictors of somatic symptoms: A five year follow up of adolescents. *Archives in Diseases in Childhood, 83,* 388–392.

Poikolainen, K., Kanerva, R., & Lonnqvist, J. (1995). Life events and other risk factors for somatic symptoms in adolescence. *Pediatrics, 96,* 59–63.

Rauste-von Wright, M., & von Wright, J. (1981). A longitudinal study of psychosomatic symptoms in healthy 11–18 year old girls and boys. *Journal of Psychosomatic Research, 25,* 525–534.

Rauste-von Wright, M., & von Wright, J. (1992). Habitual somatic discomfort in a representative sample of adolescents. *Journal of Psychosomatic Research, 36,* 383–390.

Reynolds, L. K., O'Koon, J. H., Papademetriou, E., Szczygiel, S., & Grant, K. E. (2001). Stress and somatic complaints in low-income urban adolescents. *Journal of Youth and Adolescence, 30,* 499–514.

Rhee, H. (2000). Prevalence and predictors of headaches in US adolescents. *Headache, 40,* 528–538.

Rhee, H. (2002). *Physical symptoms in adolescents: Prevalence and patterns.* Unpublished doctoral dissertation, University of North Carolina, Chapel Hill.

Rhee, H., Miles, M. S, Halpern, C. T., & Holditch-Davis, D. (2002). *Prevalence of physical symptoms and its association with age and gender.* Manuscript submitted for publication.

Rudy, T. E., Kerns, R. D., & Turk, D. C. (1988). Chronic pain and depression: Toward a cognitive-behavioral mediation model. *Pain, 35,* 129–140.

Sharrer, V. W., & Ryan-Wenger, N. M. (1991). Measurement of stress and coping among school-aged children with and without recurrent abdominal pain. *Journal of School Health, 61,* 86–91.

Silverstein, B., McKoy, E., Clauson, J., Perdue, L., & Raben, J. (1995). The correlation between depression and headache: The role played by generational changes in female achievement. *Journal of Applied Social Psychology, 25,* 35–48.

Starfield, B., Gross, E., Wood, M., Pantell, R., Allen, C., Gordon, B., et al. (1980). Psychosocial and psychosomatic diagnoses in primary care of children. *Pediatrics, 66,* 159–167.

Steptoe, A., & Butler, N. (1996). Sports participation and emotional wellbeing in adolescents. *Lancet, 347,* 1789–1792.

Stewart, W. F., Lipton, R. B., & Liberman, J. (1996). Variation in migraine prevalence by race. *Neurology, 47,* 52–59.

Tamminen, T. M., Bredenberg, P., Escartin, T., Puura, K. K., Rutanen, M., Suominen, I., et al. (1991). Psychosomatic symptoms in preadolescent children. *Psychotherapy and Psychosomatics, 56,* 70–77.

Tanaka, H., Tamai, H., Terashima, S., Takenaka, Y., & Tanaka, T. (2000). Psychosocial factors affecting psychosomatic symptoms in Japanese schoolchildren. *Pediatrics International, 42,* 354–358.

Taylor, D. C., Szatmari, P., Boyle, M. H., & Offord, D. R. (1996). Somatization and the vocabulary of everyday bodily experiences and concerns: A community study of adolescents. *Journal of the American Academy of Child and Adolescent Psychiatry, 35,* 491–499.

Unruh, A. M., Ritchie, J., & Merskey, H. (1999). Does gender affect appraisal of pain and pain coping strategies? *Clinical Journal of Pain, 15,* 31–40.

Viswanathan, V., Bridges, S. J., Whitehouse, W., & Newton, R. (1998). Childhood headache: Discrete entities or continuum? *Developmental Medicine and Child Neurology, 40,* 544–550.

Walker, L. S., Garber, J., & Greene, J. W. (1991). Somatization symptoms in pediatric abdominal pain patients: Relation to chronicity of abdominal pain and parent somatization. *Journal of Abnormal Child Psychology, 19,* 379–394.

Walker, L. S., Garber, J., & Smith, C. A. (2001). The relation of daily stressors to somatic and emotional symptoms in children with and without recurrent abdominal pain. *Journal of Consulting and Clinical Psychology, 69,* 85–91.

Walker, L. S., Garber, J., van Slyke, D. A., & Greene, J. W. (1995). Long-term health outcomes in patients with recurrent abdominal pain. Special issue: Pediatric chronic conditions. *Journal of Pediatric Psychology, 20,* 233–245.

Walker, L. S., & Greene, J. W. (1989). Children with recurrent abdominal pain and their parents: More somatic complaints, anxiety, and depression than other patient families? *Journal of Pediatric Psychology, 14,* 231–243.

Walker, L. S., Lynn, S., Garber, J., & Greene, J. W. (1993). Psychosocial correlates of recurrent childhood pain: A comparison of pediatric patients with recurrent abdominal pain, organic illness, and psychiatric disorders. *Journal of Abnormal Psychology, 102,* 248–258.

Walker, L. S., & Zeman, J. L. (1992). Parental response to child illness behavior. *Journal of Pediatric Psychology, 17,* 49–71.

Williams, K., Chambers, M., Logan, L., & Robinson, D. (1996). Association of common health symptoms with bullying in primary school children. *British Medical Journal, 313,* 17–19.

Zuckerman, B., Stevenson, J., & Baily, V. (1987). Stomachaches and headaches in a community sample of preschool children. *Pediatrics, 79,* 677–682.

Zwaigenbaum, L., Szatmari, P., Boyle, M. H., & Offord, D. R. (1999). Highly somatizing young adolescents and the risk of depression. *Pediatrics, 103,* 1203–1209.

Chapter 5

Symptom Experiences of Children and Adolescents With Cancer

SHARRON L. DOCHERTY

ABSTRACT

This paper examines nursing research focused on the symptom experiences of children and adolescents with cancer, and the extent to which the perspective and methods of developmental science have been used in this research. CINALH, MEDLINE, and PSYCHLIT were searched for publications between 1990 and 2002. The researcher or research team had to include a nurse or developmentally oriented researchers from other disciplines. Studies focused exclusively on pain were excluded because of recent published reviews. While nurse researchers have contributed influential knowledge related to symptom experiences and symptom distress in children and adolescents with cancer, this research is still in a formative but exciting stage. Two nurse researchers and their teams laid the foundation for this research through their individual studies and collaborative multisite studies.

In general, children and adolescents from 10 through 18 years of age were primarily studied; few studies focused on preschool children. Given the fact that these are rare populations, sample sizes were generally small, limiting power and generalizability. Gender, ethnicity, and socioeconomic status were rarely considered in analyses. Most studies used cross-sectional designs, although several included short-term longitudinal or repeated measure designs. To date, longitudinal designs focused on long-term outcomes have not been conducted. There were only a few qualitative studies. There was limited use of conceptual models or theories, and inadequate attention was paid to broader ecological perspectives in the children's lives. Studies included a focus on global symptoms and on individual symptoms, particularly pain and fatigue. Few focused on nausea and vomiting. Operationalization of symptom distress generally involved adapting instruments designed for adults.

A more explicit employment of a developmental science perspective in future studies would call for more longitudinal designs that conceptualize the symptom experience from the perspective of the child and that view their responses as complex and multidimensional in nature. This would necessitate measuring clusters of symptoms at multiple levels (e.g., emotional, behavioral, and biophysiological) using developmental data collection methods. Furthermore, attention needs to be paid in conceptualizing studies to ecological factors related to families, social networks, communities, and ethnicity, as well as to the ecology of the health care system, which likely influences the symptom experience of children.

Approximately 9,100 new cases of childhood cancer among children between infancy and age 14 will be diagnosed in 2002 (American Cancer Society, 2002). In children aged 1 to 14 in the United States, cancer remains the chief cause of death by disease. Importantly, mortality rates have declined 50% since the early 1970s, and the five-year survival rate for all types of childhood cancer is 77% (American Cancer Society, 2002). The dramatic change in survival rates for children afflicted with cancer, brought about by new and intensive treatments, particularly chemotherapy, has led nurse researchers and others to explore the effects of treatment on the daily lives of children and their families and to examine issues related to the long-term survivors of childhood cancer.

Symptom management has been placed at the top of the list of nursing research priorities in the area of childhood cancer (Hinds, Quargnenti, Olson, et al., 1994; National Institute of Health [NIH], 1997; Soanes, Gibson, Bayliss, & Hannan, 2000). Symptoms produced by childhood cancer treatment are not only physically stressful (Enskar, Carlsson, Golsater, & Hamrin, 1997; Collins et al., 2000), but can also cause severe emotional distress (Dolgin, Katz, Zeltzer, & Landsverk, 1989; McQuaid & Nassau, 1999). Although some children appear to adapt and cope well with the physical intensity of the side effects, others appear to be particularly vulnerable and show physical, emotional, and behavioral signs of distress. The underlying mechanism that may explain this differential response to the side effects of treatment is unknown. What is well known by practitioners and researchers is that some children and adults find the side effects of cancer treatment so aversive and debilitating that they are regarded as worse than the cancer itself (Burish, Carey, Krozely, & Greco, 1987; Gorfinkle & Redd, 1993). Emotional and behavioral difficulties associated with aggressive chemotherapeutic treatment regimens and childhood cancer itself have been shown to be related to adaptation to the disease, compliance with therapy, and eventual efficacy of the treatment in children with cancer (Dolgin et al., 1989; Hubert, Jay, Saltoun, & Hayes, 1988). Inability to withstand the side effects of cancer treatment has been described as one of the most important contributors to interruption in treatments or decreased dosages (Watson & Marvell, 1992) and has been responsible for the cessation of treatment (Nahata, Ford, & Ruymann, 1992; Pinkerton & Hardy, 1997; Wilcox, Fetting, Nettesheim, & Abeloff, 1982).

Emotional, behavioral, psychological, and physiological responses to the symptoms produced by the treatment of a disease have been called symptom distress (Rhodes & Watson, 1987). The subjective evaluation of the impact of a symptom has been defined more formally as the physical or mental anguish or suffering (Rhodes & Watson, 1987). Nursing has focused on managing these symptoms and examining their occurrence, severity, frequency, and duration (McDaniel & Rhodes, 1995). However, focusing on the symptoms themselves, rather than the individual's ability to respond to, understand, and cope with their occurrence, has had limited success (Hinds, Quargnenti, & Wentz, 1992; Watson, Rhodes, & Germino, 1987).

Over the past three decades, an impressive amount of research has been conducted on symptom distress in adults with cancer (e.g., Ehlke, 1988; Holmes, 1991; Holmes & Eburn, 1989; Kukull, McCorkle, & Driever, 1986; Lough, Lindsey, Shinn, & Stotts, 1987; McCorkle & Benoliel, 1983; McCorkle & Young, 1978; Rhodes & Watson, 1987; Young & Longman, 1983). Conversely, a limited amount of research has been conducted on symptom distress in children and adolescents with cancer. Thus, this body of knowledge is in the foundational stages.

In order to understand the symptom experiences of children and adolescents with cancer, researchers must get inside the unique culture of children and adolescents to explore how the experience of disease- and treatment-related symptoms actually appears to them (Yamamoto, Soliman, Parsons, & Davies, 1987). While children live in a social world that is, in many ways, similar to that of adults, they occupy a unique position and point of view in that world. Thus in the design and analysis of studies of symptom experiences, a researcher would necessarily need to have a sound understanding of how children distinctively experience, create meanings from, and respond to cancer treatment, as well as how they communicate these experiences to the adults in their world. The perspective of developmental science can be used as a guide to understanding how the bidirectional nature of the relationships that children and adolescents have with parents, siblings, peers, and health professionals influences these experiences. Importantly, these bidirectional relationships are structured within a unique historical, economic, and ethnic context (Magnusson & Cairns, 1996). In addition, the development of responses to disease- and treatment-related symptoms involves a complex interplay of processes across time frames, levels of analyses, and contexts. The developmental science perspective permits viewing symptom experiences from multiple levels—from subsystems of genetics, neurobiology, and hormones to those of families, social networks, communities, and cultures (Carolina Consortium on Human Development, 1996).

The purpose of this review is to examine the nursing research on symptom experiences in children and adolescents with cancer and the extent to which the perspective and methods of developmental science have been used. Because of the history of scholarship in this area, the terms *symptom distress* and *symptom experience* have often been used synonymously. Thus, for consistency in this review the term *symptom experience* will be used in place of both because it implies a broader perspective about symptoms and their impact on children and youth.

METHOD

This review focused on identifying peer-reviewed reports of studies of symptom experiences in children and adolescents with cancer from 1990 through 2002. The computer databases of MEDLINE, CINALH, and PSYCHLIT were searched for studies published after 1990, using the keywords *symptom, symptom distress, symptom experience, symptoms of treatment, treatment distress, emotional responses, stress, quality of life, fatigue, nausea,* and *vomiting*. Secondly, reference lists of obtained reports were searched for other relevant publications.

The main criterion for inclusion was that the researcher or research team had to include a nurse or developmentally oriented researchers from other disciplines if the research was to be relevant to nursing. The majority of subjects had to be between the ages of birth and 18 years and have a diagnosis of cancer, defined as any category (lymph, blood, soft tissue, nerve tissue, bone, central nervous system) of malignant cell growth (Pizzo & Poplack, 2002). However, researchers that studied parent or nurse reports of symptom experiences of children and adolescents were included.

This review included reports focusing on responses to or experiences with selected symptoms such as fatigue, and nausea and vomiting as well as those centered on the global symptom experience. Reports that focused exclusively on pain were excluded because of in-depth reviews published by Hester (1993), Sutters and Miaskowski (1992), and, more recently, Williams (1996). However, a brief description of these reviews is presented in the Results section.

Analytic Strategies

Research reports that fit the inclusion criteria were retrieved, reviewed, and critiqued using a developmental science perspective. The critique focused on the following points:

1. What frameworks were used in the design of studies focused on symptom experiences of children and adolescents with cancer? To what extent was a holistic, developmental systems perspective used to explore how the children's ecological and sociocultural background, including ethnicity, socioeconomic status (SES), and gender, as well as the ecology of the health care system, affected their symptom experience?

2. How was the symptom experience conceptualized across studies, and what methods were used to measure symptom distress or the symptom experiences of children and adolescents with cancer? Were these methods developmentally sound in terms of concepts measured, design of the tool or method, and scaling? To what extent did the measures capture the complex and interrelated nature of symptom experiences in children and adolescents with cancer? Were linkages made between distress at the psychological, biological, and physiological levels?

3. Did the samples include children and adolescents from different socioeconomic levels and ethnic groups? Were analyses conducted examining gender, SES, and ethnic group differences?

4. What designs were most commonly used in this body of research? To what extent were repeated measures or longitudinal designs used to assess stability and change in the symptom experiences of children and adolescents over time? Were factors affecting these changes and the bidirectionality of these factors considered?

Did any investigators use designs and analytic strategies that allowed for understanding the individual's symptom experience over time, such as naturalistic, qualitative designs and/or person-centered analyses?

Finally, findings were summarized to describe what is known about symptom experiences in children and adolescents with cancer and to identify areas for further research.

RESULTS

The body of empirical knowledge regarding the symptom experiences of children and adolescents with cancer can be described as in its formative stages and is characterized by a small number of researchers laying the foundation on which to build important programs of research. This foundation has been prepared by a multisite group of investigators headed by Pamela Hinds and her team from St. Jude Children's Research Hospital and Marilyn Hockenberry-Eaton and her research team at Texas Children's Hospital. These research teams have conducted studies collaboratively as well as independently. For the most part, the remainder of nurse researchers conducted isolated studies that have not yet led to programs of research. This review is organized around studies of global symptom distress, which include the study of multiple symptoms, and then around studies that focus on specific symptoms.

Studies of Global Symptom Experiences

Hinds and colleagues (Hinds, 1990; Hinds, Scholes, Gattuso, Riggins, & Heffner, 1990; Hinds et al., 1992) were the first group of researchers to conduct studies that rated the global symptom experience of children during chemotherapy. The researchers conceptualized symptom distress as an interaction of biological, physiological, social, and psychological forces. Their model illustrated how these forces combine to determine the burden of a symptom or combination of symptoms, including the degree of discomfort and extent of interference with daily function and general quality of life (Hinds et al., 1992). Using the adult-designed symptom distress scale (SDS) by McCorkel and Young (1978), a study was conducted to test the use of the SDS on a population of adolescent cancer patients (Hinds et al., 1992). The 33 adolescents were able to complete the scale quickly without any problems. Cronbach's alphas of .82 and .85 were found, indicating moderate to high internal consistency in the sample. Data were collected at 1 to 2 weeks, 6 to 7 weeks, 3 months, and 6 months after the initiation of cancer treatment. The SDS scores decreased gradually over the first 6 months of treatment. Inverse relationships between symptom distress and adolescent hopefulness and between symptom distress and self-concept were found. Feeling tired, concern with appearance, and lessened ability to get around were the three highest sources of distress.

Guided by their Adolescent Self-Sustaining Model (Hinds & Martin, 1988), Hinds and colleagues tested the effect of an educational intervention to facilitate coping on psychological (hopelessness, self-esteem, self-efficacy, and symptom distress) and clinical outcomes (treatment toxicity) in newly diagnosed adolescents with cancer (Hinds et al., 2000). This two-site study used a longitudinal experimental design with 78 adolescents (46 females and 32 males) randomly assigned to the intervention or control group. Data were collected at four measurement points spanning the first 6 months of treatment. No statistically significant differences were found between the intervention and control groups or between male and female participants.

Schneider and Workman (1999, 2000) also used the SDS in an intervention study involving virtual reality distraction in a sample of 12 children 10 to 17 years of age undergoing chemotherapy for cancer. These investigators also employed Hinds and Martin's (1988) Adolescent Self-Sustaining Model, and this was combined with the Lazarus and Folkman (1991) stress and coping model as their theoretical framework. An interrupted time series design with removed treatment was used. The intervention was effective at reducing the level of symptom distress immediately following the chemotherapy treatment as measured by the SDS but not by the State Trait Anxiety Inventory for Children-1. The distraction did not significantly lower symptom distress scores at the second time point (48 hours post chemotherapy treatment). One subject was dropped as an outlier because the individual profile graph was distinctly different from the rest of the group. A person-centered approach to data analysis, as supported by developmental science, would have kept this participant in analysis to see if he or she illuminated important information on differences in children's responses to disease- and treatment-related symptoms.

Collins and colleagues examined symptom prevalence, characteristics, and distress in one hundred fifteen 10- to 18-year-old children undergoing treatment for cancer (Collins et al., 2000). A secondary purpose of this study was to test the use of the adult-designed Memorial Symptom Assessment Scale (MSAS) for use with children and adolescents. The MSAS assesses the prevalence of a full range of both physical and psychological symptoms according to severity, frequency, and distress (Portenoy et al., 1994). The three subscales can then be combined to get a total overall symptom distress score. Twenty-two symptoms important to children and adolescents were added to the 32-item scale for this study. The 45 inpatients completed the instrument twice over a 2- to 4-day span to assess test-retest reliability. However, the variable nature of symptom experience makes this marker of reliability invalid. While the authors suggest that their analysis supports the reliability and validity of the MSAS 10–18, a major limitation is that the multidimensional assessment of frequency, intensity, and distress is negated by the calculation of a composite symptom score based upon the average of the three dimensions which equates the dimensions of severity, frequency, and distress. Additional findings from this study indicated that a high prevalence of symptoms was found overall and that symptom distress was higher among inpatients, children with solid tumors, and children who were undergoing cancer treatment. The symptoms with the highest prevalence in this sample were lack of energy, pain, drowsiness, nausea, cough, lack of appetite, and psychological symptoms (feeling sad, nervous, irritable, or worried) (Collins et al., 2000).

Several researchers have applied naturalistic qualitative approaches to the study of symptom experiences in children and adolescents. This approach allows for a more multidimensional, person-centered, holistic perspective on symptom experiences than is possible in quantitative studies using adult-adapted symptom distress scales.

Enskar et al. (1997) interviewed 10 Swedish adolescents undergoing treatment for cancer about symptoms, inconveniences, and benefits related to their disease and treatments. The researchers compared the results from the interviews to a quantitative measure of problems encountered during treatment from an earlier study (Enskar, Carlsson, Golsater, Hamrin, & Kreuger, 1997). The adolescents found the physical side effects of the treatment to be the worst aspect of having cancer. Side effects greatly influenced their ability to live life the way they wanted, and several experienced periods of wanting to discontinue treatments.

Docherty (1999) conducted 3-month longitudinal case studies of the symptom experiences of two children (7 and 12 years) and one adolescent (16 years) undergoing treatment for cancer. Three classes of data collection techniques—self-report, biobehavioral, and narrative interviews—were used to track the patterns of symptom experiences over the study period. An investigator-designed symptom diary was used for the subjects to report the occurrence and severity of fatigue, pain, worry, mood alterations, and general well-being. The subjects also completed the Pediatric Nausea, Vomiting, and Retching Guide (Geib & Wright, 1998), the Oucher pain scale (Beyer, Villarruel, & Denyes, 1995), and the Revised Children's Manifest Anxiety Scale (Reynolds & Richmond, 1978). The biobehavioral measures included twice-daily collections of salivary cortisol as a measure of adrenocortical activity in response to the stress and challenge of the symptom experience, and actigraph measures of sleep efficiency. Lastly, narrative interviews were used at four time points over the 3-month study period. Data from the interviews and biobehavioral data contradicted the low frequency of self-report symptoms. The symptom experience of these three children was characterized as cumulative and constellatory. The total global experience could not be described by the summative descriptions of isolated symptoms (Docherty & Sandelowski, 2002). Each child best expressed his or her symptom experience by means of a differing data collection method based on age, gender, culture, and temperament. This study underscores the complexity of measuring symptom distress in children of varying ages, genders, and cultures as well as different personality and coping styles.

Studies of Specific Symptoms

The research on the symptom experiences of children and adolescents with cancer also includes studies of specific symptoms. The three symptoms that have been studied in children undergoing treatment for cancer are pain, fatigue, and nausea and vomiting. In addition, emotional distress as a response to cancer and its treatment is considered an aspect of the symptom experience.

PAIN

Pain associated with the disease or treatments is an important part of the symptom experience of children. Three authors have recently published comprehensive reviews of the literature on pain in children. Hester (1993) conducted an integrative review of research on the more general topic of pain in children. This review included 142 studies conducted by nurses on such topics as prevalence of pain, children's perspectives on pain, assessment of children's pain, and management of children's pain (Hester, 1993). While it is generally well-known that nurse researchers have made significant contributions to the large knowledge base regarding pain in children, Hester (1993) described a variety of problems in the pain research regarding the validity of the studies, including lack of random selection and small samples sizes, lack of theory specification, and lack of studies conducted with preverbal children. Her review did not specifically isolate the research on pain in children with cancer; however, the description and review of the state of knowledge of the development of pain in children in general are very instructive to researchers with an interest in studying pain as a treatment symptom in children with cancer. Sutters and Miaskowski (1992) conducted a review of research on pain in children with cancer from 1977 through 1990. They grouped the 31 studies into seven main areas: pain as a presenting symptom of childhood malignancy, incidence and etiology, assessment, pharmacologic management, psychological strategies for management, coping strategies identified by children, and pain associated with terminal disease. They concluded that, in light of the large amount of pediatric pain research in general, relatively little research has focused on pediatric cancer pain. The majority of the research has centered upon pain associated with procedures. They identified the areas needing investigation as description of the pain trajectories for children with cancer, and studies of the late effects of cancer pain in children. More recently, Williams (1996), in a review of nursing research studies of pediatric oncology procedural pain from 1986 through 1996, found seven studies. She identified problematic areas related to small, nonrepresentative, biased samples and lack of focus on the influence of sociocultural factors on procedural pain in children with cancer. Williams recommended continual pain assessments including the child's emotional and psychological status, the influence of parents' and siblings' anxiety and fears, the influence of inadequate pain management, and parental reinforcement of stoicism or overreactions (Williams, 1996).

FATIGUE

Fatigue has been studied extensively in adults with cancer and is more closely related to the quality of life during cancer treatment than nausea, vomiting, and appetite loss (Schumacher et al., 2002). Until recently, research on treatment-related fatigue in children and adolescents with cancer was nonexistent. Hinds and Hockenberry-Eaton and their respective research teams initiated a multi-institutional collaborative research program to describe cancer- and treatment-related fatigue in children 7 to 12 years old and in adolescents 13 to 18 years old (Hinds, Hockenberry-Eaton, Gilger, et al., 1999; Hinds, Hockenberry-Eaton, Quargnenti, et al., 1999; Hockenberry-Eaton, Hinds, Alcoser, et al., 1998; Hockenberry-Eaton, Hinds, O'Neill, Euell, et al., 1998; Hockenberry-Eaton, Hinds, O'Neill, Alcose, et al., 1999). Parents, staff, children, and adolescents participated in focus group interviews from which the essential attributes of fatigue as well as contributing and alleviating factors were determined. Results suggested that fatigue in children and adolescents with cancer may be a universal experience and one of the most distressing symptoms experienced by this population.

In analysis of two focus group interviews with 14 children and 15 adolescents, developmental level had an important impact on how fatigue was defined (Hinds & Hockenberry-Eaton, 2001; Hockenberry-Eaton, Hinds, Alcoser, et al., 1998). While both children and adolescents described fatigue as a physical and emotional process, the adolescents described the causes of fatigue in much greater detail and were able to point out how symptoms like worry and concern contributed to fatigue. Importantly, children as young as 7 years of age were aware of the physical and emotional manifestations of fatigue (Hockenberry-Eaton, Hinds, Alcoser, et al., 1998). In another analysis of the focus group interviews with the 29 children and adolescents as well as with 31 parents and 38 staff members (advanced practice nurses, staff nurses, nurse managers, nutritionists, chaplain, physician), the essential characteristics, outcomes, and contributory and alleviating factors of fatigue were identified (Hinds, Hockenberry-Eaton, Gilger, et al., 1999). These findings were used to construct a conceptual definition and model of fatigue for each of the four study groups. These definitions and models all reflected changes in the patient's behavior or emotional state and identified cancer treatment as the causative factor. Physical sensation was emphasized in the child's definition, the dynamic sensation of physical or mental exhaustion in the adolescent's definition, loss of will and spiritual distress in the definition from the staff, and multiple causative factors in the parent's definition.

Hinds and Hockenberry-Eaton (2001) used the conceptual definitions from this study to construct a patient self-report, parent-report, and staff-report instrument to measure fatigue in children with cancer. The instrument uses a Likert-type scale to assess both intensity and bother of fatigue. The researchers in this group plan to test this instrument in future studies of the relationship between fatigue and anemia, a pharmacologic intervention, and patient sleep.

The programs of research developed by the Hinds and Hockenberry-Eaton groups are excellent exemplars of how to build a program research. They began with a qualitative, descriptive study that resulted in a clear conceptual and operational definition of fatigue in children and adolescents with cancer. These researchers then used this model to develop and test the psychometrics of the instrument. Additionally, use of a separate analysis for children and adolescents gives evidence of a developmental basis to this program of research.

NAUSEA AND VOMITING

Clinically, nausea and vomiting are the most commonly reported side effects of cancer treatment and, in conjunction with fever and pain, are the symptoms found most distressing for the child (Rostad & Moore, 1997). Few nurses have taken on the task of studying nausea and vomiting in children undergoing treatment for cancer. Lo and Hayman (1999) conducted the only published nursing study that focused on nausea and vomiting related to childhood cancer treatment. Their study examined the relationship between parent and child reports of nausea and vomiting related to acute and delayed chemotherapy. The Adapted Rhodes Index of Nausea and Vomiting was completed every 12 hours by 20 parent-child dyads. The authors noted that the reliability and validity of this instrument for use with children have been established, but this could not be found in the published literature. The authors concluded that parents' observation of their children's experience of nausea and vomiting was accurate.

Geib and Wright (1998) attempted to address one of the major barriers to the study of nausea and vomiting in children undergoing treatment for cancer. They designed and pilot-tested the Pediatric Nausea, Vomiting and Retching Guide. This tool measures frequency, duration, and severity of nausea, vomiting, and retching as well as the degree of bother related to all three symptoms. In developing this instrument, the authors reviewed other tools designed by pharmacists and other health care professionals, interviewed pediatric oncology nurses as content experts, and interviewed well and sick children to assess content validity. A repeated measures design was used in pilot-testing with 15 children. Data were also collected from parents and from nurses' notes in the medical record. Children reported that the scale was easy to complete and understand. Cronbach's alpha for the bother scale, which had several items, was .68. Statistically significant correlations were found between children's and parents' scores on most scales, and between children's ratings and nurse recordings of the frequency of vomiting and retching but not nausea or bother, which are subjective assessments of the patient. Unfortunately, the authors have not further studied this important tool.

Docherty (1999) used this tool in a repeated measures, longitudinal case study design with three children undergoing treatment for cancer and found a consistent pattern of high peaks in morning nausea and vomiting immediately following a cycle of chemotherapy with periods of respite occurring in between the cycles. The evening scores showed less respite from nausea and vomiting. Although the intensity of nausea was the same as the morning scores, the frequency was much higher. This pattern did not change over the study period. The vomiting patterns were unique in that they showed a gradual increase in the slope of the pattern over the course of the study (Docherty & Sandelowski, 2002).

Psychologists have also done important work examining the impact of nausea and vomiting on children undergoing cancer treatment. Zeltzer, LeBaron, and colleagues undertook a series of descriptive studies followed by intervention studies focusing on nausea and vomiting (LeBaron, Zeltzer, LeBaron, Scott, & Zeltzer, 1988; Zeltzer, Dolgin, LeBaron, & LeBaron, 1991; Zeltzer, LeBaron, Richie, & Reed, 1988). An important finding was that children and adolescents (5 to 18 years) could use a self-report rating scale to quantify somatic symptoms in a series of vignettes. They asked the children to rate the amount of time they thought the child in the vignettes spent having nausea and vomiting using a 0-to-10 Likert scale, as well as the extent to which the child was "bothered" by the symptoms, using a scale consisting of six faces of children showing increasing amounts of distress. Both healthy children and children with cancer as young as 5 years of age were able to understand and use a rating scale. No significant differences were found between the ratings of children and adults. For the pairs of vignettes, vomiting was consistently rated as occurring for a longer duration and producing more bother than nausea. These researchers concluded that highly distressing symptoms might be perceived as occurring for a longer duration than less distressing symptoms.

Tyc and colleagues also studied children's (6 to 18 years old) self-reports of the frequency and severity of nausea and vomiting (Tyc et al., 1993; Tyc, Mulhern, Jayawardene, & Fairclough, 1995). They found significant correlations between different dimensions of the same symptoms (nausea frequency versus severity and emesis frequency versus severity) and between similar dimensions of different symptoms. They concluded that different estimates of nausea and emesis would be obtained if raters were asked to rate their symptoms globally, rather than separately and without reference to descriptive dimensions.

One key area of study is anticipatory nausea and vomiting. Anticipatory nausea and vomiting constitute a learned conditioned response stimulated by something that occurs in association with the true stimulant, in this case chemotherapy. Through repeated pairings with chemotherapy and its aftereffects, previously neutral stimuli (e.g., the sights, sounds, and odors of the treatment setting) acquire nausea- and emesis-eliciting properties (Redd & Hendler, 1984). Anticipatory nausea and vomiting develop in approximately 33% of adult patients and usually occur after the third or fourth cycle of chemotherapy (Cotanch & Strum, 1987). Dolgin et al. (1989) found that more than 75% of newly diagnosed adolescents experienced postchemotherapy nausea and vomiting, and 36% developed anticipatory nausea and vomiting; rates were lower in children (40% and 6%, respectively). Research on anticipatory nausea and vomiting has not been conducted by nurses.

EMOTIONAL DISTRESS

Emotional responses to symptoms associated with treatment are an important factor in evaluating quality of life for children during treatment. While an impressive amount of work in this area has been conducted by developmental psychologists, only one nursing study was conducted. Hockenberry-Eaton, Kemp, and DiIorio (1994) and Hockenberry-Eaton, DiIorio, and Kemp (1995) examined the relationship between childhood cancer treatment and the stress of the treatment. Forty-four children between the ages of 6 and 13 were studied to identify perceptions of cancer stressors and protective factors during treatment. Stressors were the type of treatment received and the child's perception of the experience. Protective factors were self-perception, coping strategies, perceived social support, and family environment. Responses to stress were measured by epinephrine, norepinephrine, and cortisol levels in the urine as well as by a self-report measure of state anxiety. While epinephrine was elevated in the children during the treatment visits to the clinic, norepinephrine and cortisol remained normal. Multiple regression analyses revealed that the family environment and global self-worth were the best predictors of epinephrine levels, while social support from friends predicted norepinephrine levels and the family environment, and social support from teachers predicted state anxiety (Hockenberry-Eaton et al., 1994, 1995).

SUMMARY AND CRITIQUE

The empirical nursing research presently available on the symptom experience of children with cancer is in the beginning stages. There are two major programs of research and a number of other investigators with single studies. A number of researchers focused on the global symptom experiences of children, while many targeted specific symptoms, particularly pain and fatigue. Nurse researchers have placed limited attention on one of the most common symptoms managed by nurses—nausea and vomiting. Since most people undergoing treatment for cancer do not encounter isolated symptoms but rather clusters of symptoms (Dodd, Miaskowski, & Paul, 2001), there is a need for more studies on the global symptom experience and on clusters of symptoms. Dodd and her colleagues defined a symptom cluster as three or more concurrent symptoms that seem to be related to each other (e.g., pain, fatigue, sleep insufficiency). In a study of 93 adult patients with cancer, they found that the symptom cluster of pain, fatigue, and sleep insufficiency explained 48% of the variance in functional status, a figure greater than the sum of explained variance by each individual symptom (Dodd et al., 2001). This approach to symptom clusters was used by Docherty (1999) in a repeated measures, longitudinal, multiple case study design. More work is needed to identify appropriate measures and designs to study symptom clusters in children.

Employing the perspective of developmental science to programs of research on the symptom experiences of children and adolescents with cancer demands a fresh look at conceptual frameworks, conceptualization and measurement of the symptom experience, sampling, and design and analysis. Without a thorough reexamination of these issues and their relations to theory, researchers may become unintentionally drawn to methodologies that are not suitable for studying developmental processes (Carolina Consortium on Human Development, 1996).

Conceptual Frameworks and Perspectives

With the exception of Hinds and Martin's (1998) nursing model, few of the studies reviewed here used a conceptual framework. The framework used most was stress and coping, which has a limited developmental perspective but does include important ecological factors (Hockenberry-Eaton et al., 1994). A developmental, ecological systems framework is important for focusing research on broader factors within the hospital, home, and community environment as well as on individual characteristics such as personality and coping style that likely affect the symptom experience. In particular, research is needed to help understand how the ecological niche of the child (e.g., culture and ethnicity, family, parents, siblings, and peers) affects the symptom experience. The ecology of the health care system (e.g., the relationship of the child and family with the health care team, the presence or absence of environmental supports) also needs to be included to increase the ecological validity of designs.

The developmental science perspective necessitates viewing children not as "little adults" with abilities that are "less than" those of adults, but as a population that is different from adults and that has a different set of competencies and manners of expression (Harden, Scott, Backett-Milburn, & Jackson, 2000; James, Jenks, & Prout, 1998). A more useful approach is to conceptualize childhood not as a stage toward adulthood, but as another culture that is different than and relatively autonomous from the adult world (Harden et al., 2000; Waksler, 1991). This would suggest the need for more naturalistic, qualitative designs to truly understand how the culture of childhood intersects with the symptom experience of children and youth undergoing treatment for cancer. Several researchers approached their studies from this perspective (Enskar et al., 1997; Docherty, 1999; Hinds & Hockenberry-Eaton, 2001; Hinds et al., 1999; Hockenberry-Eaton et al., 1998).

Conceptualization and Measurement of Symptoms

An important first challenge for researchers in this field is to clarify and come to some consensus regarding conceptualizations of disease- and treatment-related symptom experiences in children and adolescents. The lack of clarity enables studies in which concepts, measurement, design, and analysis are loosely tied together. In addition, it makes summarization across studies difficult. Until the conceptual definition of symptom distress or the symptom experience of children is clarified, the conceptual frameworks used to situate and design studies and to interpret study findings will be inadequately developed. Although the term *symptom distress* is now being used in the literature on children's responses to cancer treatment more frequently, there is no consistently used definition of the concept. The terms *symptom frequency*, *symptom intensity*, *symptom distress*, and symptom experience have often been used synonymously. *Symptom occurrence* (frequency, duration, severity) and *symptom distress* (physical or emotional response) were first linked together to describe adult symptom experiences by Rhodes, Watson, Johnson, Madsen, and Beck (1987). A developmental science perspective would call for the conceptualization of symptom experiences as occurring in a bidirectional manner across levels, such as genetic, neurocognitive, and hormonal levels, with a connection between the physiologic responses to cancer and to its treatment (Gottlieb, 1996; Magnusson & Cairns, 1996). Few studies incorporated biological measures, and no studies examined the bidirectional relationship between subsystems.

While symptom experiences are understood to be highly abstract, subjective, and intangible phenomena, the findings of this review suggest that children undergoing treatment for cancer can report clinically relevant and highly consistent information about their symptom experiences (Docherty, 1999; Hinds et al., 1994; Schneider, 1999). Children as young as 7 years of age have the ability to accurately report the intensity, frequency, and bother of symptoms related to cancer treatment. However, measuring the symptom experience of children and adolescents remains a challenge to researchers. In-depth understanding of the effect of the symptom experience on the daily lives of children, the meaning that symptoms have for children, and the language they use to express their distress is still lacking (Woodgate & McClement, 1998). The more consistent use of a developmental science perspective from which to conceptualize symptom experiences of children and adolescents and to design developmentally sensitive measures would allow for a clearer understanding of the meaning of these experiences within the unique culture of childhood. The "ages and stages" conceptualization of development led to a measurement approach in which instruments originally designed for adult populations were "downsized" for use with children. Limited attention was paid in many of these adaptations to the special perspectives of children or related measurement issues. However, some researchers developed tools to measure symptom experiences, such as fatigue, based on data from focus groups with children and youth (Hinds & Hockenberry-Eaton, 2001; Hinds et al., 1999; Hockenberry-Eaton et al., 1998).

Many of the existing tools focus on unidimensional aspects of the symptom experience—measuring only one symptom or measuring only one aspect of a symptom. This makes the examination of the experience across levels and the patterning of symptoms, clustering of symptoms, or constellation of symptoms difficult, if not impossible. In addition, these ordinal measures do not permit one to weigh the importance of specific symptoms based upon the significance of each symptom to the child (Degner & Sloan, 1995). Thus interpretation of scores may be very complex and almost impossible (Hinds et al., 1992). Since two children may experience the same type, frequency, and intensity of a symptom and yet have a completely different response, this weakness is of particular importance. More complex multidimensional measures that allow individuals to clarify their perspective of the symptom experience are important in studying how a child's unique background (e.g., culture, gender, temperament) and experience contribute to symptom distress.

An additional challenge to design and measurement lies in recent research which suggests that children are reluctant to report physical and emotional symptoms and may use denial or avoidance to cope with what might otherwise be an overwhelming experience (Canning, Canning, & Boyce, 1992; Docherty, 1999; Phipps, Fairclough, & Mulhern, 1995; Worschel et al., 1992). Some children and adolescents have been found to underreport their symptom distress in an effort to keep the family caregivers from knowing about their suffering (Docherty, 1999; Kristjanson et al., 1998). Thus, multiple methods are needed to assess the symptom distress of children.

In summary, it is paramount to develop and test developmentally appropriate measures that approximate children's views regarding symptom experiences. These measures need to reflect dimensions relevant to the experiences and socioecological world of children and adolescents. James et al. (1998) described the problems inherent in using mainly "talk-centered" or "word-centered" methods such as interviews or questionnaires (Docherty & Sandelowski, 1999). Instead, they advocated the use of "task-centered activities" which employ the unique talents and interests of individual children as a better way of allowing children to express their ideas and feelings (e.g., sentence completion exercises, social network maps). These methodologies have been influenced by techniques developed in anthropology and by practitioners working with troubled children (Hill, Laybourn, & Borland, 1996) and may allow us to access children in a different, more culturally specific way.

Sampling

Sampling in this area of research is burdened with the challenge of studying a relatively rare population that is undergoing the distress of coping with cancer and its treatments. The relatively low incidence of childhood cancer resulted in studies with small samples and low power. While many of the studies lacked clear information regarding sampling, the majority used convenience samples of small numbers of white, middle-class children from clinical settings. Thus, the diversity of the samples was inadequate, and caution must be used in generalizing results to these groups. Likewise, researchers need to explore in more depth how ethnicity and socioeconomic status, as well as the geographical setting in which treatment is provided (inpatient, clinic, home), affect the child's symptom experience. Furthermore, few studies explored how gender affected the response of children to cancer and its treatments. Given the importance of gender on behavioral and emotional expression, this warrants more attention. Another issue is the focus in most studies on children over 10 years of age. Epidemiological studies have shown that the average age of the child with any type of cancer is 5 years old. There is an urgent need to develop methods to study these younger children.

The studies conducted by the research teams of Hinds and Hockenberry-Eaton are sterling examples of multisite samples that are helpful in obtaining a larger and more heterogeneous population. These researchers and others have called for a movement toward more multisite collaborative efforts in nursing research on children with cancer (Schneider, Hinds, & Pritchard, 2001), so that results would be more generalizable and have broader findings. The technology available to researchers today is making this type of research more feasible (Challinor, Miaskowski, Moore, Slaughter, & Frank, 2000; Schneider et al., 2001).

Design

The majority of the research reviewed was designed with more of an "ages and stages" conceptualization of development. In this view, children are thought of as occupying different stages of development toward becoming an adult. The idea that such differences are real has resulted in the use of cross-sectional designs that have dominated the studies in this review. Results from these types of designs must be interpreted with caution because the data represent one slice in time during the child's experience, and this slice may not be representative of the child's total experience or predictive of the child's long-term adjustment. Cross-sectional studies that explored responses of school-age children separately from adolescents and that used short-term longitudinal designs, however, are a step toward acknowledging the developmental differences that occur within childhood (Hinds et al., 1992).

The developmental science perspective would guide researchers into conceptualizing disease- and treatment-related symptom experiences of children and adolescents as a process that develops and changes across time and levels. Thus, patterns of response to childhood cancer treatment and how these patterns develop and change over time must be examined in the developing child using repeated measures and longitudinal designs. While some studies used short-term longitudinal designs, few examined symptom distress over a long enough period to determine the long-term developmental and health outcomes. The short-term longitudinal designs were also limited in that most did not include frequent enough observations with sensitive enough instruments to capture trajectories, the emergence of novelty, or patterns of change in symptoms (Shanahan, Valsiner, & Gottlieb, 1997). In addition, many studies with longitudinal data did not use longitudinal statistics that allow for the examination of process over time. The challenge in using a repeated measures design in this field of inquiry is that many children undergoing treatment for cancer undergo periods of extreme morbidity that leave them unable or unwilling to report their symptoms (Docherty, 1999; Phipps et al., 1994). Thus, the data that would describe the most intense period of the symptom experience are missing.

Developmental science also calls for the use of person-oriented designs that allow for a more powerful examination of individual differences in the symptom experience of children (Bergman & Magnusson, 1997). The study of disease- and treatment-related experiences of children and adolescents with cancer is an excellent field in which nurse researchers can begin to explore the use of person-oriented methods of analysis. The multidimensional, multilevel nature of this developmental process intuitively seems to correspond with an approach in which the focus is on change in individuals over time as compared to the variable-oriented approach in which the focus is on the relationships between variables

(Magnusson & Cairns, 1996). Understanding individual differences in response to treatment-related symptoms may allow us to target those children for whom intervention would be most efficacious. Person-centered analysis would also help in understanding characteristics of children who are usually dropped from the study as outliers. Additionally, these types of analytic designs allow for the interpretation of symptom experiences across levels and for identifying patterns by which data across multiple dimensions (and levels) can be brought together for an individual as a totality (Bergman, 1998).

Given the role of nurses in alleviating symptom distress in children, there is an urgent need for more theoretically based intervention studies to identify approaches that help reduce symptom distress in these children. Only two intervention studies were found. One was an educational intervention to facilitate coping and reduce psychological distress, symptom distress, and clinical outcomes (Hinds et al., 2000). Another study involved virtual reality distraction in a small sample of children (Schneider & Workman, 1999, 2000). Both studies were guided by Hinds and Martin's (1988) Adolescent Self-Sustaining Model.

CONCLUSION

The contribution of nurse researchers to the body of empirical knowledge regarding the symptom experiences of children and adolescents with cancer, while in its formative stages, has been significant. This is an exciting stage of knowledge development with opportunities to develop new, more developmentally sensitive studies by applying the perspective and methods of developmental science to strengthen future nursing research in this area. Methodological, sampling, and design challenges need to be faced to enable nurse researchers to understand children's responses to the symptoms produced as a result of treatment, identify vulnerable subpopulations, and test interventions that will help to reduce the distress. Searching for a clearer understanding of the types of responses children have to treatment symptoms as well as the process that occurs when children learn to respond to these symptoms may make the difference between the success and failure of the treatment. The ability to identify the "symptom-distress-vulnerable" child could possibly lead to important interventions for children undergoing childhood cancer treatment that will reduce their distress, increase their survival, and prevent long-term problems.

REFERENCES

American Cancer Society. (2002). *Cancer facts and figures—2002*. Atlanta: Author.

Bergman, L. R. (1998). A pattern-oriented approach to studying individual development: Snapshots and processes. In R. B. Cairns, L. Bergman, & J. Kagan (Eds.), *Methods and models for studying the individual* (pp. 83–121). Thousand Oaks, CA: Sage.

Bergman, L. R., & Magnusson, D. (1997). A person-oriented approach in research on developmental psychopathology. *Development and Psychopathology, 9,* 291–319.

Beyer, J., Villarrueal, A., & Denyes, M. (1995). *THE OUCHER: User's manual and technical report.* Bethesda, MD: Association for Care of Children's Health.

Burish, T. G., Carey, M. P., Krozely, M. G., & Greco, F. A. (1987). Conditioned side effects induced by cancer chemotherapy: Prevention through behavioral treatment. *Journal of Consulting and Clinical Psychology, 55,* 42–48.

Canning, E. H., Canning, R. D., & Boyce, W. T. (1992). Depressive symptoms and adaptive style in children with cancer. *Journal of the American Academy of Child and Adolescent Psychiatry, 31,* 1120–1124.

The Carolina Consortium on Human Development. (1996). Developmental science: A collaborative statement. In R. B. Cairns, G. H. Elder, & E. J. Costello (Eds.), *Developmental science* (pp. 1–6). New York: Cambridge University Press.

Challinor, J., Miaskowski, C., Moore, I., Slaughter, R., & Franck, L. (2000). Review of research studies that evaluated the impact of treatment for childhood cancers on neurocognition and behavioral and social completence: Nursing implications. *Journal of the Society of Pediatric Nursing, 5*(2), 57–74.

Collins, J. J., Byrnes, M. E., Dunkel, I. J., Lapin, J., Nadel, T., Thaler, H. T., et al. (2000). The measurement of symptoms in children with cancer. *Journal of Pain and Symptom Management, 19,* 363–377.

Cotanch, P. H., & Strum, S. (1987). Progressive muscle relaxation as antiemetic therapy for cancer patients. *Oncology Nursing Forum, 14,* 33–37.

Degner, L. F., & Sloan, J. A. (1995). Symptom distress in newly diagnosed ambulatory cancer patients and as a predictor of survival in lung cancer. *Journal of Pain and Symptom Management, 10,* 423–431.

Docherty, S. L. (1999). *Patterns of symptom distress in three children with cancer.* Unpublished doctoral dissertation, University of North Carolina, Chapel Hill.

Docherty, S. L., & Sandelowski, M. (1999). Interviewing children. *Research in Nursing and Health, 22,* 177–185.

Docherty, S. L., & Sandelowski, M. (2002). Patterns of symptom distress during the initial treatment period in an adolescent with cancer. Manuscript in preparation.

Dodd, M. J., Miaskowski, C., & Paul, S. M. (2001). Symptom clusters and their effect on the functional status of patients with cancer. *Oncology Nursing Forum, 28,* 465–470.

Dolgin, M. J., Katz, E. R., Zeltzer, L. K., & Landsverk, J. (1989). Behavioral distress in pediatric patients with cancer receiving chemotherapy. *Pediatrics, 84,* 103–110.

Ehlke, G. (1988). Symptom distress in breast cancer patients receiving chemotherapy in the outpatient setting. *Oncology Nursing Forum, 15,* 343–346.

Enskar, K., Carlsson, M., Golsater, M., & Hamrin, E. (1997). Symptom distress and life situation in adolescents with cancer. *Cancer Nursing, 20*(1), 23–33.

Enskar, K., Carlsson, M., Golsater, M., Hamrin, E., & Kreuger, A. (1997). An international account: Life situation and problems as reported by children with cancer and their parents. *Journal of Pediatric Oncology Nursing, 14*(1), 18–26.

Geib, K. B., & Wright, F. H. (1998). *Development of a nausea, vomiting, and retching instrument.* Unpublished research project submitted to the School of Nursing, University of North Carolina at Chapel Hill.

Gorfinkle, K., & Redd, W. H. (1993). Behavioral control of anxiety, distress, and learned aversions in pediatric oncology. In W. Breitbart & J. C. Holland (Eds.), *Psychiatric aspects of symptom management in cancer patients* (pp. 129–146). Washington, DC: American Psychological Association.

Gottlieb, G. (1996). Developmental psychobiological theory. In R. B. Cairns, G. H. Elder, & E. J. Costello (Eds.), *Developmental science* (pp. 63–77). New York: Cambridge University Press.

Harden, J., Scott, S., Backett-Milburn, K., & Jackson, S. (2000). Can't talk, won't talk? Methodological issues in researching children. *Sociological Research On-line, 5*(2), *http://www.socresonline.org.uk/5/2/harden.html*

Hester, N. O. (1993). Pain in children. *Annual review of nursing research* (Vol. 11, pp. 105–142).

Hill, M., Laybourn, A., & Borland, M. (1996). Engaging with primary-aged children about their emotions and well-being: Methodological considerations. *Children and Society, 10,* 129–144.

Hinds, P. S. (1990). Quality of life in children and adolescents with cancer. *Seminars in Oncology Nursing, 6,* 285–291.

Hinds, P. S., & Hockenberry-Eaton, M. (2001). Developing a research program on fatigue in children and adolescents with cancer. *Journal of Pediatric Oncology Nursing, 18*(2)(Suppl 1), 3–12.

Hinds, P. S., Hockenberry-Eaton, M., Gilger, E., Kline, N., Burleson, C., Bottomley, S., et al. (1999). Comparing patient, parent, and staff descriptions of fatigue in pediatric oncology patients. *Cancer Nursing, 22,* 277–289.

Hinds, P. S., Hockenberry-Eaton, M., Quargnenti, A., May, M., Burleson, C., Gilger, E., et al. (1999). Fatigue in 7- to 12-year-old patients with cancer from the staff perspective: An exploratory study. *Oncology Nursing Forum, 26,* 37–45.

Hinds, P. S., & Martin, J. (1988). Hopefulness and the self-sustaining process in adolescents with cancer. *Nursing Research, 37,* 336–340.

Hinds, P. S., Quargnenti, A., Bush, A. J., Pratt, C., Fairclough, D., Rissmiller, G., et al. (2000). An evaluation of the impact of a self-care coping intervention on psychological and clinical outcomes in adolescents with newly diagnosed cancer. *European Journal of Oncology Nursing, 4*(1), 6–17.

Hinds, P., Quargnenti, A., Olson, M., Gross, J., Puckett, P., Randall, E., et al. (1994). The 1992 APON Delphi study to establish research priorities for pediatric oncology nursing. *Journal of Pediatric Oncology Nursing, 11*(1), 20–30.

Hinds, P. S., Quargnenti, A. G., & Wentz, T. J. (1992). Measuring symptom distress in adolescents with cancer. *Journal of Pediatric Oncology Nursing, 9,* 84–86.

Hinds, P., Scholes, S., Gattuso, J., Riggins, M., & Heffner B. (1990). Adaptation to illness in adolescents with cancer. *Journal of Pediatric Oncology Nursing, 7*(2), 64–65.

Hockenberry-Eaton, M., DiIorio, C., & Kemp, V. (1995). The relationship of illness longevity and relapse with self-perception, cancer stressors, anxiety, and coping strategies in children with cancer. *Journal of Pediatric Oncology Nursing, 12*(2), 71–79.

Hockenberry-Eaton, M., Hinds, P. S., Alcoser, P., O'Neill, J. B., Euell, K., Howard, V., et al. (1998). Fatigue in children and adolescents with cancer. *Journal of Pediatric Oncology Nursing, 15*(3), 172–182.

Hockenberry-Eaton, M., Hinds, P., O'Neill, J., Alcoser, et al. (1999). Developing a conceptual model for fatigue in children. *European Journal of Oncology Nursing, 3*, 5–11.

Hockenberry-Eaton, M., Hinds, P. S., O'Neill, J. B., Euell, K., Howard, V., Gattuso, J., et al. (1998). Fatigue in children and adolescents with cancer. *Journal of Pediatric Oncology Nursing, 15*(3), 172–182.

Hockenberry-Eaton, M., Kemp, V., & DiIorio, C. (1994). Cancer stressors and protective factors: Predictors of stress experienced during treatment for cancer. *Research in Nursing and Health, 17*, 351–361.

Holmes, S. (1991). Preliminary investigations of symptom distress in two cancer patient populations: Evaluation of a measurement instrument. *Journal of Advanced Nursing, 16*, 439–446.

Holmes, S., & Eburn, E. (1989). Patients' and nurses' perceptions of symptom distress in cancer. *Journal of Advanced Nursing, 14*, 840–846.

Hubert, N. C., Jay, S. M., Saltoun, M., & Hayes, M. (1988). Approach-avoidance and distress in children undergoing preparation for painful medical procedures. *Journal of Clinical Child Psychology, 17*, 194–202.

James, A., Jenks, C., & Prout, A. (1998). *Theorizing childhood.* Cambridge: Polity.

Kristjanson, L. J., Nikoletti, S., Porock, D., Smith, M., Lobchuk, M., & Pedler, P. (1998). Congruence between patients' and family caregivers' perceptions of symptom distress in patients with terminal cancer. *Journal of Palliative Care, 14*(3), 24–32.

Kukull, W. A., McCorkle, R., & Driever, M. (1986). Symptom distress, psychosocial variables and lung cancer survival. *Journal of Psychosocial Oncology, 4*, 91–104.

Lazarus, R., & Folkman, S. (1991). The concept of coping. In A. Monat & R. Lazarus (Eds.), *Stress and coping: An anthology* (3rd ed., pp. 189–206). New York: Columbia University Press.

LeBaron, S., Zeltzer, L. K., LeBaron, C., Scott, S. E., & Zeltzer, P. (1988). Chemotherapy side effects in pediatric oncology patients: Drugs, age, and sex as risk factors. *Medical and Pediatric Oncology, 16*, 263–268.

Lo., L., & Hayman, L. L. (1999). Parents associated with children in measuring acute and delayed nausea and vomiting. *Nursing and Health Sciences, 1*(3), 155–161.

Lough, M. E., Lindsey, A. M., Shinn, J. A., & Stotts, N. A. (1987). Impact of symptom frequency and symptom distress on self-reported quality of life in heart transplant recipients. *Heart and Lung, 16*, 193–200.

Magnusson, D., & Cairns, R. B. (1996). Developmental science: Toward a unified framework. In R. B. Cairns, G. H. Elder, & E. J. Costello (Eds.), *Developmental science* (pp. 7–30). New York: Cambridge University Press.

McCorkle, R., & Benoliel, J. Q. (1983). Symptom distress, current concerns and mood disturbance after diagnosis of life-threatening disease. *Social Science and Medicine, 17,* 431–438.

McCorkel, R., & Young, K. (1978). Development of a symptom distress scale. *Cancer Nursing, 1,* 373–378.

McDaniel, R. W., & Rhodes, V. A. (1995). Symptom experience. *Seminars in Oncology Nursing, 11,* 232–234.

McQuaid, E. L., & Nassau, J. H. (1999). Empirically supported treatments of disease-related symptoms in pediatric psychology: Asthma, diabetes, and cancer. *Journal of Pediatric Psychology, 24,* 305–328.

Nahata, M. C., Ford, C., & Ruymann, F. B. (1992). Pharmacokinetics and safety of prochlorperazine in paediatric patients receiving cancer chemotherapy. *Journal of Clinical Pharmacy and Therapeutics, 17,* 121–123.

National Institute of Health. (1997). Management of symptoms secondary to treatment. *NIH Guide, 26*(24), 1–7.

Phipps, S., Fairclough, D., & Mulhern, R. K. (1995). Avoidant coping in children with cancer. *Journal of Pediatric Psychology, 20,* 217–232.

Phipps, S., Hinds, P. S., Channell, S., & Bell, G. L. (1994). Measurement of behavioral, affective and somatic responses to pediatric bone marrow transplantation: Development of the BASES Scale. *Journal of Pediatric Oncology Nursing, 11*(3), 109–117.

Pinkerton, C. R., & Hardy, J. R. (1997). Cancer chemotherapy and mechanisms of resistance. In C. R. Pinkerton & P. N. Plowman (Eds.), *Paediatric oncology. Clinical practice and controversies* (2nd ed., pp. 157–188). London: Chapman & Hall Medical.

Pizzo, P. A., & Poplack, D. G. (2002). *Principles and practice of pediatric oncology* (4th ed). Philadelphia: Lippincott Williams & Wilkins.

Portenoy, R. K., Thaler, H. T., Kornblith, A. B., et al. (1994). The Memorial Symptom Assessment Scale: An instrument for the evaluation of symptom prevalence, characteristics and distress. *European Journal of Cancer, 30A,* 1326–1336.

Redd, W., & Hendler, C. (1984). Learned aversions to chemotherapy treatment. *Health Education Quarterly, 10*(Suppl), 57–66.

Reynolds, C. R., & Richmond, B. O. (1978). What I think and feel: A revised measure of children's manifest anxiety. *Journal of Abnormal Child Psychology, 6*(2), 271–280.

Rhodes, W. A., & Watson, P. M. (1987). Symptom distress: The concept past and present. *Seminars in Oncology Nursing, 3,* 242–247.

Rhodes, W. A., Watson, P. M., Johnson, M. H., Madsen, R. W., & Beck, N. C. (1987). Patterns of nausea, vomiting, and distress in patients receiving antineoplastic drug protocols. *Oncology Nursing Forum, 14*(4), 35–44.

Rostad, M., & Moore, K. (1997). Childhood cancers. In C. Varricchio, M. Pierce, C. L. Walker, & T. B. Ades (Eds.), *A cancer source book for nurses* (pp. 443–437). Sudbury, MA: Jones and Bartlett.

Schneider, S. M. (1999). I look funny and I feel bad: Measurement of symptom distress. *Journal of Child and Family Nursing, 2*(5), 380–384.

Schneider, S. M., Hinds, P. S., & Pritchard, M. (2001). From single site to societal belief: The impact of pediatric oncology nursing research. *Journal of Pediatric Oncology Nursing, 18*(4), 164–170.

Schneider, S. M., & Workman, M. L. (1999). Effects of virtual reality on symptom distress in children receiving chemotherapy. *CyberPsychology and Behavior, 2*(2), 125–134.

Schneider, S. M., & Workman, M. L. (2000). Virtual reality as a distraction intervention for children receiving chemotherapy. *Pediatric Nursing, 26,* 593–597.

Schumacher, A., Wewers, D., Heinecke, A., Sauerland, C., Koch, O., van de Loo, J., et al. (2002). Fatigue as an important aspect of quality of life in patients with acute myeloid leukemia. *Leukemia Research, 26,* 355–362.

Shanahan, M. J., Valsiner, J., & Gottlieb, G. (1997). Developmental concepts across disciplines. In J. Tudge & M. J. Shanahan (Eds.), *Comparisons in human development: Understanding time and context. Cambridge studies in social and emotional development* (pp. 34–71). New York: Cambridge University Press.

Soanes, L., Gibson, F., Bayliss, J., & Hannan, J. (2000). Establishing nursing research priorities on a paediatric haematology, oncology, immunology and infectious disease unit: A Delphi Survey. *European Journal of Oncology Nursing, 4,* 108–117.

Sutters, K. A., & Miaskowski, C. (1992). The problem of pain in children with cancer: A research review. *Oncology Nursing Forum, 19,* 465–471.

Tyc, V., Mulhern, R., Fairclough, D., Ward, P. M., Relling, M. V., & Longmire, W. (1993). Chemotherapy induced nausea and emesis in pediatric cancer patients: External validity of child and parent emesis ratings. *Journal of Developmental & Behavioral Pediatrics, 14,* 236–249.

Tyc, V., Mulhern, R., Jayawardene, M., & Fairclough, D. (1995). Chemotherapy induced nausea and emesis in pediatric cancer patients: An analysis of coping strategies. *Journal of Pain and Symptom Management, 10,* 338–347.

Waksler, F. C. (1991). *Studying the social worlds of children.* Basingstoke: Falmer Press.

Watson, M., & Marvell, C. (1992). Anticipatory nausea and vomiting among cancer patients: A review. *Psychology and Health, 6,* 97–106.

Watson, P. M., Rhodes, V. A., & Germino, B. B. (1987). Symptom distress: Future perspectives for practice, education and research. *Seminars in Oncology Nursing, 3,* 313–315.

Wilcox, P. M., Fetting, J. H., Nettesheim, K. M., & Abeloff, M. D. (1982). Anticipatory vomiting in women receiving cyclophosphamide, methotrexate, and 5-FU adjuvant chemotherapy for breast carcinoma. *Cancer Treatment Reports, 66,* 1601–1604.

Williams, H. (1996). The silent ones: A review of sampling issues and biases pertinent to the area of pediatric oncology procedural pain. *Journal of Pediatric Oncology Nursing, 13,* 31–39.

Woodgate, R., & McClement, S. (1998). Symptom distress in children with cancer: The need to adopt a meaning-centered approach. *Journal of Pediatric Oncology Nursing, 15*(1), 3–12.

Worschel, F. F., Rae, W. A., Olson, T. K., et al. (1992). Selective responsiveness of chronically ill children to assessments of depression. *Journal of Personality Assessment, 59*, 605–615.

Yamamoto, K., Soliman, A., Parsons, J., & Davies, O. L. (1987). Voices in unison: Stressful events in the lives of children in six countries. *Journal of Child Psychology, 28*, 855–864.

Young, K. J., & Longman, A. J. (1983). Quality of life and persons with melanoma: A pilot study. *Cancer Nursing, 7*, 219–225.

Zeltzer, L., Dolgin, M. J., LeBaron, S., & LeBaron, C. (1991). A randomized, controlled study of behavioral intervention for chemotherapy distress in children with cancer. *Pediatrics, 88*, 34–42.

Zeltzer, L. K., LeBaron, S., Ritchie, D., & Reed, D. (1988). Can children understand and use a rating scale to quantify somatic symptoms? Assessment of nausea and vomiting as a model. *Journal of Consulting and Clinical Psychology, 56*, 567–572.

Chapter 6

Growing Up With Chronic Illness: Psychosocial Adjustment of Children and Adolescents With Cystic Fibrosis

BECKY CHRISTIAN

ABSTRACT

This chapter reviews the published research from 1980 through 2001 on the psychosocial adjustment of children and adolescents with cystic fibrosis. The inclusion criteria were that research was conducted by nurses and researchers from related disciplines that focused on the psychosocial adjustment of children (6 to 12 years) and/or adolescents (13 to 22 years) with cystic fibrosis (CF). Three computerized databases were used for retrieval: Cumulative Index of Nursing and Allied Health Literature (CINAHL), Medline, and PsycINFO. Of the 74 citations published from 1980 through 2001, only 20 studies met the inclusion criteria, including 7 nursing research studies and 13 studies published by nonnurses in related disciplines. Key findings from this review were that the focus of nursing research was on the social consequences of chronic illness, while the non-nursing research focused on self-concept, self-worth, and psychiatric symptoms of anxiety, worry, and behavior problems. Only two programs of research were identified. Developmental science was used as a guiding frame-work for the critique of the research. Recommendations for future research include developmentally sensitive longitudinal studies to track developmental change and stability over time, as well as research that captures individual developmental differences.

Growing up with a chronic illness such as cystic fibrosis (CF) is a challenge for children and adolescents. Children with chronic illness must cope with stressful situations related to their disease and treatments as well as with the interpersonal situations related to managing their chronic illness (Grey & Sullivan-Bolyai, 1999; Stein, 1992; Thompson & Gustafson, 1996). Sources of stress for children with chronic illness include physical and functional limitations, difficulty in adhering to treatment regimens, school absences, social isolation, and limited opportunities to interact with peers. Many children's stressors with chronic conditions develop in the context of coping with peer responses to their illness-related differences (Eiser, 1993). When the demands of illness and treatment are combined with the developmental demands of childhood and adolescence, problems with psychosocial adjustment are likely to occur. Efforts by children and adolescents to integrate their chronic illness into their social environment of peers and school threaten to mark them as different, disrupting their ability to manage their chronic illness. Faced with integrating the demands of the chronic illness into their everyday lives, children with chronic illness such as CF are at risk for psychosocial adjustment problems (Thompson & Gustafson, 1996).

With the marked change in the CF illness trajectory and the increased survival rates over the past 30 years, children with CF are now living longer and growing up into adulthood (Cystic Fibrosis Foundation, 1999). Consequently, children and adolescents with CF face new developmental challenges as they attempt to integrate their chronic illness into their everyday lives. As a result of this transformation in the course of CF, research has lagged behind and has not addressed the central issues related to psychosocial adjustment. Indeed, much of the past CF research has focused on parental adjustment to CF, the impact of CF on the family, or mother reports of children's adjustment to CF, instead of the perspectives of children (Angst, 2001; Christian, 1993; Quittner, DiGirolamo, Michel, & Eigen, 1992; Thompson & Gustafson, 1996). Further, there is lack of developmentally appropriate research on children and adolescents with CF.

Although a substantial body of literature exists on psychosocial adjustment to chronic illness in children, few studies have explored *children's* perceptions of growing up with a chronic illness (Faux, 1998). The majority of research has been descriptive or epidemiological in nature, combining developmental age groups and using parents as informants. Many studies have used a noncategorical approach to the study of chronic illness by combining different chronic illnesses to focus on the adaptation process in general, even though this prevents the examination of illness-specific patterns, identification of targets for intervention, and the exploration of different mechanisms for adaptation. Further, most studies have been limited to cross-sectional designs that do not capture developmental change and stability of adjustment over time (Thompson & Gustafson, 1996). Much of the research has focused on other chronic illnesses with a higher prevalence, such as asthma and diabetes. Clearly, with the change in the CF illness trajectory, children with CF are at risk for psychosocial adjustment problems, but the long-term consequences of chronic illness on the quality of life of children with CF are only beginning to be addressed. This chapter examines the published research from nursing and related disciplines on the psychosocial adjustment of children and adolescents with CF. The aim is to explore the use of developmental perspectives in research on children and adolescents with CF to improve sensitivity to key developmental issues they face growing up with this disease.

METHOD

The nursing and related literature from 1980 through 2001 was searched for published studies about the psychosocial adjustment of children and adolescents with CF. Three computerized databases were used for retrieval of the literature: Cumulative Index of Nursing and Allied Health Literature (CINAHL), Medline, and PsycINFO. The literature was searched using the following keywords: *child* (6 to 12 years) *and/or adolescents with cystic fibrosis with psychosocial adjustment; psychological adjustment; psychological well-being; adaptation, psychological; coping;* and *support, psychological.*

The inclusion criteria for the review were that the research focused on the psychosocial adjustment of children (6 to 12 years) and/or adolescents (13 to 22 years) with cystic fibrosis (CF). Family studies and parent reports of the child or adolescent's psychosocial adjustment were excluded unless the perspective of the child or adolescent was also reported. Research reviews, instrument development articles, abstracts, and unpublished dissertations were excluded.

The following criteria were used to evaluate the use of a developmental science perspective (Magnusson & Cairns, 1996) in the studies in this review: (a) the conceptual framework used a developmental, systems, or ecological framework to explore the interaction between children and adolescents and their environmental context; (b) the design focused on developmental change and stability as well as the importance of timing of developmental transitions; (c) the sample included distinct developmental age groups; (d) the measures were developmentally appropriate for children and adolescents in the sample; (e) the data analysis employed appropriate statistical methods to determine stability and change over time; and (f) the discussion incorporated an analysis of developmental issues to explain findings and identify limitations.

FINDINGS

Of the 74 citations on psychosocial adjustment of children and adolescents with CF published from 1980 through 2001 that were retrieved and reviewed, only 20 met the inclusion criteria (7 studies were redundant across the three databases). Studies were categorized as nursing or non-nursing research based on the discipline of the primary author. Seven research studies published by nurses and 13 research studies published by non-nurses in related disciplines were retrieved.

Nursing Research

Among the seven published nursing studies, five used qualitative methods with in-depth interviews and two studies used mixed methods, combining descriptive correlational designs with semistructured interviews. No intervention studies conducted by nurses were retrieved. There was only one program of research.

Using mixed methods, Patton, Ventura, and Savedra (1986) explored the stress and coping of adolescents ($n = 17$) in the daily management of CF and compared coping behaviors with a normative sample of healthy adolescents ($n = 467$). They reported that adolescents with CF experienced three types of stressors: problems communicating with health care providers and school personnel, restrictions in participating in school activities, and difficulty acquiring close friends. They concluded that adolescents with CF demonstrated similar coping behaviors to healthy adolescents when they were able to maintain participation in social activities. The authors incorporated an appropriate developmental perspective to explain how adolescents managed stress and coped with CF. However, the use of a cross-sectional design limited their ability to assess coping with respect to timing of developmental transitions and changes in the chronic illness trajectory. The adolescent CF sample and a normative group of healthy adolescents were used for developmental comparisons. Both the measures and statistics were appropriate for this sample, although they did not enhance an understanding of developmental change because the design was cross-sectional. However, the authors did incorporate developmental issues in their explanation of findings.

In a combined sample of school-age children and adolescents (8 to 17 years) with three groups of chronic illnesses—CF ($n = 16$), diabetes ($n = 16$), and spina bifida ($n = 15$)—social support and coping with the everyday demands of chronic illness were compared to the functioning of 15 healthy children (Ellerton, Stewart, Ritchie, & Hirth, 1996). Children with CF were found to have smaller social networks and less peer support when compared to healthy children. All children identified family as the most important source of support. Children with chronic illness used support-seeking strategies to cope in everyday situations. Further, their limited social networks contributed to loneliness and social isolation. Thus, the identified stressors of chronic illness developed within the context of peer relationships and the social consequences of the chronic illness. The authors integrated a developmental perspective into their conceptualization of social support; stress and coping were used as the framework to guide the study. However, by combining developmental age groups and using a cross-sectional design, it is impossible to determine developmental changes over time in relation to social support from peers and changes in coping strategies. Further, by using a noncategorical approach to chronic illness and including three different chronic illness groups within the sample, illness-specific characteristics and adaptations related to the level of functional disability (which could vary across chronic illnesses, thereby affecting the level and type of social support) were not addressed. Both the measures and statistics were appropriate for this sample. However, the explanation of findings was facilitated by the incorporation of developmental issues into the discussion.

In a retrospective life history exploration of how adolescents ($n = 5$) and young adults ($n = 5$) with CF (16 to 25 years) manage disease-related information, Admi (1995) found that disclosure of the CF diagnosis and dealing with the potential stigma associated with a chronic illness were based on the individual's ability to deal with the information and the type of relationship with others. Thus, the social consequences of disclosure of the CF diagnosis were key considerations in managing information for adolescents and adults. The sample combined retrospective accounts of adolescents and young adults in an attempt to capture the process of managing information across developmental stages. However, the combination of adolescents with young adults in the sample ignores the important developmental changes that occur in relation to the cognitive, social, and emotional development from adolescence to adulthood that would influence the willingness to disclose potentially stigmatizing information. Further, these adolescents and adults would vary in their ability to understand and process their memories of managing disease-related information, as well as in changes in their perspectives that would filter the importance and significance of past events. Thus, even though a longitudinal design was used, the addition of a developmental framework in the conceptualization and explanation of findings would improve understanding about how development affects disclosure and would capture how the disclosure process changes over time and across contexts.

The work of Christian and D'Auria represents the only program of research identified from this review of the nursing literature. Christian and D'Auria used a grounded theory approach in three studies to explore how children and adolescents (6 to 22 years) with CF view growing up with a chronic illness (Christian & D'Auria, 1997; Christian, D'Auria, Hall, & White, 2001; D'Auria, Christian, & Richardson, 1997; D'Auria, Christian, Henderson, & Haynes, 2000). They identified middle childhood as the most vulnerable period for growing up with CF. Three critical transitions in adjusting to CF emerged: (a) from home to elementary school, when they first experienced the social consequences of having a chronic illness; (b) early adolescence, when many experienced acute exacerbations of CF; and (c) late adolescence, when they realized that self-care management had a direct relationship to their illness course.

Contextual issues of peer relationships and chronic illness-related differences were also critical factors in these retrospective, qualitative studies of children and adolescents with CF. When adolescents (12 to 18 years) with CF ($n = 20$) retrospectively described their chronic illness experience as children, they identified the central phenomenon as reducing a sense of difference during the transition from home to elementary school (Christian & D'Auria, 1997). In the social context of school and peers, they discovered their CF-related differences and began to use three protective strategies to reduce their sense of difference from peers: (a) keeping secrets, (b) hiding visible differences, and (c) discovering a new baseline. Thus, when children are different from peers and do not understand the social meaning of their illness, peer acceptance is jeopardized.

In a second qualitative study, the perceptions of 20 school-age children (6 to 12 years) were obtained to explore the unfolding nature of the chronic illness experience during middle childhood (D'Auria et al., 1997). These children recognized that they did not understand the meaning of their CF diagnosis. They struggled with puzzling out the meaning of the diagnosis, being teased, telling others, and keeping up with their peers. As with Admi's (1995) findings, disclosing and managing disease-related information became a critical issue for these children and adolescents.

The influence of peer relationships and social interactions continued to be a primary issue in adjustment to CF. In a third qualitative study, 15 adolescents with CF during late adolescence (17 to 22 years), described the process of discovering the course of the CF chronic illness trajectory (D'Auria et al., 2000). With the progressive changes in CF and repeated school absences, these adolescents found new opportunities for creating peer relationships with a new company of friends with CF that they met during hospitalization. These CF peers helped them develop a self-identity and sense of belonging, as well as learn to incorporate CF into their lives. In a small pilot study (Christian et al., 2001), adolescents with CF who experienced more peer rejection had more difficulty with disclosure of CF to peers, while those with greater self-worth had more social acceptance and positive feelings about physical appearance. However, these efforts at peer socialization have been hindered by recent recommendations to prevent cross-infection among individuals with CF (Tyrrell, 2001).

Further, the ongoing developmental struggle to integrate CF management into everyday life was captured in an in-depth, single-case study of an adolescent with CF awaiting lung transplantation (Christian, D'Auria, & Moore, 1999). As the severity of his CF worsened, he struggled with the competing demands of decreased pulmonary function, meeting developmental needs, and achieving psychologic readiness for lung transplantation. He tried to maintain his quality of life by balancing the demands of his chronic illness with participation in activities with peers. By delaying his lung transplant, he was able to continue to be an active participant and maintain his quality of life.

Each of these four studies focused on a specific age group, allowing examination of developmental variability as well as the interplay of chronic illness management and the changing developmental demands over time. The authors incorporated a socioecological, developmental framework to conceptualize these studies. Qualitative, retrospective designs allowed the authors to explore developmental transitions and changes in the chronic illness trajectory over time from an individual perspective. The samples were limited to distinct developmental age groups, and the authors incorporated developmental issues into their explanation of findings. A longitudinal design would represent an improvement in these studies and provide the opportunity to capture stability and change over time across development and change in the chronic illness trajectory.

Few intervention studies have focused on the psychosocial adaptation of children with chronic illness (Deatrick, 1998), and no nursing intervention studies of children or adolescents with CF were found in this review. Currently, Christian and D'Auria (1998) are conducting a multisite, longitudinal intervention study with a two-group, repeated measures experimental design to test the effectiveness of an intervention to improve the physiologic, psychosocial, and functional health status of school-age children (8 to 12 years) early in the course of CF. The Building Life Skills in Children With Cystic Fibrosis intervention program was based on the three qualitative studies discussed earlier. The intervention program is a problem-solving and social skills intervention designed to assist school-age children with CF learn to manage the health and developmental demands of their chronic illness and achieve a more satisfactory quality of life. The four modules include strategies to deal with child-identified problems related to (a) finding out, (b) telling others, (c) teasing, and (d) keeping up (Christian, 2001). Preliminary findings ($N = 101$) suggest critical linkages among the psychosocial, physiologic, and functional health status of school-age children with CF (Christian, D'Auria, & Belyea, 2001). That is, an exploration of the psychosocial impact of CF on the quality of life of these children with CF demonstrated significant associations between loneliness and lower social acceptance, poorer global self-worth, greater functional disability, and greater perceived illness effects.

SUMMARY AND CRITIQUE

A strength of the nursing studies was that they targeted the children's and adolescents' views of adjustment, rather than parent reports. This change from parent to child reports represents an improvement over previous research in that it validates the distinct contribution of children's perspectives, attempts to capture children's developmental understanding of their chronic illness, and identifies areas that are problematic to them and thus important for maintaining their quality of life. Thus, these findings should guide the development of appropriate psychosocial interventions for children and adolescents with CF.

The majority of studies focused on adolescents, while only one study was specific to the psychosocial adjustment of school-age children (D'Auria et al., 1997). However, two studies combined developmental age groups in the same sample: one study of both children and adolescents (Ellerton et al., 1996) and another with both adolescents and adults (Admi, 1995). The combination of different developmental age groups within the same sample and the lack of comparison by age group prevents the identification of specific developmental patterns and the effects of children's interactions with the environment. Only a few studies addressed how developmental transitions are affected by CF.

All of the nursing researchers used theoretical frameworks to guide their research. The majority used a socioecological or systems framework combined with developmental perspectives to guide research and interpret their findings. Other nursing studies used developmental theory in combination with stress and coping theory (Patton et al., 1986); social support with stress and coping theory (Ellerton et al., 1996); or social psychological theory (Admi, 1995). However, few studies incorporated a broad ecological perspective such as culture and socioeconomic status. In addition, gender differences were not explored in these studies. It is important to note that for all the nursing studies, psychosocial adjustment to CF was explored within the context of growing up with a chronic illness, including the social consequences. Taken as a group, they illustrate common themes about how children and adolescents incorporate CF into their everyday lives. Particularly important were problems with peer relationships and disclosing the chronic illness diagnosis, and the need for social support. The findings of all these nursing studies stress the importance of the social context of peers and schools for the psychosocial adjustment of children and adolescents with CF.

Methodologically, knowledge development would be enhanced by building upon the findings of the qualitative studies to design intervention studies that target key developmental transitions and link them with changes in the chronic illness trajectory. Another critical improvement would be to use longitudinal designs to track developmental change and stability over time, with a particular emphasis on key developmental transitions such as puberty. Further, it is essential to use samples that are developmentally congruent in order to capture the unfolding nature of development, ongoing life changes, and changes in the illness course. Given that the sample sizes for these studies was very small, it is essential that future studies have larger samples to be more representative of the population; this may require multisite studies.

Non-Nursing Research

In contrast to the nursing studies, 12 of the 13 studies retrieved from non-nursing disciplines used correlational designs. Of these, 5 used descriptive-correlational designs; 6 used mixed methods combining self-report measures with standardized diagnostic, clinical interviews; and 1 used a longitudinal design with self-report measures and standardized diagnostic, clinical interviews. Many studies compared children with CF to normal children. There was one small intervention study with multiple baseline comparisons. Only the work of Thompson and colleagues represented a distinct program of research within the non-nursing disciplines. The 13 non-nursing studies were categorized into three groups based on design and focus: psychosocial problems, psychiatric symptoms, and intervention research.

PSYCHOSOCIAL PROBLEMS: SELF-CONCEPT, SELF-ESTEEM, AND SELF-WORTH

The majority of non-nursing studies of children and adolescents with CF used cross-sectional, correlational designs to explore self-concept and self-worth. The findings were equivocal. That is, studies reported a range of findings, from identified problems of self-concept and self-worth to no differences, as well as similarities to normative data.

No differences in self-concept and self-efficacy were found between school-age children and adolescents with chronic illness and healthy controls. Using a developmental framework, Cappelli and colleagues (1989) used mixed methods to explore adolescents' perspectives of the impact of chronic illness on their lives. They studied matched groups of adolescents (11 to 18 years) with CF ($n = 31$) and diabetes ($n = 31$) when compared to healthy controls ($n = 31$). No differences were found in coping strategies, self-efficacy, social support, and depression. However, significant group differences were found on the semistructured interview. Sources of stress for adolescents with CF related to concerns about parental reactions to their health and concerns about the future, and they rated their health as significantly worse than their peers. However, the discussion of findings would have been strengthened if it had been framed in relation to development. Kashani, Barbero, Wilfley, Morris, and Shepperd (1988) also found no differences in self-concept and hopelessness with a combined sample of children and adolescents with CF (n = 30, 7 to 17 years) and a matched healthy control group (n = 30).

In contrast, other studies reported significant problems with self-concept and self-esteem for children and adolescents with CF. In a study of school-age and adolescent boys with CF (n = 23, 7 to 15 years), lower self-concept was associated with poor maternal adherence to CF treatment (Johnson, Gershowitz, & Stabler, 1981). However, the authors did not use a developmental framework to guide their study or incorporate developmental issues into the discussion of findings. Sawyer, Rosier, Phelan, and Bowes (1995) reported significant gender differences in self-image between adolescent males (n = 24) and females (n = 25) with CF (14 to 18 years). Although both males and females with CF exhibited extensive growth delay, females had significantly more problems related to self-esteem and body image when compared to males with CF and normative data. It is important to note that the authors conceptualized the study within a developmental science perspective by focusing on age, gender, and developmental differences. In addition, they interpreted the findings by incorporating a developmental perspective into their discussion. Moreover, these findings of identified problems with low self-esteem and low self-worth were supported by several studies of psychiatric diagnoses of children and adolescents with CF (discussed in the next section) (Thompson, Gustafson, George, & Spock, 1994; Thompson, Gustafson, Gil, Godfrey, & Murphy, 1998; Thompson, Gustafson, Hamlett, & Spock, 1992; Thompson, Hodges, & Hamlett, 1990).

Further confounding any conclusions, comparisons of self-concept to normative data indicated that the self-concepts of children and adolescents with CF were within normal range. Smith, Treadwell, and O'Grady (1983) reported that mean scores for self-concept in adolescents with CF (n = 26, 12 to 18 years) were at the 30th percentile when compared to a normative sample of adolescents, and no significant differences in life event changes were noted. However, when adolescents were grouped by CF severity, those adolescents (n = 10) with moderate to severe CF had a significantly greater number of negative life events when compared with those with better health status (n = 12). These authors included a developmental science perspective in their interpretation, presentation of limitations, and implications for clinical practice. Simmons and colleagues (1987) found that school age-children (6 to 11 years) with CF (n = 108) demonstrated higher self-concept and perceived health locus of control when compared to published norms. Using the Child Behavior Checklist (CBCL), parents reported that 23% of the children with CF demonstrated behavior problems. The authors discussed their findings using a developmental science perspective in relation to gender differences. They also addressed the need for a longitudinal study to determine the developmental changes from preschool to school-age children with CF.

PSYCHIATRIC SYMPTOMS: ANXIETY, WORRY, AND BEHAVIOR PROBLEMS

The development of psychiatric symptoms and diagnoses in children and adolescents with CF was the focus of several non-nursing studies. Pearson, Pumariega, and Seilheimer (1991) examined the development of psychiatric symptoms in two groups of patients with CF: a combined group of school-age children and adolescents ($n = 61$, 8 to 15 years), as compared to a combined group of older adolescents and adults ($n = 36$, 16 to 40 years). However, the authors noted that no direct comparisons of the two groups were possible because different measures were used. As expected, more symptoms of eating disorders were found in the younger group, while more symptoms of depression and anxiety were reported in the older adolescents and adults. These authors did use a developmental science perspective to interpret their findings. However, cross-sectional designs combining early and middle adolescents with school-age children, as well as middle to late adolescents with young and middle-aged adults confounded their ability to capture developmental issues and change.

Psychosocial adjustment has also been explored in several mixed-method studies that combined child and parent self-report measures with standardized diagnostic, clinical interviews. Kashani and colleagues (1988), using a combined age sample of children and adolescents with CF ($n = 30$, 7 to 17 years) and a matched healthy control group ($n = 30$), found no significant differences for symptoms and number or type of diagnoses using the diagnostic interview for children and adolescents. However, children with CF reported significantly more somatic complaints than the healthy controls. Using the CBCL, parents rated children with CF as having significantly more internalizing behavior problems, although there was no difference in the number of behavior problems. The authors reported that those with CF had a marginal tendency for lower social competence and used more externalizing behaviors, although neither score was statistically significant. A developmental science perspective was not used to guide the study or interpret the findings.

Other evidence of increased behavior problems in school-age children with CF has been reported (Simmons et al., 1987). Graetz, Shute, and Sawyer (2000) found that behavior problems in adolescents with CF ($n = 35$, 11 to 18 years) were predicted by family nonsupportive behaviors. In addition, adolescents reported that family members provided more tangible support, while friends provided more companionship support. No conceptual framework was used to guide the study, and the authors did not incorporate a developmental science perspective into their discussion of findings.

Thompson and colleagues, as part of their program of research focused on chronically ill children, included children and adolescents with CF. In an early study, Thompson et al. (1990) used a cross-sectional design with matched groups of children and adolescents with CF (7 to 14 years) ($n = 43$), those with psychiatric referrals ($n = 43$), and healthy children and adolescents ($n = 43$) to examine psychosocial adjustment using standardized diagnostic, clinical interviews. Children and adolescents with CF did not have more symptoms of psychological disturbance when compared to healthy children. However, children and adolescents with CF did demonstrate internalizing behavior problems of poor self-image, worry, and anxiety similar to those in the psychiatric-referred group. This study did not employ a conceptual model nor use a developmental science perspective in the interpretation of findings. Combining two different developmental age groups in a cross-sectional design limited the ability of the study to explore developmental processes over time. However, the authors did explore age differences in adjustment among groups in statistical analysis.

Continuing their program of research, Thompson and colleagues (1992) explored psychosocial adjustment in children with CF ($n = 45$, 7 to 12 years) and found that 60% of the children had a mother reported behavior problem and 62% met the criteria for a DSM-III diagnosis using a standardized diagnostic, clinical interview with the child. Children reported more internalizing (anxiety) and externalizing (oppositional disorder) behavior problems, and there was 66% congruence between child-reported and mother-reported behavior problems. Further, children's perceptions of self-worth were lower in those with self-reported distress, as well as in children with poor adjustment by mother report. Using a transactional stress and coping model to guide the conceptualization of the study, this systems model was consistent with a developmental science perspective. However, the authors did not use a developmental perspective to explain their findings.

In a longitudinal follow-up study of children and adolescents with CF ($n = 41$, 7 to 14 years), Thompson et al. (1994) found that levels of psychosocial adjustment remained stable over 12 months when children were grouped by good and poor adjustment. However, in relation to individual change, there was little stability in the type of child behavior problems and child-reported symptoms. In addition, children's lower perceptions of self-worth were associated with maternal distress. The authors used their transactional stress and coping model to guide the conceptualization of the study. The use of a longitudinal design represents an improvement over other studies in this review by providing a developmental perspective for addressing the process of adjustment. However, the combination of two developmental age groups in the sample limits the ability to determine specific developmental patterns associated with differences in levels of cognitive, emotional, and social development.

Illness-specific patterns of adjustment were identified in a study of two groups of children (7 to 12 years) with CF ($n = 40$) and sickle cell disease ($n = 40$) (Thompson et al., 1998). While both groups most frequently exhibited anxiety disorders, children with CF also had a higher rate of oppositional disorders. Children with CF demonstrated significant associations between low self-worth, low self-efficacy, and high levels of perceived stress with high levels of symptoms. Although the authors used their transactional stress and coping model to guide the conceptualization of the study, they did not include a developmental perspective for the interpretation of findings. Rather, they suggested that it would be important in the future to add a developmental perspective to explore the interrelationships among illness tasks and the process of adaptation.

INTERVENTION STUDIES

Among the non-nursing studies, only one small intervention study was conducted. Hains, Davies, Behrens, and Biller (1997) used a multiple baseline across-subjects design to examine the effectiveness of a cognitive behavioral intervention to improve coping in adolescents ($n = 5$, 13 to 15 years) with CF who were referred for therapy. There was no control group. The sample may have been biased, since the CF health care team ratings of anxiety in adolescents were used rather than an objective measure. These adolescents exhibited decreased anxiety, an increased use of positive coping strategies, a reduction in the use of negative coping strategies with CF-related problems, and a decrease in functional disability after intervention. On follow-up at 3 months, three to four adolescents maintained decreased functional disability and stable anxiety levels. These results are promising, although the intervention must be replicated on a larger scale with a control group. Even though a longitudinal design was used, a developmental science perspective was not used for conceptualizing the study or interpreting the findings.

SUMMARY AND CRITIQUE

There was wide variability in the use of conceptual frameworks in these non-nursing studies. In their program of research, three of the four studies by Thompson and colleagues clearly specified the use of a transactional stress and coping model to guide their studies (Thompson et al., 1994; Thompson et al., 1998; Thompson et al., 1992). This framework incorporates a broad perspective of the child and family. Cappelli and colleagues (1989) used a developmental framework to conceptualize their study of adolescents with CF and social functioning. Although no conceptual framework was identified in four additional studies, the authors did use psychosocial developmental perspectives to explain and interpret findings (Smith et al., 1983; Simmons et al.,1987; Pearson et al., 1991; Sawyer et al., 1995). However, some studies did not use an ecological, development model in the design or developmental perspectives in interpreting their findings. Because chronic illness in children and adolescents occurs in the context of development, this represents a major weakness. The use of an ecological, developmental framework to guide research and interpret findings would provide a more holistic view of the developing child and adolescent in the context of their environment.

As noted earlier, most of these studies used descriptive correlational designs. Only two studies used longitudinal designs (Hains et al., 1997; Thompson et al., 1998). Clearly, there is a need for more longitudinal research in this area. Developmentally sensitive longitudinal studies are important in tracking developmental change and stability over time. Moreover, the fact that only one small intervention study (Hains et al., 1997) has been done highlights critical directions for future research.

Various sample configurations were used: five studies focused specifically on adolescents, four studies used school-age children, four studies combined samples of both children and adolescents, and one study compared school-age children, adolescents, and adults. Many of these studies also used multiple comparison groups of different chronic illnesses (e.g., CF, diabetes, asthma, sickle cell disease, psychiatric-referred) with healthy children or normative data. Given the quantitative design of the studies, the sample sizes were small.

Most of the studies used standardized instruments to collect data, and most also used both child and mother assessments of children's adjustment. However, many used the Child Behavior Checklist, which Perrin, Stein, and Drotar (1991) caution may not be valid in children with chronic disease. The use of diagnostic, clinical interviews demonstrated more sensitivity in capturing the psychosocial adjustment problems than the standardized psychological measures used in a majority of the non-nursing studies. Clearly, the identification of psychiatric symptoms and diagnoses across studies suggests the vulnerability of children and adolescents with CF to long-term psychosocial problems and the implications for quality of life.

Although the findings of these non-nursing studies of the psychosocial adjustment of children and adolescents with CF were equivocal, it is important to note that variables of self-concept, self-worth, and self-esteem remain critical indicators of adjustment. Some of the variability of findings may be explained by methodologic flaws. For example, most of these studies used small sample sizes with multiple independent variables and parametric statistics. Over a third combined developmental-age groups of children and adolescents as well as adults in one sample, and so were unable to determine specific differences in levels of cognitive, emotional, and social development.

THEORETICAL AND METHODOLOGICAL CONSIDERATIONS

Although all studies were concerned with psychosocial adjustment, studies from nursing and non-nursing disciplines were singularly different. Nursing studies focused on children's or adolescents' perspectives of CF and used primarily qualitative methods with two mixed-methods designs. In contrast, the majority of the non-nursing studies used quantitative, cross-sectional, correlational designs; many combined parent and child reports with a standardized diagnostic, clinical interview with the child. No intervention studies were retrieved from the published nursing literature, and only one small intervention study was identified in the non-nursing literature. Moreover, there were few longitudinal studies. To improve CF research, designs must target developmental change over time (Thompson et al., 1994) and permit tracking of changes in the chronic illness trajectory to inform interventions that can improve quality of life. Research designs that incorporate a developmental science perspective require an integration of experimental, comparative, and longitudinal designs (Magnusson & Cairns, 1996).

A primary difference between the nursing and non-nursing studies was related to the use of theoretical frameworks, particularly ecological, developmental frameworks. All of the nursing studies used conceptual frameworks that encompassed aspects of development. Still, broader eco-logical aspects such as culture, socioeconomic status, and gender were rarely considered. In contrast, the conceptual frameworks in the non-nursing studies varied. Several authors used ecological system perspectives combined with transactional stress and coping models, while some did not have a clear conceptual framework. Interestingly, both programs of research from nursing (Christian & D'Auria) and related disciplines (Thompson and colleagues) were conceptualized using developmental sci-ence perspectives.

The qualitative nursing research provided rich descriptions of the impact of CF on the lives of children and adolescents. Developmental theory was used to explain and interpret the findings in all of the nursing studies. Paired with the use of developmental theory to explain psychoso-cial adjustment, these studies were able to integrate the chronic illness experience within a social context. In contrast, only four non-nursing studies (Smith et al., 1983; Simmons et al., 1987; Pearson et al., 1991; Sawyer et al., 1995) used developmental theory to interpret their findings. Clearly, the use of developmental theory and a developmental science perspective would have enhanced the interpretation of findings and the ability to draw conclusions. The use of a developmental science perspective allows the researcher to explore the psychological significance of variables within the social and environmental context (Magnusson & Cairns, 1996). Thus, research in this area would be strengthened by the addition of a developmental science framework for conceptualization of research, as well as for the interpretation of findings.

Methodologically, one of the critical design flaws evident in much of the research was the small sample sizes and the use of combined age groups within the samples. Perhaps this within-group variability accounted for the lack of sensitivity in obtaining statistical significance in some of the studies. Moreover, children and adolescents are confronted with different developmental issues and life experiences in addition to managing their chronic illness. Thus, a developmental perspective in the configuration of samples would enhance the researcher's ability to interpret findings. In addition, larger samples in the quantitative studies would improve the representativeness of the sample and the generalizability of findings.

SUMMARY AND RECOMMENDATIONS FOR FUTURE RESEARCH

Research on the psychosocial adjustment of children and adolescents with CF over the past twenty years has continued to be a central focus across disciplines. With the dramatic changes in illness trajectory and increased life span coupled with changing treatment modalities, research focused on children and adolescents with CF presents new challenges for health care. A developmental science perspective should be used to enhance conceptualization of research and knowledge development in this area. Without developmental sensitivity, it is difficult to determine if psychosocial adjustment problems are related to developmental demands or to the impact of the chronic illness. For knowledge development in this area, it is critical that nursing and related disciplines build upon research across disciplines. Moreover, programmatic research will contribute to knowledge development across disciplines.

Research needs to address the social consequences of chronic illness with consideration given to the changing course of the illness and related treatment modalities. Although nursing research has begun to address the social consequences of living with CF, it would be advantageous for researchers across disciplines to collaborate in their efforts to explore the impact of CF over time by using longitudinal designs. More research is needed that addresses individual developmental differences and that uses designs that can capture developmental process and change.

The lack of intervention research continues to be problematic in the CF literature. There is a need for intervention research by multidisciplinary teams to address the psychosocial adjustment as well as the physiologic and functional health status needs of children and adolescents. Based on this review, the next step for nurse researchers should be using the findings of qualitative studies as the basis for developing appropriate interventions. New intervention strategies to teach children and adolescents how to maintain a satisfactory quality of life need to be developed and tested. Of critical importance is the need for cost-effective interventions that help children and adolescents with CF manage the demands of their chronic illness in the social contexts of peers and school (Christian, 2001). Special attention needs to be given to interventions that are developmentally appropriate to promote children's understanding of CF and their own feelings associated with the chronic illness and its treatment. If they can achieve meaningful outcomes in their everyday lives, such as being able to make friends or participate more fully in physical activities, children are more likely to take better care of their health, adhere to treatment more, and improve their functional and physiologic health. Thus, children and adolescents with CF need intervention programs that can teach them strategies for managing their chronic illness in the social context of their everyday lives. Future research on children and adolescents with CF must incorporate the social contexts of school and peers to help children achieve a more satisfactory quality of life while meeting the relentless demands of CF and development. Ultimately, the goal of this research is to improve the quality of life of children and adolescents growing up with CF.

ACKNOWLEDGMENTS

The author wishes to acknowledge support from Grant P30 NR 03962, Center for Research on Chronic Illness, and Grant R01 NR04576, both from the National Institute of Nursing Research, National Institutes of Health.

REFERENCES

Admi, H. (1995). Nothing to hide and nothing to advertise: Managing disease-related information. *Western Journal of Nursing Research, 17,* 484–501.

Angst, D. B. (2001). School age children. In M. Bluebond-Langer, B. Lask, & D. B. Angst (Eds.), *Psychosocial aspects of cystic fibrosis* (pp. 125–138). London: Arnold.

Cappelli, M., McGrath, P. J., Heick, C. E., MacDonald, N. E., Feldman, W., & Rowe, P. (1989). Chronic disease and its impact: The adolescent's perspective. *Journal of Adolescent Health Care, 10,* 283–288.

Christian, B. J. (1993). Quality of life and family relationships in families coping with their child's chronic illness. In S. G. Funk, E. M. Tornquist, M. T. Champagne, & R. A. Wiese (Eds.), *Key aspects of caring for the chronically ill: Hospital and home* (pp. 304–312). New York: Springer.

Christian, B. J. (2001, May). *Building life skills for children with cystic fibrosis.* Paper presented at the spring science workgroup: Increasing Nursing Research Opportunities in Cystic Fibrosis, sponsored by the National Institute for Nursing Research, NIH, Bethesda, MD.

Christian, B. J., & D'Auria, J. P. (1997). The child's eye: Memories of growing up with cystic fibrosis. *Journal of Pediatric Nursing, 12,* 3–12.

Christian, B. J., & D'Auria, J. P. (1998). *Building life skills in children with cystic fibrosis.* Unpublished grant submitted to the National Institute for Nursing Research, NIH, Grant number R01 NR04576.

Christian, B. J., D'Auria, J. P., & Belyea, M. J. (2001, April). *Psychosocial adjustment, physiologic and functional health status of school-age children with cystic fibrosis.* Poster presented at biennial meeting of the Society for Research in Child Development, Minneapolis, MN.

Christian, B. J., D'Auria, J. P., Hall, E., & White, M. (2001, February). *Perceived illness experience and self-esteem with cystic fibrosis.* Paper presented at the 15th Annual Conference of the Southern Nursing Research Society, Baltimore, MD.

Christian, B. J., D'Auria, J. P., & Moore, C. B. (1999). Playing for time: Adolescent perspectives of lung transplantation for cystic fibrosis. *Journal of Pediatric Health Care, 13,* 120–125.

Cystic Fibrosis Foundation (1999). *Cystic Fibrosis Foundation national CF patient registry 1998 annual data report.* Bethesda, MD: Author.

D'Auria, J. P., Christian, B. J., Henderson, Z. G., & Haynes, B. (2000). The company they keep: The influence of peer relationships on adjustment to cystic fibrosis during adolescence. *Journal of Pediatric Nursing, 15,* 175–182.

D'Auria, J. P., Christian, B. J., & Richardson, L. F. (1997). Through the looking glass: Children's perceptions of growing up with cystic fibrosis. *Canadian Journal of Nursing Research, 29,* 99–112.

Deatrick, J. A. (1998). Integrative review: Intervention models for children who have chronic conditions and their families. In M. E. Broome, S. Feetham, K. Knafl, & K. Pridham (Eds.), *Children and families in health and illness* (pp. 221–235). Thousand Oaks, CA: Sage.

Eiser, C. (1993). *Growing up with a chronic disease: The impact on children and their families.* London: Jessica Kingsley.

Ellerton, M. L., Stewart, M. J., Ritchie, J. A., & Hirth, A. M. (1996). Social support in children with a chronic condition. *Canadian Journal of Nursing Research, 28,* 15–36.

Faux, S. A. (1998). Historical overview of responses of children and their families to chronic illness. In M. E. Broome, S. Feetham, K. Knafl, & K. Pridham (Eds.), *Children and families in health and illness* (pp. 179–195). Thousand Oaks, CA: Sage.

Graetz, B. W., Shute, R. H., & Sawyer, M. G. (2000). An Australian study of adolescents with cystic fibrosis: Perceived supportive and nonsupportive behaviors from families and friends and psychological adjustment. *Journal of Adolescent Health, 26,* 64–69.

Grey, M., & Sullivan-Bolyai, S. (1999). Key issues in chronic illness research: Lessons from the study of children with diabetes. *Journal of Pediatric Nursing, 14*, 351–358.

Hains, A. A., Davies, W. H., Behrens, D., & Biller, J. A. (1997). Cognitive behavioral interventions for adolescents with cystic fibrosis. *Journal of Pediatric Psychology, 22*, 669–687.

Johnson, M. R., Gershowitz, M., & Stabler, B. (1981). Maternal compliance and children's self-concept in cystic fibrosis. *Journal of Developmental and Behavioral Pediatrics, 2*, 5–8.

Kashani, J. H., Barbero, G. J., Wilfley, D. E., Morris, D. A., & Shepperd, J. A. (1988). Psychological concomitants of cystic fibrosis in children and adolescents. *Adolescence, 23*, 873–880.

Magnusson, D., & Cairns, R. B. (1996). Developmental science: Toward a unified framework. In R. B. Cairns, G. H. Elder, Jr., & E. J. Costello (Eds.), *Developmental science* (pp. 7–30). New York: Cambridge University Press.

Patton, A. C., Ventura, J. N., & Savedra, M. (1986). Stress and coping responses of adolescents with cystic fibrosis. *Children's Health Care, 14*, 153–156.

Pearson, D. A., Pumariega, A. J., & Seilheimer, D. K. (1991). The development of psychiatric symptomatology in patients with cystic fibrosis. *Journal of the American Academy of Child and Adolescent Psychiatry, 30*, 290–297.

Perrin, E. C., Stein, R. E. K., & Drotar, D. (1991). Cautions in using the Child Behavior Checklist: Observations based on research about children with a chronic illness. *Journal of Pediatric Psychology, 16*, 411–422.

Quittner, A. L., DiGirolamo, A. M., Michel, M., & Eigen, H. (1992). Parental response to cystic fibrosis: A contextual analysis of the diagnostic phase. *Journal of Pediatric Psychology, 17*, 683–704.

Sawyer, S. M., Rosier, M. J., Phelan, P. D., & Bowes, G. (1995). The self-image of adolescents with cystic fibrosis. *Journal of Adolescent Health, 16*, 204–208.

Simmons, R. J., Corey, M., Cowen, L., Keenan, N., Robertson, J., & Levison, H. (1987). Behavioral adjustment of latency age children with cystic fibrosis. *Psychosomatic Medicine, 49*, 291–301.

Smith, M. S., Treadwell, M., & O'Grady, L. (1983). Psychosocial functioning, life change, and clinical status in adolescents with cystic fibrosis. *Journal of Adolescent Health Care, 4*, 230–234.

Stein, R. E. K. (1992). Chronic physical disorders. *Pediatrics in Review, 13*, 224–229.

Thompson, R. J., Jr., & Gustafson, K. E. (1996). *Adaptation to chronic childhood illness.* Washington, DC: American Psychological Association.

Thompson, R. J., Jr., Gustafson, K. E., George, L. K., & Spock, A. (1994). Change over a 12-month period in the psychological adjustment of children and adolescents with cystic fibrosis. *Journal of Pediatric Psychology, 19*, 189–203.

Thompson, R. J., Jr., Gustafson, K. E., Gil, K. M., Godfrey, J., & Murphy, L. M. (1998). Illness specific patterns of psychological adjustment and cognitive adaptational processes in children with cystic fibrosis. *Journal of Clinical Psychology, 54*, 121–128.

Thompson, R. J., Jr., Gustafson, K. E., Hamlett, K. W., & Spock, A. (1992). Psychological adjustment of children with cystic fibrosis: The role of child cognitive processes and maternal adjustment. *Journal of Pediatric Psychology, 17,* 741–755.

Thompson, R. J., Jr., Hodges, K., & Hamlett, K. W. (1990). A matched comparison of adjustment in children with cystic fibrosis and psychiatrically referred and non-referred children. *Journal of Pediatric Psychology, 15,* 745–759.

Tyrrell, J. (2001). Growing up with cystic fibrosis: The adolescent years. In M. Bluebond-Langner, B. Lask, & D. Angst (Eds.), *Psychosocial aspects of cystic fibrosis* (pp. 139–149). London: Arnold.

Chapter 7

Children's Psychological Responses to Hospitalization

JUDITH A. VESSEY

ABSTRACT

The data-based literature addressing children's psychological responses to hospitalization was reviewed using methods outlined by Cooper (1989). Using a developmental science perspective, early research was reviewed and a model of variables that contribute to children's responses was constructed. This model consists of three major foci, including maturational and cognitive variables (developmental level, experience, coping style), ecological variables (family and hospital milieu), and biological variables (inborn factors and pathophysiology). Coping serves as the overarching framework for examining these variables and their contributions to children's responses to hospitalization. A variety of theoretical perspectives from the social sciences have been used, with psychoanalytic and stress and adaptation theories predominating. The majority of the research used simple case study, descriptive, or pre- and post-test designs. Methodologic issues were common. Little qualitative work has been done. Future research directions call for studies to adopt new theoretical and empirical models that are methodologically rigorous and clinically relevant and that embrace the precepts of developmental science.

Understanding children's psychological responses to hospitalization is central to pediatric nursing care. It requires identifying antecedent events and mediating factors and their relationships to these responses, and designing interventions that help children have growth-promoting experiences while mitigating unhealthy responses. This chapter reviews the data-based nursing literature and synthesizes the accumulated knowledge on children's psychological responses to hospitalization from the perspective of developmental science.

Developmental science is "an integrated, holistic model for individual functioning and development" (Magnusson, 1995, p. 19). Specifically, children's psychological responses to hospitalization are not temporally bound, linear cause-and-effect reactions to a situational event. Rather, their responses are partially determined by inborn attributes, gender, previous experiences, and family and cultural dynamics. During hospitalization children's responses are further shaped by an ongoing dynamic and complex interplay among cognitive, biological, and ecological factors, such as their age, symptom management, parental presence, and the hospital environment. Moreover, children's responses are mediated by their ability for psychological adaptation, often termed coping. Coping abilities are in turn partially shaped and refined by the ecology of the hospitalization experience. After hospitalization, children's responses to the experience are continually refined by concurrent and future developmental processes, social and ecological encounters, and the interactions among them. Therefore, children's early experiences with hospitalization have enduring consequences, affecting individuals' responses to hospitalization throughout their lifetimes (Elder, 1998).

Although children's psychological responses to hospitalization constantly evolve and differentiate in light of new developmental inputs, for this synthesis it is conceptually useful to view children's responses in terms of process and outcome. Guided by the compilation of conceptual descriptions used in this body of research, *psychological responses to hospitalization* are considered to be multidimensional in nature. They result from emotional and cognitive challenges and the biobehavioral responses to these challenges that accompany hospitalization. Responses may be demonstrated in any developmental domain (e.g., self-control, autonomy, socialization, physiologic functions), range from psychologically distressful to beneficial, and evolve across three temporal periods. *Immediate responses* occur during hospitalization. *Posthospital responses* evolve during the period immediately following hospitalization or during institutional rehabilitation but prior to resumption of normal activities of daily living. *Prolonged responses* are relatively stable and emerge after discharge from the hospital and institutional rehabilitation and after the child has returned to physiologic stability. Psychological responses are operationalized by investigators through behavioral observation, self-report, third party report, or standardized physiological or psychological measures (Thompson, 1985).

A historical overview sets the stage for a discussion of the current state of the science. The concept of coping serves as an overarching framework for exploring three groups of variables and their relationships—developmental and cognitive, biological, and ecological—espoused in the developmental science framework (Cairns, Costello, & Elder, 1997; Magnusson, 1995; Magnusson & Cairns, 1996). The diverse conceptual and methodological underpinnings of this body of research and the linkages among them are critiqued and gaps and disparities are identified. Lastly, directions for future study are proposed.

METHOD

Criteria for Inclusion

In order to allow for the greatest representation of the topic and for generalization for later analysis and synthesis (Cooper, 1989), the identified target population was all studies that were conducted by nurses (primary or coauthor/investigator) or that appeared in the nursing literature in which children's psychological response to hospitalization was a major variable (e.g., dependent, independent, intervening). Inclusion criteria required that the article be original research and published in a refereed data-based journal.[1] Relevant early unpublished dissertations (prior to 1980) also were included if they were obtainable, since these early studies provided the foundation for this area of study. Unpublished research after 1980 and articles published in electronic journals were omitted because of identification and retrieval difficulties. Because of the impact of culture on children's behavioral responses, only studies using samples from Western nations and Australia were included.

All research was included except for anecdotal case study reports. Studies needed to include the variable "children's responses to hospitalization" or a related concept (e.g., emotional upset, coping) anywhere along the pre- to posthospitalization trajectory. Hospitalizations for surgery (including day procedures), acute problems, or exacerbations of long-term medical problems were included; excluded were hospitalizations for psychiatric conditions. All age cohorts of children were included except pre-

---

[1]Wherever possible, research conducted by nurses and published in non-nursing journals is included. It is acknowledged that this area is underrepresented because of identification difficulties.

term infants. Populations of children with marked cultural or developmental differences, including new immigrants, the terminally ill, or those with cognitive deficits or multiple developmental delays, were also excluded.[2] Previous reviews of nursing studies in topical areas such as pain, psychological preparation, and parental and sibling responses were limited to their influence on children's psychological responses to hospitalization.

Search Strategies

The accessible literature base was identified using search strategies that included keyword and author searches of journals indexed in relevant databases: CINAHL (1982 to 2001), Medline (1966 to 2001), PsycINFO (1887 to 2001), and Dissertation Abstracts (1931 to 1980). Manual searches of indexed pediatric nursing and nursing research journal tables of contents (1970 to 2001) and searches of identified literature in review articles (Barnard & Neal, 1977; Fletcher, 1981; Lambert, 1984; Lipman & Hayman, 2000; McClowry, 1988; O'Conner-Von, 2000; Olson, Heater, & Becker, 1990; Ryan-Wenger, 1994; Thompson, 1985; Vernon, Foley, Sipowcz, & Schulman, 1965; Vernon & Thompson, 1993) were also conducted. The earliest nursing study identified was from 1955. Although attempts were made to be as inclusive as possible, the conclusions drawn from the retrieved nursing studies might not be totally representative of the target population.

Critique Method

A total of 65 studies were identified. These were reviewed chronologically to ascertain how each contributed to nursing knowledge on children's psychological responses to hospitalization. Factors influencing children's responses were identified (e.g., prior experience, rooming-in, symptom distress). How subsequent studies built upon earlier findings was then tracked. Studies were initially coded as to the type of research, major variables included, conceptual framework used, and design and analytic

---

[2]Although this criterion was established a priori, it is noted that with the exception of a body of literature on terminally ill children, no studies were identified that specifically address these populations.

techniques employed. A determination of the study's theoretical and methodological congruence and overall quality was then made.

Studies were then evaluated according to the precepts of developmental science. Specifically, each study was analyzed as to whether it embraced a holistic perspective and the complexity its conceptualizations. Emphasis was placed on examining the interactions among biological, cognitive, and ecological factors influencing children's psychological responses to hospitalization. In addition to standard design analysis, attention was paid to the developmental, ecological, and temporal aspects of the study. Of specific concern was whether the study design, instrumentation, and interventions were developmentally appropriate and sensitive for the populations being studied, whether they allowed for individual differences to be identified, and whether the design and analytic techniques were appropriate for understanding change over time. Where possible, attempts were made to identify linkages among multilevel measures.

FINDINGS: THE STATE OF THE SCIENCE

Historical Overview

Anecdotal reports of children's untoward psychological responses to hospitalization appeared in the health care literature as early as the mid-19th century (West, 1954/1845). However, seminal works by Spitz (1945), who documented the negative impact of maternal child separation, and Prugh, Staub, Sands, Kirschbaum, and Lenihan (1953), who identified the deleterious effects of the hospital environment, were not published until a full century later. By the mid-1960s, the impact of hospitalization on children's psyche became a public policy issue (Shore, 1965) and the focus of numerous transdisciplinary research studies (Carty, 1977; Davenport & Werry, 1970; Holt, 1968; Mahaffy, 1965; Sipowcz & Vernon, 1965; Vernon et al., 1965; Vernon, Schulman, & Foley, 1966).

Most early studies focused on psychological upset, or negative responses children demonstrate during or in response to hospitalization (McClowry, 1988; Thompson, 1985). Changes in observable behaviors within activities of daily living were emphasized. Common variables included sleep disturbances (e.g., insomnia, night terrors), nutrition (e.g., refusal to eat), elimination (e.g., nocturnal enuresis), socialization with peers or family members (e.g., fear of separation, whining, clinging, in-creased aggression), overconcern with body functioning, fear of death, and generalized anxiety. Many of these responses were characterized as behavioral regression or the loss of previously mastered skills. Little atten-tion was focused on whether hospitalization could be an emotionally maturing experience, despite early studies (Prugh, 1965; Vernon et al., 1966) demonstrating that maturation occurred for subgroups of children. The early adoption of a deficit model significantly influenced the develop-ment of this field of inquiry.

Major intervening variables shown to affect children's psychological responses to hospitalization included age, separation, length of hospitaliza-tion, hospital milieu, type and severity of illness and symptomatology, previous adaptive capacity, perceptions of the experience, parent-child relationships, and parental equilibrium. To determine the children at great-est risk, the contributions of these variables to children's psychological responses began to be further explicated in numerous transdisciplinary descriptive and intervention studies.

Areas investigated by nurse researchers in the 1960s to the early 1980s included illness-related variables such as pain (Schultz, 1971; Stew-art, 1977), loss of control (McCaffery, 1971), and body integrity fears (Miles, 1969). Contextual variables such as parental separation and room-ing-in (Bransetter, 1969a, 1969b; Fagin, 1966; Godfrey, 1955; Hennessey, 1976; McGillicuddy, 1976), parental participation (Meng, 1980), restraint (Holt, 1968), psychological preparation (Abbott, Hansen, & Lewis, 1970; Bailey, 1967; McGrath, 1979; Visintainer & Wolfer, 1975; Wolfer & Visintainer, 1975, 1979), play (Clatworthy, 1981; Lockwood, 1970; Vredevoe, Kim, Dambacher, & Call, 1969), and parental reactions (Visin-tainer & Wolfer, 1975; Wolfer & Visintainer, 1975, 1979) also were examined descriptively or through intervention studies. The role of coping as an overarching framework for determining the gravity of responses also was promulgated (Rose, 1972). Collectively, these studies serve as the foundation for understanding children's psychological responses to hospitalization.

A Model of Key Concepts

Over the past two decades, nurse researchers have continually advanced the science in these areas by examining the effects of numerous variables, using a variety of theoretical perspectives, and refining methodologies. When considered from the perspective of developmental science, these approaches helped describe and explain children's psychological responses to hospitalization. Figure 7.1 delineates these variables and their basic relationships. This schematic does not, however, list all the contributing variables or depict the intracategory (e.g., parental response and culture) and intercategory (e.g., prior experiences and disease process) connections among the variables or capture the temporal and holistic components of these relationships.

This model serves as a guide to examining the contributions of nurses to the state of the science on children's psychological responses to hospitalization. Because these responses are mediated by children's coping abilities, this concept is first explored. This is followed by an exploration of its relationship to cognitive/maturational, ecological, and biological factors. Lastly, intervention work using specific coping strategies is described.

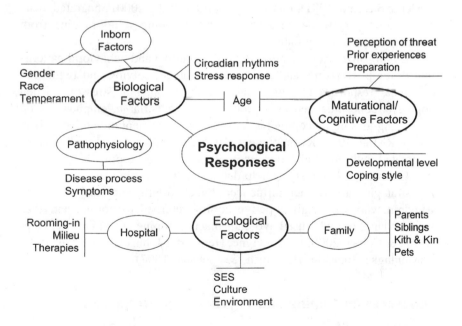

FIGURE 7.1   Variables that contribute to children's psychological responses depicted according to three developmental science domains.

Coping: An Overarching Framework

The concept of coping serves as an overarching framework for a discussion of children's responses to hospitalization. Coping, a form of psychological adaptation, can be defined as an individual's constantly changing emotional and behavioral efforts to gain mastery over environmental and internal stressors. The concept of coping has been deconstructed into "coping styles" and "coping strategies," each with distinct theoretical origins. Throughout the literature the term *coping* is often used generically with little distinction made between coping styles or strategies or with an amalgam of the two. This definitional ambiguity has led to difficulty in interpreting study findings.

Coping styles are relatively fixed patterns of behavior that describe an individual's adaptation to stressors. Coping styles, derived from Lazarus's (1966) model of cognitive appraisal of coping, are trait variables and not highly amenable to change. Coping styles were initially deconstructed into three types—inactive, orienting (precoping), and active (Rose, 1972; Tesler & Savedra, 1981). LaMontagne (1984, 1987, 2000) integrated locus of control theory to create a continuum of coping styles ranging from avoidant-inactive to vigilant-active.

Coping strategies are more flexible cognitive and behavioral patterns that develop over time and are used in problem solving and regulating emotional responses to situational and developmental stressors. When coping is conceptualized as a process or state variable, emphasis is on examining the child's coping mode, function, and orientation (Caty, Ellerton, & Richie, 1984; Ryan-Wenger, 1996). As children deal with stresses associated with hospitalization, they are said to be "coping."

Children's coping styles help determine their coping strategies. Coping strategies are further influenced by children's appraisal of threat. Children who used vigilant-active coping returned to normal activities sooner than those who used avoidant-inactive coping (LaMontagne, Hepworth, & Cohen, 2000; LaMontagne, Hepworth, Johnson, & Cohen, 1996; LaMontagne, Johnson, Hepworth, & Johnson, 1997).

Influences on Coping and Psychological Responses

The specific variables correlated with children's coping behaviors and psychological outcomes to hospitalization (McClowry, 1988; Vessey, 1998) as presented in Figure 7.1 are discussed below.

MATURATIONAL AND COGNITIVE FACTORS

Early studies of children's psychological responses to hospitalization indicate that a curvilinear relationship between age and potential for upset exists. Six months to 6 years was the period of greatest vulnerability (Vernon et al., 1965). Further study began to reveal that each developmental period has vulnerabilities that influence how situational stressors are perceived and behavioral responses are manifested (Scavnicky-Mylant, 1987; Stevens, 1986). Prior experiences mediate developing cognitive schema about illness and hospitalization (Yoos, 1994) and their impact over time. Unfortunately, most studies focused on a single age group (e.g., school age) and paid superficial attention to individual differences or the impact of prior experience. Little empirical evidence is available in the *nursing* literature as to the impact of hospitalization on infants and adolescents or the role of experience.

Individual differences may further explain children's psychological responses to hospitalization. Early on, Holt (1968) noted that children's distant memories of hospitalization were highly selective and reflected individual differences in personality, family situations, and meanings assigned to the experience. McClowry's (1990) study demonstrated that children's temperament explained over 50% of the variance in their post-hospitalization behaviors. However, a study attempting to lessen children's behavioral distress to repeated lumbar punctures by using a cognitive-behavioral intervention failed to demonstrate any relationship between temperament and distress (Broome, Rehwaldt, & Fogg, 1998).

ECOLOGICAL INFLUENCES

Two sets of ecological influences, the child's family and the hospital milieu, specifically influence children's coping abilities, and subsequently their psychological responses to hospitalization. Children's most significant ecological context is their family. Parental reactions to their child's hospitalizations affect children's responses to hospitalization and vice versa. The widely promulgated, but weakly supported, emotional contagion hypothesis posits that parental stress is communicable and readily transferred to the child (Thompson, 1985). Regardless of whether this hypothesis is true, anxious parents are less able to provide emotional support, thus interrupting the normal parental role and creating confusion for the child. Other variables—illness acuity and prognosis, length of stay, symptomatology—further influence both child and parental anxiety and coping abilities

(Curley, 1988; Curley & Wallace, 1992; LaMontagne, Wells, Hepworth, Johnson, & Manes, 1999; Melnyk, 2000; Tiedeman, 1997). Parental stresses associated with their child's repeated hospitalizations are qualitatively different from stresses experienced with a single hospitalization for a limited problem (Burke, Costello, & Handley-Derry, 1989; Burke, Kauffmann, Costello, & Dillon, 1991). Less evidence is available on the contributions siblings make to a child's coping abilities and response to hospitalization.

Preliminary findings suggest differences in responses depending on a child's cultural background (Carty, 1977; Glazebrook & Sheard, 1994) or residence (frontier, rural, or urban) (Strickland, Leeper, Jessee, & Hudson, 1987). Other ecological factors, including the family's religiosity and socioeconomic status, have rarely been addressed. The effect of friends and pets is also underinvestigated (Stevens, 1986).

The hospital milieu has undergone significant changes in response to evidence on the effects of the physical environment (Godfrey, 1955; Prugh, 1965), parental presence (Fagin, 1966; McGillicuddy, 1976), and effective symptom management (Abu-Saad & Hamers, 1997; Broome & Huth, in press). Supportive nursing behaviors also positively influence children's responses to hospitalization. Unfortunately, nursing's role frequently is insufficiently described or so embedded in the description of the setting or intervention that empirical evidence of nursing's contributions to children's adjustment is obfuscated.

Nursing intervention studies using diverse theoretical frameworks and interventions have decreased anxiety and stress and improved coping abilities in children and parents. For example, positive robust results were reported by Melnyk (1994, 1995) and colleagues (Melnyk, Alpert-Gillis, Hensel, Cable-Beiling, & Rubenstein, 1997), who used regulation and control theory and informational interventions with parents; Curley and Wallace (1992), who used the double ABCX Model of Crisis as a framework for modifying staff interactions with families; and Burke and colleagues (Burke, Handley-Derry, Costello, Kauffmann, & Dillon, 1997; Burke, Harrison, Kauffmann, & Wong, 2001), who used stress point interventions with parents and children. Other nursing intervention studies involved therapeutic play (Clatworthy, 1981; Lockwood, 1970), psychological preparation (Demarest, Hook, & Erickson, 1984; Månsson, Björkhem, & Wiebe, 1993; McGrath, 1979; Schmidt, 1990; Visintainer & Wolfer, 1975; Wolfer & Visintainer, 1975, 1979), or caregiving with children and families (Pederson, 1996). These interventions generally resulted in less psychological upset and better adjustment during the immediate pre- to posthospitalization period; however, prolonged effects are poorly documented.

BIOLOGICAL INPUTS AND RESPONSES

No significant gender effects have been detected (Cormier, 1979; Tiedeman, 1997; Youssef, 1981). When available, race, although rarely reported, is inextricably embedded with socioeconomic status and family culture, so that no valid information may be garnered as to its unique contribution.

Influencing Behavioral Responses by Enhancing Coping Strategies

A body of transdisciplinary intervention studies has sought to strengthen children's and/or their parents' coping abilities. The most popular framework, stress inoculation,[3] explored techniques designed to help individuals identify their coping styles and assist them with risk appraisal, perception modification, and response selection (Meng & Zastowny, 1982; Poster, 1983). These techniques included relaxation (Hennesey, 1976; White, Williams, Alexander, Powell-Cope, & Conlon, 1990); desensitization, distraction, and modeling (Demarest et al., 1984); cognitive rehearsal (Visintainer & Wolfer, 1975; Wolfer & Visintainer, 1975, 1979; Zastowny, Kirschenbaum, & Meng, 1986); play (Clatworthy, 1981; Ellerton, Caty, & Ritchie, 1985; Lockwood, 1970); or combined methodologies (Pederson, 1996).

Many of these stress inoculation techniques serve as the foundation for psychological preparation—those interventions specifically designed to help children anticipate, deal with, and gain mastery over the events they will experience. Psychological preparation is necessary but not sufficient for effective coping. These concepts are inextricably intertwined. Coping is used in the psychological preparation literature as both a process and an outcome variable, whereas psychological preparation is a process variable in many coping studies.

Studies proved efficacious that helped children combine cognitive and emotional resources to actively participate in activities designed to desensitize threat and gain mastery over intrusive experiences (e.g., play,

---

[3]Also referred to as "stress immunization" or "psychological immunization."

behavioral rehearsal) as a method of coping (Clatworthy, 1981; Demarest et al., 1984; Lockwood, 1970; McGrath, 1979; Schmidt, 1990; Visintainer & Wolfer, 1975; Wolfer & Visintainer, 1975, 1979). Similar findings were noted in studies seeking to ameliorate parental stress directly or indirectly by providing them with the skills they needed to prepare their children (Abrams, 1982; Burke et al., 1997; Mahaffy, 1965; Visintainer & Wolfer, 1975; Wolfer & Visintainer, 1975, 1979; Zastowny et al., 1986).

Little data are available on the relationship between coping skills and styles and physiologic arousal (e.g., pain). Pain studies, arguably the most well-developed body of pediatric nursing research, have focused more on assessment than on intervention or outcomes (Abu-Saad & Hamers, 1997; Broome & Huth, in press; Vessey & Carlson, 1996). Other symptoms (e.g., nausea, fatigue) and biological variables (e.g., interrupted circadian rhythms, physiology of stress) that affect psychological functioning are largely absent from pediatric nursing research literature, despite being explicated in studies of adults (LaMontagne, Hepworth, Johnson, & Deshpande, 1994).

Measuring Coping

Nurse researchers have contributed a small body of methodological work. Using limited theoretical perspectives, they have attempted to operationalize both coping styles and coping strategies used by hospitalized children (Ryan-Wenger, 1994). Rose's (1972) observational method for measuring coping was grounded in Murphy and Moriarity's (1976) work on individual differences. It was later modified to study school-age children undergoing surgery (Savedra & Tesler, 1981; Tesler & Savedra, 1981). LaMontagne's (1984, 1987) work on the effect of temperament on coping styles resulted in the Preoperative Mode of Coping Interview, adapted from Cohen and Lazarus's (1973) avoidance-vigilance framework of adult coping.

Coping strategies have received greater attention. The Transactional Model of Stress and Coping (Lazarus, 1966) provided theoretical underpinning for the Children's Coping Strategies Checklists (Ritchie, Caty, & Ellerton, 1988; Ritchie, Caty, Ellerton, & Arklie, 1990) and the Schoolagers' Coping Strategies Inventory (Ryan, 1989; Ryan-Wenger, 1990). Lastly, Child Drawing: Hospital is an instrument that uses projective drawings to measure children's emotional status throughout hospitalization (Clatworthy, Simon, & Tiedeman, 1999).

SUMMARY AND CRITIQUE

Developmental Science Perspectives

Key concepts central to developmental science are that (a) the individual develops and functions as an integrated organism, (b) the individual develops and functions in continuously ongoing interactions with his or her environment, and (c) biological, ecological, and cognitive/behavioral factors dynamically interact with each other during these processes (Magnusson, 1995). Exploration of these concepts mandates multisystem, complex research approaches (Cairns, 2000). To date, nursing research on children's psychological responses to hospitalization has not significantly used these concepts. In part it is an issue of timing. When the trajectory of nursing research on children's psychological responses to hospitalization was initiated four decades ago, developmental science had not yet been conceived. However, most newer studies also fail to embrace the developmental science perspective.

Theoretical and Conceptual Underpinnings

Numerous theoretical frameworks adapted from grand and midrange theories are used to study children's psychological responses to hospitalization. Some programs of research (e.g., the works of Burke, LaMontagne, Ritchie, Ryan-Wenger, and their colleagues) have a strong theoretical grounding. A potpourri of conceptually disparate theories guides others. Lastly, a small group is atheoretical, with the research question derived directly from clinical practice.

THEORIES FROM THE SOCIAL SCIENCES

Studies conducted in the 1960s and 1970s that focused on the effects of separation and its amelioration by rooming-in used theoretical frameworks rooted in the psychoanalytic (e.g., Freud, Erikson) and ethological (e.g., Bowlby) traditions. As attention shifted to psychological preparation in the 1970s and early 1980s, cognitive developmental theories (Piaget) were used to explain how children developed concepts of their bodies, illness, and hospitalization (Bibace & Walsh, 1981). Behavioral theory combined with theories of stress was heavily used in descriptive studies and was foundational to the stress-inoculation interventions.

Numerous stress and coping theories have been used. Murphy's (1974) concepts of coping provided the theoretical underpinnings for Rose's (1972) work on coping processes of hospitalized children and for descriptive studies (Tesler & Savedra, 1981). As previously noted, Lazarus and colleague's (Lazarus, 1966; Cohen & Lazarus, 1973) stress and adaptation theory also was widely embraced. Information-processing theories (e.g., self-regulation and control) were adopted by Melnyk (1994, 1995) and colleagues (1997) to look at parental and child coping. Finally, McCubbin and Patterson's (1983) double ABCX Model of Crisis was used in intervention studies designed to moderate parental stress through mutual participation (Curley, 1988; Curley & Wallace, 1992).

As the importance of individual differences was recognized, theories about explicating their influence on psychological outcomes of hospitalization were adopted. These included temperament theory, attributional theories (e.g., locus of control), and theories about the contributions of experience (LaMontagne, 1984, 1987; LaMontagne et al., 2000; McClowry, 1988).

NURSING THEORY

Nursing theories are virtually absent in studies of children's responses to hospitalization, suggesting that their utility in describing, explaining, or predicting the phenomena of interest is not readily evident to investigators. Although grand theories were evolving during the same time that the first nursing intervention studies in this area were initiated, it was psychological theories of stress and coping that were embraced by investigators. No doubt this was due to their obvious (although untested) utility.

Most of the theoretical perspectives used did not have a developmental approach. The most frequently used theoretical perspective, Lazarus's (1966) model of cognitive appraisal, was derived to explain adult behavior and pays little regard to the effects of growth, maturation, experience, or ecological factors (e.g., parental behavior, hospital milieu) on developing coping styles and processes. As a result, available knowledge only explains children's psychological responses to hospitalization at their current psychological disposition and does not explain the ontogeny of these responses.

Another area of concern is the influence of early assumptions made about hospitalized children on their responses to hospitalization. The psychological upset of hospitalized children was often considered a maladaptive process. When this assumption colored a study's design, it became impossible to determine whether children who displayed psychological upset were engaging in healthy, active adaptation to stressful situations or suffering from trauma, and what the long-term ramifications might be. Without a longitudinal perspective, interventions that effectively prevent signs of short-term behavioral upset may be insufficient or possibly even harmful.

Children's responses to hospitalization were usually considered outside the nexus of biological, cognitive, and ecological forces. The assumption was made that hospitalized and nonhospitalized children came from similar backgrounds. This limits understanding of how a child's ecology (e.g., family culture, environment) mediates response patterns. Moreover, focusing only on hospitalization, rather than including other variables such as illness severity, chronicity, and symptomatology, does little to inform us about biological influences. Finally, the relationships between a child's developing metacognitive abilities and coping behaviors from within the context of experience (Yoos, 1994) need to be considered.

Methodological Considerations

Collectively, studies addressing children's psychological responses to hospitalization lack scientific rigor. These methodological issues are critically discussed elsewhere (Barnard, 1983; Denyes, 1983; McClowry, 1988; Melnyk, 2000; O'Conner-Von, 2000; Thompson, 1985; Vernon et al., 1965; Vernon & Thompson, 1993). Common problem areas identified in this and previous reviews are listed in Table 7.1. Insufficient information about methodological details, including interventions, renders most studies irreproducible.

DESIGN ISSUES

The earliest nursing research examining children's responses to hospitalization used case study (Barnes, Bandak, & Beardslee, 1990; Caty, Ellerton, & Ritchie, 1984), descriptive, or correlational designs (Thompson, 1985). The emphasis was on describing children's psychological responses to hospitalization at single points of time and in response to specific stressors (Riffee, 1981). Case studies, primarily published in the *Maternal-Child Nursing Journal*, provided limited insight on this topic (Barnes et al., 1990).

TABLE 7.1   Common Methodological Weaknesses of Research Investigating Children's Psychological Responses to Hospitalization

- Inappropriate use of theory, confounding theoretical implications
- Insufficient sampling: use of convenience samples, limited age span, failure to address cultural issues, etc.
- Inadequate description of procedures
- Failure to use control groups
- Failure to control observer bias
- Insufficient concern with appropriateness, reliability, and/or validity of measures
- Insufficient statistical analyses
- A narrow range of designs employed

A small body of intervention research on ameliorating children's negative responses during hospitalization and in the immediate posthospital period usually used two- or three-group pretest, post-test designs. These designs emphasized short-term negative psychological sequelae, rather than any maturation that may have resulted from hospitalization. Newer studies have embraced more complex methodologies and have examined more intriguing questions, such as the influence of development (McClowry, 1990; LaMontagne et al., 2000) and the role of parental behaviors and family functioning (Burke et al., 2001; Melnyk, 2000). Reliability and validity problems in design are common. These include the failure to provide information about manipulation checks, Hawthorne effect issues, measurement blinding, and so on.

Few qualitative studies were conducted in nursing to investigate children's views of hospitalization, despite the presence of such work in other disciplines (Barowsky, 1978; Beuf, 1979). Exceptions were Barnes's (1975a, 1975b) work in children's responses to the intensive care unit and the elegant work of Ritchie, Caty, and Ellerton (1984), who identified concerns of ill and healthy preschoolers. Studies by Burke and colleagues (1991, 1998) of stressors of parents with chronically ill children focused on the parents but provided insights into children's responses as well. Whether the lack of qualitative studies is due to children being viewed as incapable or unreliable reporters of their own reality or to a historical lack of research diversification and sophistication within nursing can only be speculated. However, failing to explore this phenomenon holistically and from the child's vantage point has no doubt limited the development of assessment instruments or interventions (Woodgate, 2001).

Few studies used methodologies that could capture the complexity and dynamics of the bio-psycho-social interactions involved in the hospitalization experience. For example, the design of most intervention studies has focused on only one aspect of coping, either problem solving or regulation of emotional responses. Emphasis on single variables restricts understanding of the interplay and bidirectionality of these factors. When results are only available for sample aggregates, information that might be garnered from examining outliers is lost.

The lack of person-centered, longitudinal study designs and the use of static points of measurement negate the temporal dimension of development and prohibit the identification of longer-term psychological responses (Elder, 1998). For example, negative behavioral change can persist or increase in the weeks following hospitalization (Melnyk, 2000). However, preliminary evidence suggests that, despite initial psychological upset, hospitalization may promote a sense of mastery and accomplishment over the long term (Månsson, Fredikzon, & Rosberg, 1992; Peterson & Shigetomi, 1982). Such concerns underscore the need for longitudinal designs.

SAMPLING

Study samples do not reflect the universe of sick children, with the preschool and school-age period being overrepresented and infants and adolescents rarely being included. Half the intervention studies used a sample of school-age children undergoing tonsillectomies and adenoidectomies, no doubt because there was a sufficiently large pool of demographically similar children. Concomitantly, studies often fail to differentiate the cognitive and developmental differences of subgroups of children within a single study. The same intervention would be applied to children from ages 3 to 16 with varying levels of hospitalization experience. As previously noted, minimal attention was given to demographic variables such as race/ethnicity, religiosity, culture, socioeconomic status, or rural/metropolitan locale.

MEASUREMENT

Investigators have examined children's psychological responses at various levels of abstraction (e.g., from global mood disorders to specific behaviors such as enuresis) and have operationalized responses accordingly. The majority of instruments used focused on the psychological dimensions of stress and coping. Instruments commonly used and developed outside of nursing include the Hospital Fears Rating Scale, the Manifest Upset Scale, the Observer Rating Scale of Anxiety, and the Post-Hospital Behavior Questionnaire. All were designed to capture the psychological distress rather than the psychological benefit of hospitalization. The psychometric properties of these instruments vary considerably. Most were normed on relatively narrow samples and have limited reliability and validity. With some exceptions (Carty, 1977), investigators did not use instruments that were normed outside of the hospitalization experience or that could measure social and emotional maturity.

Of special concern is the failure to refine early instruments and techniques in more recent research. For example, one of the first standardized instruments that codified children's psychological responses was the 28-item, six-factor, Post-Hospital Behavior Questionnaire (Vernon, Schulman, & Foley, 1966). This tool was widely adopted by nurse researchers (Abrams, 1982; Kennedy & Riddle, 1989; McGrath, 1979; Schmidt, 1990; Visintainer & Wolfer, 1975; Wolfer & Visintainer, 1975, 1979), despite its lack of psychometric properties or its appropriateness for the changing hospital environment with its greater emphasis on developmentally appropriate support (Vernon & Thompson, 1993).

Failure to capture relevant information because of poor instrumentation particularly affects intervention studies on psychological preparation. Generally, these studies measured anxiety abatement and improved cooperation at points during hospitalization but did not assess process issues such as what the children learned, the extent to which they expressed concerns, and the level of trust with providers (O'Conner-Von, 2000; Thompson, 1985). The advent of video technologies in the 1980s and 1990s provided a mechanism for reducing observer bias and collecting direct information from the child. However, with a few exceptions (e.g., Månsson et al., 1993; Ritchie et al., 1988), these were not used.

Biological responses have rarely been incorporated into studies of children's psychological responses to hospitalization. Thus, biological and immunological markers of stress, such as cortisol, catecholamines, or cytokines, were underutilized. When physiologic measures were used, the study presumed cause and effect rather than examining the bidirectionality and interconnectedness with cognitive and ecological variables (Cairns, Elder, & Costello, 1997). Psychological and physiological methods of measuring stress frequently yield contradictory information. These questions beg investigation, which today's burgeoning literature on biobehavioral interactions could illuminate. Such information, now obtainable from developmental psychobiology where animal models are used to manipulate biological, social, and environmental interconnections of stress responses, could help elucidate our understanding of children's psychological responses to hospitalization (Magnusson, 1995).

Early studies reported poor correlations between physiological and psychological measures in determining "successful" outcomes (Thompson, 1985). Other studies failed to show a difference in the cortisol levels of children with varying anxiety levels (Barnes, Kenney, Call, & Reinhart, 1972) or interventions comparing nonpharmacological and pharmacological preparation for surgery (Månsson, Fredikzon, & Rosberg, 1992). The most common measures, first voiding after surgery (Mahaffy, 1965; McGrath, 1979), vital signs (Mahaffy, 1965; McGrath, 1979), or enumeration of active sweat glands (Dabbs, Johnson, & Leventhal, 1968; Johnson & Dabbs, 1967), were used but were discarded because of their high reactivity or lack of measurement sensitivity. Although recent monitoring technologies have fewer measurement problems, they have rarely been used.

DATA ANALYSIS TECHNIQUES

Simple analytic strategies are the norm for this body of research, although, during the past decade, more complex analytic techniques (e.g., regression or path analyses) have been used. These techniques have generally sought to disentangle the contributions of numerous variables to psychological upset. Statistical analyses also focused on the sample aggregate, rather than the individual. Intergenerational studies were limited to the child-parent dyad and did not extend to the larger kin network.

The absence of other analytic techniques mirrors the simplicity (or insufficiency) of the designs adopted. An attempt to conduct a comprehensive meta-analysis of the psychological preparation literature was foiled by methodological problems and lack of necessary data in the majority of published studies (Vessey & Carlson, 1993). Meta-analyses of other variables, such as distraction as a pain intervention (Kleiber & Harper, 1999), have been published.

Interdisciplinary Collaboration

Cairns (2000) notes that because developmental science is a metatheory of developmental principles designed to guide disparate areas of developmental inquiry, we need interdisciplinary research that transcends individual disciplines and institutional barriers. Virtually all nursing research on children's psychological responses to hospitalization incorporates theory and methods first espoused by other disciplines, primarily psychology. A number of studies also reflect true interdisciplinary involvement. Unfortunately, there are few sustained programs of research on children's psychological responses to hospitalization. Despite the salience of the topic to pediatric nursing practice, significant barriers to conducting such research exist, including difficulty accessing samples, a limited number of reliable and valid instruments, and limited funding opportunities (Vessey, 1998).

AREAS FOR FUTURE STUDY

Nursing research that addresses children's psychological responses to hospitalization continues to evolve. Since the mid-1960s, nursing research has contributed to the increasingly complex body of knowledge on identifying children's psychological responses to hospitalization and the factors that influence them. Still, there is a great need to revisit the children's responses to hospitalization and related themes. Nursing must reexamine "what we know," or more precisely, "what we think we know" about children's responses to hospitalization within the framework proposed by developmental science and within the current contexts of health care delivery.

For example, much of the intervention research was conducted between the 1970s and early 1990s using stress inoculation techniques. Stress inoculation requires that interventions take place in advance and in a relatively anxiety-free situation (Poster, 1983). This is difficult to achieve in today's hospital milieu, which includes shorter inpatient stays, children being treated outside of pediatric units, different staffing patterns, and greater family involvement in care (regardless of their desire or preparation) juxtapositioned against greater patient acuity, more invasive procedures performed in outpatient settings, and more (but not necessarily correctly) informed families. The collective impact of these factors brings into question the effectiveness and efficacy of knowledge from older intervention studies, already problematic because of their paucity and methodological limitations. New intervention work must meld the advances in developmental theory with the clinical realities of patient care.

Children's responses to hospitalization evolve from reciprocal interactions with the social and physical environments and in response to internal biological, cognitive, and psychological forces and, thus, cannot be explained by studying contributing factors in isolation from each other. The next generation of studies needs solid theoretical frameworks that embrace precepts from developmental-psycho-biology and that are of sufficient methodological complexity to capture the interplay of numerous seemingly disparate variables. Creating metatheory by articulating theoretical knowledge across domains will help identify the ontogeny of children's responses to hospitalization.

Methodologies that promote understanding of how disparate variables work together in affecting children's responses to hospitalization are needed. Developmental science proposes that events that help establish behavior patterns are usually different from those needed to maintain it. Hospitalization is often a landmark event a child's life course and helps shape the ontogeny of the child's responses to illness and health care. Although the developmental impact of an event is dependent on when it occurs during an individual's life (Elder, 1998), little is known about the real contribution of age. For this reason, it is critically important that children's psychological responses to hospitalization be examined from the perspective of timing and its relationship to age as well as to previous experience, socialization, personality, biological factors, and ecological circumstances. This will require complex designs that examine the bidirectionality of responses and longitudinal studies that assess the long-term impact of hospitalization, particularly long-term critical care hospitalizations, on children's development.

Methodologies need to address the individualized behavioral styles of children and also of their families. Newer, sophisticated designs (e.g., action research, qualitative designs), instrumentation (e.g., continual physiological measurement), and analyses (e.g., person-oriented analyses of outliers, metasynthesis) need to be explored. Person-centered designs and analyses will add information about the outliers—children who either cope very well or who are developmentally devastated as a result of hospitalization.

Newer data collection technologies (e.g., videotaping), when used with sophisticated study designs, also may help in capturing complex interrelated phenomena over time. All of these techniques will require testing and validation against traditional techniques (Cairns, 2000) to see if they can advance our knowledge of children's psychological responses to hospitalization.

New intervention studies that consider individual differences are needed to determine how to help children with varying strengths transcend the stressors of hospitalization and capitalize on their resilience, thus promoting emotional maturation. Only then can efficacious interventions that are also culturally sensitive, clinically efficient, reproducible, and cost-effective be tested and adopted. In addition, the current health care climate demands that health services research be conducted to demonstrate the cost-effectiveness of interventions that prevent or ameliorate poor psychological outcomes.

Interdisciplinary collaborative research on children's psychological responses to hospitalization is sorely needed. The need for programs of nursing research on children's responses to hospitalization that embrace the precepts of developmental science; are designed from an ecological, systems model; are methodologically rigorous; and have clinical relevance cannot be overstated in today's health care climate. Results are needed to create individualized milieus that allow children and families to transcend situational crises of hospitalization and illness and flourish emotionally.

ACKNOWLEDGMENTS

The assistance of Wanda Anderson, Boston College Reference Librarian, and Melissa Rumsey, Research Assistant, in identifying and procuring references is gratefully acknowledged. Support for this study was provided by Boston College Undergraduate Research Assistants Program.

REFERENCES

Abbott, N. C., Hansen, P., & Lewis, K. (1970). Dress rehearsal for the hospital. *American Journal of Nursing, 70,* 2360–2362.

Abrams, L. (1982). Resistance behaviors and teaching media for children in day surgery. *AORN Association of Operating Room Nurses, 35,* 244–258.

Abu-Saad, H. H., & Hamers, J. P. (1997). Decision-making and paediatric pain: A review. *Journal of Advances in Nursing, 26,* 946–952.

Bailey, T. F. (1967). Puppets teach young patients. *Nursing Outlook, 15,* 36–37.

Barnard, K. E. (1983). Nursing research related to infants and young children. *Annual Review of Nursing Research, 1,* 3–25.

Barnard, K. E., & Neal, M. V. (1977). Maternal-child nursing research: Review of the past and strategies for the future. *Nursing Research, 26,* 193–200.

Barnes, C. M. (1975a). School-age children's recall of the intensive care unit. *ANA clinical sessions, San Francisco, 1974.* New York: Appleton-Century-Crofts.

Barnes, C. M. (1975b). Levels of consciousness indicated by responses of children to phenomena in the intensive care unit. *Maternal-Child Nursing Journal, 4,* 215–285.

Barnes, C. M., Bandak, A. G., & Beardslee, C. I. (1990). Content analysis of 186 descriptive case studies of hospitalized children. *Maternal-Child Nursing Journal, 19,* 281–296.

Barnes, C. M., Kenney, F. M., Call, T., & Reinhart, J. B. (1972). Measurement in management of anxiety in children for open-heart surgery. *Pediatrics, 9,* 250–259.

Barowsky, E. I. (1978). Young children's perceptions and reactions to hospitalization. In E. Gellert (Ed.), *Psychological aspects of pediatric care* (pp. 37–50). New York: Grune and Stratton.

Beuf, A. (1979). *Biting off the bracelet. A study of children in hospitals.* Philadelphia: University of Pennsylvania Press.

Bibace, R., & Walsh, M. (Eds.). (1981). *Children's conceptions of health, illness, and bodily functions.* San Francisco: Jossey-Bass.

Bransetter, E. (1969a). The young child's response to hospitalization: Separation anxiety or lack of mothering care? *American Journal of Public Health, 59,* 92–97.

Bransetter, E. (1969b). The young child's response to hospitalization: Separation anxiety or lack of mothering care? *Communicating Nursing Research, 2,* 13–25.

Broome, M. E., & Huth, M. (in press). Nursing management of the child in pain. In N. Schechter, C. Berde, & M. Yaster (Eds.), *Pain in infants, children and adolescents* (2nd ed.). Philadelphia: Lippincott, Williams and Wilkins.

Broome, M. E., Rehwaldt, M., & Fogg, L. (1998). Relationships between cognitive behavioral techniques, temperament, observed distress, and pain reports in children and adolescents during lumbar puncture. *Journal of Pediatric Nursing, 13,* 48–54.

Burke, S. O., Costello, E. A., & Handley-Derry, M. H. (1989). Maternal stress and repeated hospitalization of children who are physically disabled. *Children's Health Care, 18,* 82–90.

Burke, S. O., Handley-Derry, M. H., Costello, E. A., Kauffmann, E., & Dillon, M. C. (1997). Stress-point intervention for parents of repeatedly hospitalized children with chronic conditions. *Research in Nursing and Health, 20,* 475–485.

Burke, S. O., Harrison, M. B., Kauffmann, E., & Wong, C. (2001). Effects of stress-point intervention with families of repeatedly hospitalized children. *Journal of Family Nursing, 7,* 128–158.

Burke, S. O., Kauffmann, E., Costello, E. A., & Dillon, M. C. (1991). Hazardous secrets and reluctantly taking charge: Parenting a child with repeated hospitalizations. *Image: Journal of Nursing Scholarship, 23,* 39–45.

Burke, S. O., Kauffmann, E., Costello, E., Wiskin, N., & Harrison, M. B. (1998). Stressors in families with a child with a chronic condition: An analysis of qualitative studies and a framework. *Canadian Journal of Nursing Research, 30,* 71–95.

Cairns, R. B. (2000). Developmental science: Three audacious implications. In L. R. Bergman, R. B. Cairns, L. Nilsson, & L. Nystedt (Eds.), *Developmental science and the holistic approach* (pp. 49–72). Mahway, NJ: Lawrence Erlbaum Associates.

Cairns, R. B., Elder, G. H., & Costello, E. J. (1997). The making of developmental science. In R. B. Cairns, G. H. Elder, & E. J. Costello (Eds.), *Developmental science* (pp. 223–234). New York: Lawrence Erlbaum Associates.

Carty, R. M. (1977). Identification of behavioral responses of preschool-age children before, during, and after hospitalization in a pediatric intensive care unit (Doctoral dissertation, Catholic University of America, 1977). *Dissertation Abstracts International, 38,* 1380–1381B.

Caty, S., Ellerton, M. L., & Ritchie, J. A. (1984). Coping in hospitalized children: An analysis of published case studies. *Nursing Research, 33,* 277–282.

Clatworthy, S. (1981). Therapeutic play: Effects on hospitalized children. *Children's Health Care, 9,* 108–113.

Clatworthy, S., Simon, K., & Tiedeman, M. E. (1999). Child drawing: Hospital-instrument designed to measure the emotional status of hospitalized school-aged children. *Journal of Pediatric Nursing, 14,* 2–9.

Cohen, F., & Lazarus, R. S. (1973). Active coping processes, coping dispositions, and recovery from surgery. *Psychosomatic Medicine, 35,* 375–389.

Cooper, H. M. (1989). *Integrating research: A guide for literature reviewers* (2nd ed.). Newbury Park, CA: Sage.

Cormier, P. P. (1979). Identification of typologies derived from child behaviors in the hospital as predictors of psychological upset. *Journal of Psychiatric Nursing and Mental Health Services, 17*(6), 28–35.

Curley, M. A. Q. (1988). Effects of the nursing mutual participation model of care and parental stress in the pediatric intensive care unit. *Heart and Lung, 17,* 682–688.

Curley, M. A. Q., & Wallace, J. (1992). Effects of the nursing mutual participation model of care on parental stress in the pediatric intensive care unit—a replication. *Journal of Pediatric Nursing, 17,* 377–385.

Dabbs, J. M., Johnson, J. E., & Leventhal, H. (1968). Palmar sweating: A quick and simple measure. *Journal of Experimental Psychology, 78,* 347–350.

Davenport, H. T., & Werry, J. S. (1970). The effect of general anesthesia, surgery and hospitalization upon the behavior of children. *American Journal of Orthopsychiatry, 40,* 806–824.

Demarest, D. S., Hooke, J. F., & Erickson, M. T. (1984). Preoperative intervention for the reduction of anxiety in pediatric surgery patients. *Children's Health Care, 12,* 179–183.

Denyes, M. J. (1983). Nursing research related to school-age children and adolescents. *Annual Review of Nursing Research, 1,* 27–53.

Elder, G. H. (1998). The life course as developmental theory. *Child Development, 69,* 1–12.

Ellerton, M., Caty, S., & Ritchie, J. A. (1985). Helping young children master intrusive procedures through play. *Children's Health Care, 13,* 167–173.

Fagin, C. M. (1966). *The effects of maternal attendance during hospitalization on the posthospital behavior of young children.* Philadelphia: F. A. Davis.

Fletcher, B. (1981). Psychological upset in posthospitalized children: A review of the literature. *Maternal-Child Nursing Journal, 10,* 185–193.

Glazebrook, C. P., & Sheard, C. E. (1994). A prospective study of factors associated with delayed discharge in school-age children undergoing ward-based minor surgery. *International Journal of Nursing Studies, 31*(6), 487–497.

Godfrey, A. E. (1955). A study of nursing care designed to assist hospitalized children and their parents in their separation. *Nursing Research, 4,* 52–70.

Hennessey, J. A. (1976). Hospitalized toddlers; responses to mothers' tape recordings during brief separations. *Maternal-Child Nursing Journal, 5,* 69–91.

Holt, J. L. (1968). Discussion of the method and clinical implications from the study "Children's recall of a pre-school age hospital experience after an interval of five years." *Communicating Nursing Research, 1,* 56–81.

Johnson, J. E., & Dabbs, J. M. (1967). Enumeration of active sweat glands: A simple physiological indicator of psychological changes. *Nursing Research, 16,* 273–275.

Kennedy, C., & Riddle, I. I. (1989). The influence of the timing of preparation on the anxiety of preschool children experiencing surgery. *Maternal-Child Nursing Journal, 18,* 117–132.

Kleiber, C., & Harper, D. C. (1999). Effects of distraction on children's pain and distress during medical procedures: A meta-analysis. *Nursing Research, 48,* 44–49.

Lambert, S. A. (1984). Variables that affect the school-age child's reaction to hospitalization and surgery: A review of the literature. *Maternal-Child Nursing Journal, 13*(1), 1–18.

LaMontagne, L. L. (1984). Children's locus of control beliefs as predictors of preoperative coping behavior. *Nursing Research, 33,* 76–79.

LaMontagne, L. L. (1987). Children's preoperative coping: Replication and extension. *Nursing Research, 36,* 163–167.

LaMontagne, L. L. (2000). Children's coping with surgery: A process-oriented perspective. *Journal of Pediatric Nursing, 15,* 307–312.

LaMontagne, L. L., Hepworth, J. T., & Cohen, F. (2000). Effects of surgery type and attention focus on children's coping. *Nursing Research, 49,* 245–252.

LaMontagne, L. L., Hepworth, J. T., Johnson, B., & Cohen, F. (1996). Children's preoperative coping and its effects on postoperative anxiety and return to normal activity. *Nursing Research, 45,* 141–147.

LaMontagne, L. L., Hepworth, J. T., Johnson, B., & Deshpande, J. K. (1994). Psychophysiological responses of parents to pediatric critical care stress. *Clinical Nursing Research, 3,* 105–118.

LaMontagne, L. L., Johnson, J. E., Hepworth, J. T., & Johnson, B. D. (1997). Attention, coping, and activity in children undergoing orthopaedic surgery. *Research in Nursing and Health, 20,* 487–494.

LaMontagne, L. L., Wells, N., Hepworth, J. T., Johnson, B. D., & Manes, R. (1999). Parent coping and child distress behaviors during invasive procedures for childhood cancer. *Journal of Pediatric Oncology Nursing, 16,* 3–12.

Lazarus, R. S. (1966). *Psychological stress and the coping process.* New York: McGraw-Hill.

Lipman, T. H., & Hayman, L. L. (2000). Celebrating 25 years of pediatric nursing research: Progress and prospects. *MCN: American Journal of Maternal-Child Nursing, 25,* 331–335.

Lockwood, N. L. (1970). The effects of situational doll play upon the preoperative stress reactions of hospitalized children. *ANA clinical sessions, Miami* (pp. 120–133). New York: Appleton-Century-Crofts.

Magnusson, D. (1995). Individual development: A holistic, integrated model. In P. Moen, G. H. Elder, & K. Luscher (Eds.), *Examining lives in context* (pp. 19–60). Washington, DC: American Psychological Association.

Magnusson, D., & Cairns, R. B. (1996). Developmental science: Toward a unified framework. In R. B. Cairns, G. H. Elder, & E. J. Costello (Eds.), *Developmental science* (pp. 7–30). New York: Lawrence Erlbaum Associates.

Mahaffy, P. R. (1965). The effects of hospitalization on children admitted for tonsillectomy and adenoidectomy. *Nursing Research, 14,* 12–19.

Månsson, M. E., Björkhem, G., & Wiebe, T. (1993). The effect of preparation for lumbar puncture on children undergoing chemotherapy. *Oncology Nursing Forum, 20,* 39–45.

Månsson, M. E., Fredikzon, B., & Rosberg, B. (1992). Comparison of preparation and narcotic-sedative premedication in children undergoing surgery. *Pediatric Nursing, 18,* 337–342.

McCaffery, M. (1971). Children's responses to rectal temperatures: An exploratory study. *Nursing Research, 20,* 32–45.

McClowry, S. G. (1988). A review of the literature pertaining to the psychosocial responses of school-aged children to hospitalization. *Journal of Pediatric Nursing, 3,* 296–311.

McClowry, S. G. (1990). The relationship of temperament to pre- and posthospitalization behavioral responses of school-age children. *Nursing Research, 39,* 30–35.

McCubbin, H. I., & Patterson, J. M. (1983). Family transitions: Adaptation to stress. In H. I. McCubbin & C. R. Figley (Eds.), *Stress and the family: I. Coping with normative transitions* (pp. 5–25). New York: Brunner/Mazel.

McGillicuddy, M. C. (1976). A study of the relationship between mothers' rooming-in during their children's hospitalization and changes in selected areas of children's behavior (Doctoral dissertation, New York University, 1976). *Dissertation Abstracts International, 37,* 700-B.

McGrath, M. M. (1979). Group preparation of pediatric surgical patients. *Image, 11,* 52–62.

Melnyk, B. M. (1994). Coping with unplanned childhood hospitalization: Effects of informational interventions on mothers and children. *Nursing Research, 43,* 50–55.

Melnyk, B. M. (1995). Coping with unplanned childhood hospitalization: The mediating functions of parental beliefs. *Journal of Pediatric Psychology, 20,* 299–312.

Melnyk, B. M. (2000). Intervention studies involving parents of hospitalized young children: An analysis of the past and future recommendations. *Journal of Pediatric Nursing, 15,* 4–13.

Melnyk, G. M., Alpert-Gillis, L. J., Hensel, P. B., Cable-Beiling, R. C., & Rubenstein, J. S. (1997). Helping mothers cope with a critically ill child: A pilot test of the COPE intervention. *Research in Nursing and Health, 20,* 3–14.

Meng, A. L. (1980). Parents' and children's reactions toward impending hospitalization for surgery. *Maternal-Child Nursing Journal, 9*(20), 83–98.

Meng, A. L., & Zastowny, T. R. (1982). Preparation for hospitalization: A stress inoculation training program for parents and children. *Maternal-Child Nursing Journal, 11,* 87–94.

Miles, M. S. (1969). Body integrity fears in a toddler. *Nursing Clinics of North America, 4,* 39–51.

Murphy, L. B. (1974). Coping, vulnerability, and resilience in childhood. In G. V. Coelho, D. A. Hamburg, & J. E. Adams (Eds.), *Coping and adaptation* (pp. 69–99). New York: Basic Books.

Murphy, L. B., & Moriarity, A. E. (1976). *Vulnerability, coping, and growth.* New Haven: Yale University Press.

O'Conner-Von, S. (2000). Preparing children for surgery—an integrative research review. *AORN Journal, 71,* 334–343.

Olson, R. K., Heater, B. S., & Becker, A. M. (1990). A meta-analysis of the effects of nursing interventions on children and parents. *MCN: American Journal of Maternal-Child Nursing, 15,* 104–108.

Pederson, C. (1996). Promoting parental use of nonpharmacologic techniques with children during lumbar punctures. *Journal of Pediatric Oncology Nursing, 13,* 21–30.

Peterson, L., & Shigetomi, C. (1982). One-year follow-up on elective surgery child patients receiving pre-operative preparation. *Journal of Pediatric Psychology, 7,* 43–38.

Poster, E. C. (1983). Stress immunization: Techniques to help children cope with hospitalization. *Maternal-Child Nursing Journal, 12,* 119–134.

Prugh, D. G. (1965). Emotional aspects of the hospitalization of children. In M. F. Shore (Ed.), *"Red is the color of hurting." Planning for children in the hospital* (pp. 17–36). Bethesda: National Institute of Mental Health.

Prugh, D. G., Staub, E., Sands, H. H., Kirschbaum, R. M., & Lenihan, E. A. (1953). A study of the emotional reactions of children and families to hospitalization and illness. *American Journal of Orthopsychiatry, 23,* 70–106.

Riffee, D. M. (1981). Self-esteem changes in hospitalized school-age children. *Nursing Research, 30,* 94–97.

Ritchie, J. A., Caty, S., & Ellerton, M. L. (1984). Concerns of acutely ill, chronically ill, and healthy preschool children. *Research in Nursing and Health, 7,* 265–274.

Ritchie, J. A., Caty, S., & Ellerton, M. L. (1988). Coping behaviors of hospitalized preschool children. *Maternal-Child Nursing Journal, 17,* 153–171.

Ritchie, J. A., Caty, S., Ellerton, M. L., & Arklie, M. M. (1990). Descriptions of preschoolers' coping with fingerpricks from a transactional model. *Behavioral Assessment, 12,* 213–222.

Rose, M. H. (1972). The effects of hospitalization on the coping behaviors of children. In M. V. Batey (Ed.), *Communicating nursing research.* Boulder, CO: Western Interstate Commission for Higher Education.

Ryan, N. M. (1989). Stress-coping strategies identified from school age children's perspective. *Research in Nursing and Health, 12,* 111–122.

Ryan-Wenger, N. M. (1990). Development and psychometric properties of the Schoolager's Coping Strategies Inventory. *Nursing Research, 39,* 344–349.

Ryan-Wenger, N. M. (1994). Coping behavior in children: Methods of measurement for research and clinical practice. *Journal of Pediatric Nursing, 9,* 183–195.

Ryan-Wenger, N. M. (1996). Children, coping, and the stress of illness: A synthesis of the research. *Journal of the Society of Pediatric Nurses, 1,* 126–138.

Savedra, M., & Tesler, M. (1981). Coping strategies of hospitalized school-age children. *Western Journal of Nursing Research, 3,* 371–384.

Scavnicky-Mylant, M. L. (1987). The hospitalized school-age child's capacity for an appraisal of threat. *Western Journal of Nursing Research, 9,* 503–526.

Schmidt, C. K. (1990). Pre-operative preparation: Effects on immediate pre-operative behavior, post-operative behavior, and recovery in children having same-day surgery. *Maternal-Child Nursing Journal, 19,* 321–330.

Schultz, N. V. (1971). How children perceive pain. *Nursing Outlook, 19,* 670–673.

Shore, M. F. (Ed.) (1965). *"Red is the color of hurting." Planning for children in the hospital.* Bethesda: National Institute of Mental Health.

Sipowcz, R. R., & Vernon, D. T. A. (1965). Psychological responses of children to hospitalization: A comparison of hospitalized and non-hospitalized twins. *American Journal of Disease of Children, 109,* 228–231.

Spitz, R. A. (1945). Hospitalism. *The Psychoanalytic Study of the Child, 1,* 53–74.

Stevens, M. (1986). Adolescents' perception of stressful events during hospitalization. *Journal of Pediatric Nursing, 1,* 303–313.

Stewart, M. L. (1977). Measurement of clinical pain. In A. K. Jacox (Ed.), *Pain: A source book for nurses and other health professionals* (pp. 107–137). Boston: Little, Brown.

Strickland, M. P., Leeper, J. D., Jessee, P., & Hudson, C. (1987). Children's adjustment to the hospital: A rural/urban comparison. *Maternal-Child Nursing Journal, 16,* 251–259.

Tesler, M., & Savedra, M. (1981). Coping with hospitalization: A study of school-age children. *Pediatric Nursing, 7*(2), 35–38.

Thompson, R. H. (1985). *Psychosocial research on pediatric hospitalization and health care. A review of the literature.* Springfield, IL: Charles C. Thomas.

Tiedeman, M. E. (1997). Anxiety responses of parents during and after the hospitalization of their 5- to 11-year-old children. *Journal of Pediatric Nursing, 12,* 110–119.

Vernon, D. T. A., Foley, J. M., Sipowcz, R. R., & Schulman, J. L. (1965). *The psychological responses of children to hospitalization and illness.* Springfield, IL: Charles C. Thomas.

Vernon, D. T. A., Schulman, J. L., & Foley, J. M. (1966). Changes in children's behavior after hospitalization. *American Journal of Diseases of Childhood, 111,* 581–593.

Vernon, D. T. A., & Thompson, R. H. (1993). Research on the effect of experimental interventions on children' behavior after hospitalization: A review and synthesis. *Journal of Developmental and Behavioral Pediatrics, 14,* 36–44.

Vessey, J. A. (1998). Historical overview of responses of children and their families to acute illness. In M. E. Broome, K. Knafl, K. Pridham, & S. Feetham (Eds.), *Children and families in health and illness* (pp. 99–114). Thousand Oaks, CA: Sage Publications.

Vessey, J. A., & Carlson, K. L. (1993, April). *A meta-analysis of the research on psychological preparation for hospitalization.* Paper presented at the annual meeting of Nursing Care of Children and Their Families, Society for Pediatric Nurses, San Francisco.

Vessey, J. A., & Carlson, K. L. (1996). Nonpharmacological interventions to use with children in pain. *Issues in Comprehensive Pediatric Nursing, 19,* 169–182.

Visintainer, M. A., & Wolfer, J. A. (1975). Psychological preparation for surgical pediatric patients: The effect of children's and parents' stress responses and adjustment. *Pediatrics, 56,* 187–202.

Vredevoe, D. L., Kim, A. C., Dambacher, B. M., & Call, J. D. (1969). Aggressive post-operative play responses of hospitalized preschool children. *Nursing Research, 4,* 1, 4–5.

West, C. (1954). *How to nurse sick children.* London: Longman. (Original work published 1854).

White, M. A., Williams, P. D., Alexander, D. J., Powell-Cope, G. M., & Conlon, M. (1990). Sleep onset latency and distress in hospitalized children. *Nursing Research, 39,* 134–139.

Wolfer, J. A., & Visintainer, M. A. (1975). Pediatric surgical patients' and parents' stress responses and adjustment as a function of psychological preparation and stress-point nursing care. *Nursing Research, 24,* 244–255.

Wolfer, J. A., & Visintainer, M. A. (1979). Prehospital psychological preparation for tonsillectomy patients: Effects on children's and parents' adjustment. *Pediatrics, 64,* 646–655.

Woodgate, R. (2001). Adopting the qualitative paradigm to understanding children's perspectives of illness: Barrier or facilitator? *Journal of Pediatric Nursing, 16,* 149–161.

Yoos, H. L. (1994). Children's illness concepts: Old and new paradigms. *Pediatric Nursing, 20,* 134–145.

Youssef, M. M. S. (1981). Self-control behaviors of school-age children who are hospitalized for cardiac diagnostic procedures. *Maternal-Child Nursing Journal, 10,* 219–284.

Zastowny, T. R., Kirschenbaum, D. S., & Meng, A. L. (1986). Coping skills training for children. Effects on distress before, during, and after hospitalization for surgery. *Health Psychology, 5,* 231–247.

Chapter 8

Children Living With Chronic Illness: An Examination of Their Stressors, Coping Responses, and Health Outcomes

JANET L. STEWART

ABSTRACT

This chapter reviews nursing research from the last decade on children and adolescents coping with chronic illnesses. Studies were identified by searches of MEDLINE and CINAHL and were included if at least one primary author was a nurse, the primary informants were children, and the focus of the study was on children's responses to illness and/or developmental stressors. Synthesis of the reviewed studies yielded typologies of illness-related and developmental stressors faced by chronically ill children, the coping strategies they commonly employed, and indices of their adjustment to illness. Although there was considerable agreement across illnesses, age ranges, and methodologies, the lack of explicitly employed developmental models or other theoretical perspectives means that very little is known about the processes by which individual characteristics, stressors, coping strategies, and outcomes are related. Recommendations for future research include the development and testing of conceptual models that will promote our understanding of how children's medical, psychosocial, and developmental outcomes can be improved, and a more systematic approach to understanding how children's maturing cognitive abilities affect their appraisal of stress and utilization of coping strategies in response to the demands of chronic illness.

The potential for serious medical illnesses to profoundly affect children's psychological functioning has generated considerable research interest in nursing as well as in the broader health disciplines over the last 30 years.

This interest has heightened as improvements in treatment for many childhood diseases have shifted attention away from the singular stress of acute life threat and toward the range of psychosocial demands engendered by prolonged illness (Kliewer, 1997; Thompson & Gustafson, 1996).

An early, and to some degree persistent, focus of research has been characterizing and quantifying chronically ill children's risk of negative psychological outcomes as compared to their non-ill peers. Two separate meta-analyses of comparative studies (Bennett, 1994; Lavigne & Faier-Routman, 1992) concluded that as a group, children with chronic illness are at increased risk for adjustment problems. However, they both noted considerable intragroup and intradisorder variability in the degree of adjustment difficulties that children exhibited, and they suggest that the relationship between childhood chronic illness and adjustment is neither simple nor direct. These and other researchers have advocated that future studies move beyond determining group differences in order to identify the specific personal, environmental, and illness-related factors that influence children's adjustment (Bennett, 1994; Lavigne & Faier-Routman, 1992; Wallander & Thompson, 1995). Children's cognitive appraisal of stressors and the coping processes they use to manage them are essential personal factors to be considered in any model of children's adjustment to chronic illness.

Prominent theorists from the health psychology discipline have advocated that the psychological consequences of childhood illnesses are most appropriately considered within a framework of adjustment, which implies a broad range of psychological functioning and incorporates both situational and temporal variability as children develop. Within this framework, children respond to the stresses associated with illness in both positive and negative ways that impact their concurrent psychoemotional functioning as well as their trajectory toward positive adult functioning (Wallander & Thompson, 1995). Cognitive processes, particularly children's appraisal of illness-related stressors and mobilization of coping strategies, may well be the most significant factors influencing children's adjustment within the context of serious illness (Thompson & Gustafson, 1996; Wallander & Marullo, 1993).

Traditionally, researchers have evoked "stage" models of cognitive development, particularly Piaget's representation of a constrained, age-dependent progression through levels of increasingly sophisticated thinking, to predict the quantity and quality of children's cognitive appraisals of illness (e.g., Bibace & Walsh, 1980). The application of such models, while providing a basic orientation to children's ways of thinking, has not fully explained how children come to understand and respond to the stresses associated with serious illness. It is increasingly recognized that children's experiences within the context of illness contribute to the development of more sophisticated domain-specific cognitive capacities than would be predicted by age alone (Chi & Ceci, 1987; Crisp, Ungerer, & Goodnow, 1996).

Pediatric nursing research has long recognized the importance of studying children's responses to chronic illness, with the most compelling goal of improving physical, psychological, and social outcomes for ill children and their families (Thomas, 1987). This review synthesizes findings from recent nursing research studies in order to determine what is currently known about children's and adolescents' responses to chronic illness, to examine the developmental scientific bases of the selected studies, and to identify problematic methodological and conceptual issues arising in the study of children with chronic illness. The intersection of illness-related demands and developmental changes across childhood and adolescence necessitates that childhood chronic illness research address developmentally relevant constructs and ultimately contribute to a developmental science that incorporates the study of non-normative stressors such as medical illness. Therefore, the reviewed nursing research studies will also be examined for the degree to which developmental science is considered in their conceptualization, design, implementation, and interpretation of findings.

METHODS

To locate the research studies included in this review, two electronic health publication databases (MEDLINE and CINAHL) were searched by the keyword phrase, "child and chronic illness," as well as by individual childhood chronic illnesses (e.g., asthma, cancer, epilepsy, etc.). (Unless otherwise specified, the term *child* is used to include school-age children and adolescents, i.e., children 6 to 18 years old.) Chronic illnesses included medical conditions with a chronic trajectory of illness and/or treatment, and excluded congenital anomalies, mental retardation, and sequelae of prematurity. Studies were selected for consideration if (a) at least one author could be identified as a nurse; (b) the research focus and primary informants were children (vs. parents, families, or caregivers); (c) the study utilized a noncategorical sample (subjects with different chronic illnesses) or one limited to a single disease; and (d) the focus of the study was on children's responses to illness and/or developmental stressors. Initially, studies published since 1994 were examined, and then previously published studies that contributed to the conceptualization and design of the same authors' more recent studies were included for review. Ultimately a few studies were included from the late 1980s, but the majority of studies were published within the last 10 years.

A total of 40 empirical studies were identified and retained in the current review (see Table 8.1). Including only those studies that used children as primary informants eliminated a considerable body of nursing research focusing on parental and family perspectives on childhood chronic illness. However, a serious deficit in knowledge generated from the child's perspective is one of the major limitations of the literature on childhood chronic illness (Amer, 1999b; Hayes, 1997), and therefore this criterion was deemed appropriate for a review of what is known about children's coping responses. The criterion of children as primary informants also set the lower limit on the age of children included in studies, since most studies relied on measurement approaches not validated with children younger than 7 or 8.

These 40 studies represent a heterogeneous pool of illness types, child ages, methodologies, variables, and frameworks. With two notable exceptions, the collective studies do not evolve from identifiable programs of research, but represent single or limited approaches to a given problem. Conceptual and empirical findings from the individual studies are organized within the following categories:

1. The nature of the identified stressors: What are children responding *to*?
2. Children's coping responses: *How* do children respond?
3. Child outcomes: What are the *consequences* from children's stressors and coping responses?
4. Intervention approaches: What works to improve children's adjustment?

The series of studies conducted by two independent nurse scientists and their colleagues will then be examined in depth as exemplars of evolving programs of research with the potential to improve the lives of children and adolescents with chronic illness. An evaluation of the degree to which

TABLE 8.1 Elements of the Reviewed Studies

Study	Sample Characteristics	Methods	Stressors/ Demands	Coping Responses	Outcomes/ Markers of Adjustment	Intervention(s)	Developmental Focus
Admi (1996)	◆ 16–25 yrs old ◆ categorical (cystic fibrosis) ◆ n = 10	◆ Grounded theory analysis of retrospective life-history interviews ◆ Longitudinal design	◆ Demands of illness & management regimen ◆ Intrusion of illness into normal life ◆ Unpredictable illness trajectory ◆ Negative peer reactions	◆ Selective disclosure ◆ Problem solving ◆ Focus on continuity of daily life ◆ Social support (parents)	◆ Definition of self as ordinary		◆ Approaches for managing intrusion into normal life changed with maturation ◆ Understanding of illness & treatment improved with maturation
Amer (1999)	◆ 7–16 yrs old ◆ quasi-categorical (IDDM & short stature) ◆ n = 27	◆ Content analysis of individual interviews	◆ Self-management demands ◆ Activity limitations ◆ Visible differences ◆ Disclosure ◆ Peer conflicts	◆ Downward comparison ◆ Compensatory personal attributes	◆ Self-esteem ◆ Mastery	◆ Bibliotherapy	

(continued)

TABLE 8.1 (*continued*)

Study	Sample Characteristics	Methods	Stressors/ Demands	Coping Responses	Outcomes/ Markers of Adjustment	Intervention(s)	Developmental Focus
Boland & Grey (1996)	◆ 8–12 yrs old ◆ categorical (diabetes) ◆ n = 43	◆ Self-report questionnaires ◆ Age comparisons	◆ Uncontrollable nature of illness-related stressors ◆ Intensive medical regimen	◆ Cognitive, behavioral, & emotional strategies ◆ Frequency & effectiveness	◆ Metabolic control	◆ Self-care	◆ Limited sample to single developmental stage ◆ Age-related differences in coping & outcomes
Boland, Grey, Mezger, & Tamborlane (1999)	◆ 12–20 yrs old ◆ categorical (diabetes) ◆ n = 40	◆ Self-report questionnaires ◆ Correlational design ◆ Longitudinal design	◆ Demanding medical regimen ◆ Changes in school calendar ◆ Family environment	◆ Self-care activities	◆ Metabolic control ◆ Quality of life		◆ School context provides structure & promotes self-care activities

TABLE 8.1 (*continued*)

Study	Sample Characteristics	Methods	Stressors/ Demands	Coping Responses	Outcomes/ Markers of Adjustment	Intervention(s)	Developmental Focus
Christian & D'Auria (1997)	◆ 12–18 yrs old ◆ categorical (cystic fibrosis) ◆ n = 20	◆ Grounded theory analysis of individual retrospective interviews	◆ Negative peer reactions ◆ Visible differences ◆ Normative school transitions	◆ Selective disclosure & social support seeking ◆ Problem solving	◆ Reduced sense of difference		◆ Social ecological framework ◆ Illness trajectory as challenge to developmental tasks of middle childhood & adolescence
D'Auria, Christian, & Richardson (1997)	◆ 6–12 yrs old ◆ categorical (cystic fibrosis) ◆ n = 20	◆ Grounded theory analysis of individual interviews	◆ Limited comprehension ◆ Negative peer reactions ◆ Activity limitations	◆ Maintaining secrecy ◆ Controlled self-presentation ◆ Problem solving	◆ Understanding personal & social meaning of illness		◆ Social implications of illness in middle childhood

(continued)

TABLE 8.1 (continued)

Study	Sample Characteristics	Methods	Stressors/ Demands	Coping Responses	Outcomes/ Markers of Adjustment	Intervention(s)	Developmental Focus
Ellerton, Stewart, Ritchie, & Hirth (1996)	◆ 8–17 yrs old ◆ non-categorical ◆ n = 47	◆ Comparative design (age group, type of stressor)	◆ Activity restrictions ◆ Demands of illness & treatment ◆ Peer conflicts ◆ Academic pressures	◆ Social support (peers, family)			◆ Age group comparisons ◆ Overlap between illness-related & everyday stressors for children with chronic illness
Grey, Boland, Yu, et al. (1998)	◆ 13–20 yrs old ◆ categorical (diabetes) ◆ n = 52	◆ Correlational & predictive design	◆ Increasingly intensive medical regimens ◆ Family environment	◆ Typology of coping behaviors	◆ Metabolic control ◆ Self-efficacy ◆ Depression ◆ Quality of life		◆ Family environment as developmentally relevant

TABLE 8.1 (*continued*)

Study	Sample Characteristics	Methods	Stressors/ Demands	Coping Responses	Outcomes/ Markers of Adjustment	Intervention(s)	Developmental Focus
Grey, Boland, Davidson, et al. (1998, 2000)	◆ 12–20 yrs old ◆ categorical (diabetes) ◆ n = 75	◆ Randomized clinical trial	◆ Increasingly intensive medical regimens	◆ Cognitive & behavioral strategies specific to illness context	◆ Metabolic control ◆ Acute illness complications ◆ Self-efficacy ◆ Quality of life	◆ Small group ◆ Cognitive strategies training	
Grey, Cameron, et al. (1991)	◆ 8–18 yrs old ◆ categorical (diabetes) ◆ n = 103	◆ Comparative design (by age/ maturational group)	◆ Self-care demands ◆ Stressful life events	◆ Typology of coping behaviors ◆ Self-care activities	◆ Metabolic control ◆ Social role performance ◆ Self-perception ◆ Anxiety ◆ Depression		◆ Adolescents at risk for diminished adjustment & poor metabolic control

(continued)

TABLE 8.1 *(continued)*

Study	Sample Characteristics	Methods	Stressors/Demands	Coping Responses	Outcomes/Markers of Adjustment	Intervention(s)	Developmental Focus
Grey, Cameron, et al. (1994)	◆ 8–16 yrs old ◆ categorical (newly diagnosed diabetes) ◆ n = 68	◆ Comparative design (non-ill peer group)	◆ Illness demands ◆ Stressful life events	◆ Typology of coping behaviors ◆ Self-care activities	◆ Overall health status ◆ Social role performance ◆ Self-perception ◆ Anxiety ◆ Depression		
Grey, Cameron, et al. (1995)	◆ 8–14 yrs old ◆ categorical (diabetes) ◆ n = 89	◆ Comparative design (healthy peer group) ◆ Longitudinal design			◆ Overall health status ◆ Social role performance ◆ Self-perception ◆ Anxiety ◆ Depression		◆ Non-ill peer group represents developmental trajectory for adjustment
Grey, Lipman, et al. (1997)	◆ 8–16 yrs old ◆ categorical (diabetes) ◆ n = 89	◆ Longitudinal design ◆ Predictive design		◆ Typology of coping behaviors ◆ Self-care activities	◆ Metabolic control ◆ Social role performance ◆ Self-perception		◆ Age-related differences in coping & outcomes ◆ Age/coping interactions

TABLE 8.1 (*continued*)

Study	Sample Characteristics	Methods	Stressors/ Demands	Coping Responses	Outcomes/ Markers of Adjustment	Intervention(s)	Developmental Focus
Haase & Rostad (1994)	◆ 5–17 yrs old ◆ categorical (cancer) ◆ n = 7	◆ Phenomenologic analysis of individual interviews & projective drawings	◆ Uncertainties surrounding completing therapy ◆ Reminders of aversive treatments	◆ Social support (peers, family) ◆ Hope ◆ Future orientation	◆ Sense of normalcy		
Haines et al. (2000)	◆ 12–15 yrs old ◆ categorical (diabetes) ◆ n = 14	◆ Randomized controlled clinical trial	◆ Illness-related stressors	◆ Cognitive-behavioral strategies	◆ Anxiety ◆ Diabetes-related stress ◆ Coping strategy use	◆ Small group ◆ Cognitive-behavioral training	◆ Limited age sample
Hinds & Martin, 1988; Hinds, Martin, & Vogel, 1987	◆ 12–18 yrs old ◆ categorical (cancer) ◆ n = 58	◆ Grounded theory analysis of individual interviews		◆ Cognitive-behavioral strategies	◆ Hope ◆ Cognitive comfort ◆ Personal competence		

(*continued*)

213

TABLE 8.1 *(continued)*

Study	Sample Characteristics	Methods	Stressors/ Demands	Coping Responses	Outcomes/ Markers of Adjustment	Intervention(s)	Developmental Focus
Hinds et al. (1999, 2000)	◆ 12–21 yrs old ◆ categorical (cancer) ◆ n = 78	◆ Randomized clinical trial	◆ Serious health threat ◆ Treatment demands	◆ Cognitive strategies to reduce distress & increase comfort ◆ Monitoring vs blunting	◆ Hopefulness ◆ Hopelessness ◆ Self-esteem ◆ Self-efficacy ◆ Symptom management	◆ Identification, modeling, & rehearsal of positive coping strategies	◆ Coping in adolescence directed at achieving developmental goal of autonomy ◆ Interaction of medical & developmental stressors put adolescents at increased risk
Horner (1998)	◆ 6–18 yrs old ◆ categorical (asthma) ◆ n = 12	◆ Grounded theory analysis of family group & individual interviews	◆ Unfamiliarity of illness & regimen ◆ Interference with normal activities ◆ Negotiating responsibility	◆ Problem-solving ◆ Visualization	◆ Self-care ◆ Shared responsibility		◆ Responsibility for self-care reflects both maturity and experience

TABLE 8.1 *(continued)*

Study	Sample Characteristics	Methods	Stressors/ Demands	Coping Responses	Outcomes/ Markers of Adjustment	Intervention(s)	Developmental Focus
Horner (1999)	◆ 11–14 yrs old ◆ categorical (asthma) ◆ n = 25	◆ Grounded theory analysis of focus group interviews	◆ Illness symptoms	◆ Help-seeking ◆ Problem-solving	◆ Self-care ◆ Mastery ◆ Self-esteem ◆ Normalcy		◆ Limited age sample
Instone (2000)	◆ 6–12 yrs old ◆ categorical (HIV) ◆ n = 12	◆ Grounded theory analysis of projective drawings	◆ Stigma ◆ Social isolation ◆ Life threat	◆ Selective disclosure ◆ Social support seeking	◆ Emotional distress		◆ Children's capacity to understand influenced the degree of family communication
Kieckhefer & Spitzer (1995)	◆ 6–14 yrs old ◆ categorical (asthma) ◆ n = 75	◆ Structured interviews ◆ Longitudinal design	◆ Knowledge & conceptualization of health & illness	◆ Self-management behaviors ◆ Shared responsibility	◆ Self-efficacy in illness management		◆ Age & cognitive abilities set upper limits for comprehension & explanation

(continued)

TABLE 8.1 (*continued*)

Study	Sample Characteristics	Methods	Stressors/ Demands	Coping Responses	Outcomes/ Markers of Adjustment	Intervention(s)	Developmental Focus
Magyary & Brandt (1996)	◆ 7–13 yrs old ◆ non-categorical ◆ n = 65	◆ Quasi-experimental	◆ Family environment ◆ Impact of illness	◆ Self-monitoring ◆ Self-care activities ◆ Problem solving ◆ Relaxation ◆ Positive self-talk	◆ Therapeutic adherence ◆ Self-responsibility ◆ Self-efficacy ◆ Knowledge ◆ Mastery	◆ Family, child group, and parent-group sessions ◆ Cognitive self-management training	◆ School as developmentally normative context for child coping
McNelis et al. (2000)	◆ 8 to 13 yrs old ◆ categorical (asthma) ◆ n = 134	◆ Longitudinal, correlational design		◆ Negative vs. positive behaviors	◆ Attitude toward illness ◆ Satisfaction with family relationships ◆ Self-concept		
Neville (1998)	◆ 14–22 yrs old ◆ categorical (cancer) ◆ n = 60	◆ Correlational design	◆ Uncertainty	◆ Social support	◆ Psychological distress		

TABLE 8.1 (continued)

Study	Sample Characteristics	Methods	Stressors/ Demands	Coping Responses	Outcomes/ Markers of Adjustment	Intervention(s)	Developmental Focus
Rehm & Franck (2000)	◆ 7–15 yrs old ◆ categorical (HIV/AIDS) ◆ n = 9	◆ Ethnographic & grounded theory analyses of individual interviews	◆ Intensive medical regimen ◆ Stigma ◆ Cross-generational infection	◆ Active adherence ◆ Social support seeking ◆ Selective disclosure ◆ Spiritual beliefs	◆ Normalcy ◆ Social/ emotional well-being		◆ School as most important developmental marker of normalcy
Ritchie (2000)	◆ 12–17 yrs old ◆ categorical (cancer) ◆ n = 45	◆ Comparative design (by age group)	◆ Dependency ◆ Physical changes ◆ Disruption of social activities & peer relationships	◆ Maintaining hopefulness ◆ Self-esteem			◆ Illness as threat to adolescent developmental task of self esteem

(continued)

TABLE 8.1 *(continued)*

Study	Sample Characteristics	Methods	Stressors/ Demands	Coping Responses	Outcomes/ Markers of Adjustment	Intervention(s)	Developmental Focus
Ritchie (2001)	◆ 12–18 yrs old ◆ categorical (cancer) ◆ n = 45	◆ Content analysis of self-reported emotional supporters	◆ Limited social support systems ◆ Illness demands ◆ Feeling different	◆ Emotional social support seeking	◆ Satisfaction with social support		◆ Emotional support linked to mastery of social tasks of adolescence
Ryan-Wenger & Walsh (1994)	◆ 8–13 yrs old ◆ categorical (asthma) ◆ n = 78	◆ Comparative design (by age)	◆ Individual appraisals of difficulties encountered before, during, & after illness episode	◆ Relaxation ◆ Cognitive & behavioral distraction ◆ Problem solving ◆ Social support seeking ◆ Prayer			◆ Age-related differences in coping frequency & effectiveness

TABLE 8.1 (continued)

Study	Sample Characteristics	Methods	Stressors/Demands	Coping Responses	Outcomes/Markers of Adjustment	Intervention(s)	Developmental Focus
Rydstrom, Englund, & Sandman (1999)	◆ 6–16 yrs old ◆ categorical (asthma) ◆ n = 14	◆ Phenomeno-logic analysis of individual interviews	◆ Activity limitations ◆ Social isolation ◆ Guilt ◆ Loneliness	◆ Information seeking ◆ Social support seeking ◆ Self-care	◆ Sense of balance ◆ Mastery		◆ Desire for normalcy may increase medical risk ◆ Illness sets limits on development of identity
Sartain, Clarke, & Heyman (2000)	◆ 8–14 yrs old ◆ non-categorical	◆ Grounded theory analysis of individual interviews & projective drawings	◆ Unpredictable treatment course ◆ "Biographical disruption"	◆ "Biographical accommodation" ◆ Social support from similar others			
Sawin, Lannon, & Austin (2001)	◆ 8–16 yrs old ◆ categorical (epilepsy) ◆ n = 20	◆ Quasi-experimental (pre-test/ post-test)	◆ Illness severity		◆ Positive attitude toward illness	◆ Attendance at illness-specific camp	

(continued)

TABLE 8.1 (continued)

Study	Sample Characteristics	Methods	Stressors/ Demands	Coping Responses	Outcomes/ Markers of Adjustment	Intervention(s)	Developmental Focus
Stewart (2003)	◆ 9–12 yrs old ◆ categorical (cancer) ◆ n = 11	◆ Grounded theory analysis of individual interviews	◆ Not understanding ◆ Unpredictability ◆ Ambiguity		◆ Fear & worry ◆ Focus on the routine & ordinary ◆ Getting used to cancer & treatment		◆ Formulation of cognitive schema central to managing illness experience
Thies & Walsh (1999)	◆ 8–16 yrs old ◆ non-categorical ◆ n = 79	◆ Content analysis of structured interviews ◆ Comparative design (age group)	◆ Disruption in desired activities ◆ Peer relationships ◆ Threats to personal identity	◆ Behavioral and emotional responses	◆ Emotional distress		◆ Appraisal of stress and coping response as hierarchical developmental phenomena

220

TABLE 8.1 *(continued)*

Study	Sample Characteristics	Methods	Stressors/ Demands	Coping Responses	Outcomes/ Markers of Adjustment	Intervention(s)	Developmental Focus
Weekes & Kagan (1994)	◆ 8–18 yrs old ◆ categorical (cancer) ◆ n = 13	◆ Qualitative analysis of semi-structured interviews ◆ Longitudinal design	◆ Aversive treatments ◆ Visible differences ◆ Activity limitations ◆ Interruption in peer relationships ◆ Uncertain outcome	◆ Positive thinking ◆ Hope ◆ Distraction ◆ Reframing ◆ Selective attention	◆ Sense of normalcy		
Yeh (2001)	◆ 4–17 yrs old ◆ categorical (cancer) ◆ n = 34	◆ Qualitative analysis of individual interviews, focus groups, & observational data ◆ Age group comparisons	◆ Intrusive procedures ◆ Protective family communication patterns ◆ Social isolation ◆ Extended dependency ◆ Uncertain future	◆ Cognitive, behavioral, & emotional responses	◆ Adaptation, represented by return to normal life		◆ Characterization of stressors & responses by age group ◆ Developmental significance of normalcy for middle childhood

(continued)

221

TABLE 8.1 (*continued*)

Study	Sample Characteristics	Methods	Stressors/ Demands	Coping Responses	Outcomes/ Markers of Adjustment	Intervention(s)	Developmental Focus
Yoos & McMullen (1996)	◆ 6–18 yrs old ◆ categorical (asthma) ◆ n = 28	◆ Qualitative analysis of semi-structured interviews ◆ Demographic comparisons	◆ Limitations and restrictions imposed by illness ◆ Intrusive symptoms and treatments		◆ Worry ◆ Sense of difference ◆ Acceptance of illness as part of life		◆ Age-related changes in focus from physical symptoms and negative feelings to reconciliation and acceptance

the reviewed studies address developmental issues is interwoven within the presentation of findings and discussed collectively in the section on conceptual and methodological research issues.

RESULTS

The Nature of Chronically Ill Children's Stressors

Although the reviewed studies represent considerable heterogeneity in the types of illnesses studied, the age range of the samples, and the methodologies employed, there is considerable agreement as to the nature of the stressors faced by children with chronic illness. These stressors can be organized into three categories: those that are common to most if not all childhood chronic illnesses, those that affect only children with particular illnesses, and those that arise from the co-occurrence of illness-related demands and developmental changes normative to maturation across childhood and adolescence. The demands faced by children with chronic illness affect multiple life domains, including biological changes, management regimens, social stressors, and disruptions in normal routines and activities (Amer, 1999b). Unlike many demands encountered by children in everyday contexts, illness-related stressors tend to be uncontrollable in nature and therefore seldom avoidable (Boland & Grey, 1996; Thies & Walsh, 1999).

The most commonly cited stressor for children with chronic illness in the reviewed studies was the intrusiveness of the illness into everyday life, particularly illness symptoms and the rigor of illness-management regimens that require frequent medications and/or treatments, self-care skills, and constant monitoring for reactions and side effects (Admi, 1996; Amer, 1999a; Boland & Grey, 1996; Ellerton, Stewart, Ritchie, & Hirth, 1996; Grey, Cameron, Lipman, & Thurber, 1994; Rehm & Franck, 2000). In addition to their toll on children's physical and emotional stamina, the demands of the illness and rigorous management regimens reverberated into two important areas of children's lives. First, they constrained children's participation in normal, everyday activities such as sports, recreation, and school (Admi, 1996; Amer, 1999a, D'Auria, Christian, & Richardson, 1997; Ellerton et al., 1996; Horner, 1998; Rehm & Franck, 2000; Sartain, Clarke, & Heyman, 2000; Weekes & Kagan, 1994; Yoos & McMullen, 1996). Furthermore, the visibility of self-care regimens, such as taking medications or monitoring blood glucose levels during the school day, amplified children's differences from their peers (Amer, 1999a; D'Auria et al., 1997; Weekes & Kagan, 1994). Another major stressor identified across childhood chronic illnesses was uncertainty, manifested primarily as unfamiliar and novel experiences, especially at diagnosis, the unpredictable nature of the illness trajectory, and uncertain outcomes (Admi, 1996; Haase & Rostad, 1994; Stewart & Mishel, 2000; Stewart, 2003; Weekes & Kagan, 1994; Weekes, 1995).

Additional stressors were identified as being unique to certain illness contexts. Whereas the social stigma associated in the past with many childhood illnesses persists to varying degrees, the stigma associated with HIV infection remains unparalleled (Instone, 2000; Rehm & Franck, 2000). The stress of the severe stigma of childhood HIV infection is compounded by the high degree of life threat and the likelihood that multiple family members are infected with the illness, which have implications for how much children are told about the nature of their illness (Instone, 2000; Rehm & Franck, 2000). Likewise, the frequency of aversive procedures and treatment side effects is commonly noted as a major stressor, specifically for children with cancer (Weekes & Kagan, 1994; Yeh, 2001).

Perhaps the most important aspect of chronic illness in childhood is the high potential for an intersection of illness demands and developmental tasks. Whether the onset of illness occurs in infancy or later in childhood or adolescence, by virtue of its chronic nature there are inevitably times in which heightened illness demands overlap with age- or maturation-related transitions and thereby intensify their impact on children's lives. These co-occurrences of illness and developmental demands most often affect the social domain, particularly as they relate to peer conflicts and affiliative relationships (Amer, 1999a; Weekes & Kagan, 1994). School entry and transitions between school settings present extraordinary challenges to children whose illness demands and self-care regimens are intensifying, including negative consequences of disclosure to peers and nonfamily adults (Christian & D'Auria, 1997; D'Auria et al., 1997). The potential negative effects of illness-related stressors such as body image changes and prolonged dependency on parents on children's self-esteem are intensified by the developmental salience of self-definition during childhood and adolescence (Ritchie, 2000; Yeh, 2001). Sartain et al. (2000) have eloquently characterized this phenomenon as "biographical disruption," in which the onset or increased demands of illness during childhood constitute an "assault on the self" (p. 914). Children's recognition of their differences from peers, and their desire to minimize these differences, can lead them to ignore their prescribed regimens and put themselves at increased medical risk (Rydstrom, Englund, & Sandman, 1999). For children who perceive their illness as particularly disruptive, seasonal changes in lifestyle dictated by the school calendar can additionally threaten their self-care regimen (Boland, Grey, Mezger, & Tamborlane, 1999).

The other major domain in which illness and development intersect for children is the cognitive domain of knowledge and how children come to understand their illness and appraise the stressors generated by it (Thies & Walsh, 1999; Yoos & McMullen, 1996). As noted previously, children may develop extraordinary expertise specific to their illness, but age and cognitive maturation do place some constraints on comprehension (Kieckhefer & Spitzer, 1995). When the onset of illness is in infancy or early childhood, children's understanding of what it means to have an illness will reflect what they've been told, what they've experienced, and their evolving developmental capacities. Parents and other adults may overestimate children's understanding of illness and provide developmentally inappropriate explanations (D'Auria et al., 1997), or they may underestimate children's capacities and limit communication about the illness, particularly in highly stigmatizing or life-threatening conditions (Instone, 2000).

In summary, the most common stressors for children with chronic illnesses identified in the reviewed studies include rigorous treatment regimens that create intrusive medical and self-care demands, disruptions in everyday activities, self- and peer awareness of physical differences, and varying degrees of social stigma. These illness-related stresses intersect with children's changing capacities and ongoing developmental tasks and result in significant personal and social challenges, particularly in the domains of peer relationships and knowledge, communication, and disclosure about the illness. Although the specific illness and developmental contexts that generated these stresses varied across studies, as did the methodologies used to illicit children's descriptions, there is remarkable agreement as to the nature and magnitude of the impact that chronic illnesses create in children's lives.

Chronically Ill Children's Coping Responses

Definitions of what constitutes coping vary widely among different theoretical perspectives, with predominant characterizations of coping as thought processes, behaviors, and/or efforts at emotional regulation (Sandler, Wolchik, MacKinnon, Ayers, & Roosa, 1997). The most pragmatic way to synthesize the findings from the reviewed research is to present a typology of coping mechanisms as they were identified across the various studies. Most of the findings come from descriptive studies that characterized children's cognitive, behavioral, and/or emotional responses to chronic illness, whereas some studies compared children's coping in different contexts (e.g., everyday vs. illness) or sought to identify relationships between specific coping strategies and adjustment outcomes.

One of the most commonly cited coping strategies used by children with chronic illness was seeking social support from peers, family members, and professionals. There is some evidence that girls are more likely to identify social support as a coping strategy than boys, although both boys and girls considered social support one of the most effective means of managing illness-related stressors (Neville, 1998; Ryan-Wenger & Walsh, 1994). As described in the broader social support literature, for children with chronic illness social support takes on several dimensions, particularly affirmation, emotional comfort and presence during difficult times, information, and distraction from illness concerns in the form of play (Ellerton et al., 1996; Horner, 1998; Ritchie, 2001; Rydstrom et al., 1999). The most frequently identified sources of social support were family members, especially mothers but also fathers and siblings, although the inclusion of friends increased the size and varied the functions of social networks as children matured into adolescence (Boland & Grey, 1996; Ellerton et al., 1996; Haase & Rostad, 1994; Ritchie, 2001). The degree to which children turned to friends for social support varied not only by age but also by context, and seeking help from friends was more likely in everyday than in illness situations (Ellerton et al., 1996; Gray, Cameron, & Thurber, 1991). Seeking social support, particularly from peers, could be significantly challenged by the stigma associated with being ill, so that children sometimes chose instead to keep secrets, selectively disclosing their illness only to friends who had proven their sensitivity and loyalty, or to limit their support seeking for illness-related demands to other ill children (Admi, 1996; Christian & D'Auria, 1997; D'Auria et al., 1997; Rehm & Franck, 2000).

Many of the coping mechanisms commonly described by children fit into the category of problem solving, characterized as active attempts to manage specific demands imposed by chronic illness. The use of problem solving was frequently identified in both medical and social contexts

(Christian & D'Auria, 1997; D'Auria et al., 1997; Grey et al., 1994; Horner, 1998, 1999; Ryan-Wenger & Walsh, 1994). For example, children with asthma described a systematic sequence of problem-solving steps used to manage an episode of difficult breathing, consisting of identifying and ameliorating the asthma trigger, using self-medication, altering physical activity, and monitoring and evaluating the effectiveness of self-care strategies (Horner, 1999). Children with cystic fibrosis used problem-solving strategies such as pacing themselves and tailoring self-care strategies to reduce the intrusion of their illness and treatment regimen into their school day (Admi, 1996; Christian & D'Auria, 1997; D'Auria et al., 1997). Closely related to problem solving were the strategies of seeking information, actively adhering to prescribed medical regimens, and conscientiously complying with self-care behaviors to minimize exacerbations of illness symptoms (Horner, 1998; Rehm & Franck, 2000; Rydstrom et al., 1999; Yeh, 2001).

As noted previously, many of the demands faced by children with chronic illness are not typically within their control; that is, it is not always possible to take direct action to alter or manage a given stressor. Fortunately, children were able to identify and employ a robust repertoire of coping strategies to manage the social and emotional impact of such stressors. These types of strategies have been characterized in the broader coping literature as emotion-focused coping (Lazarus & Folkman, 1984) or as secondary control strategies that alter one's responses to a stressor that cannot be controlled (Weisz, 1990). Cognitive and behavioral strategies such as relaxation and distraction were commonly noted, as well as emotional ventilation, selective attention, reframing, and positive thinking (Boland & Grey, 1996; Grey et al., 1994; Hinds & Martin, 1988; Ryan-Wenger & Walsh, 1994; Weekes & Kagan, 1994; Yeh, 2001). Children also used comparison with others to support their positive self-appraisal: downward comparison to assert that they were doing better than other ill children, as well as favorable comparison with peers in domains unaffected by their illness (Admi, 1996; Amer, 1999a). Another interesting strategy noted by Amer (1999a) was that some children developed "compensatory attributes" (p. 94), personal interests and abilities that offset physical or social deficits created by the illness. Boland and Grey (1996) found that the use of such cognitive control strategies was associated with better outcomes in children with diabetes, presumably because they matched well with the uncontrollable nature of the stressors these children faced.

A fourth category of coping strategies described by children with chronic illness can broadly be defined as spiritual. Specifically, children identified prayer, reliance on spiritual faith, and keeping their focus on the future as mechanisms for managing illness-related demands (Haase & Rostad, 1994; Rehm & Franck, 2000; Ritchie, 2000; Ryan-Wenger & Walsh, 1994; Weekes & Kagan, 1994). Maintaining a positive future orientation was closely related to hopefulness, which combined with a focus on everyday life to support children's sense of their lives as manageable (Admi, 1996; Haase & Rostad, 1994; Hinds et al., 1999; Ritchie, 2000; Weekes & Kagan, 1994).

Very few of the reviewed studies have taken into consideration that coping takes place across varying contexts, that children may have limited control in stressful situations, or that children's changing cognitive capacities and experiences across time might result in an evolving trajectory of coping (Eisenberg, Fabes, & Guthrie, 1997; Ryan-Wenger, 1992; Thies & Walsh, 1999). Only a few of the reviewed studies explicitly addressed the question of whether maturation and development played a role in the types of strategies children used to cope with chronic illness. Those that considered age-related differences in coping provided mixed results. Ryan-Wenger and Walsh (1994) compared the use of coping strategies across a fairly narrow age span (8 to 13 years old) and found no differences by age in children's report of the frequency or effectiveness of the coping strategies employed. Yeh (2001) described age-related changes in observable and self-reported coping behaviors in children with cancer from 7 to 17 years old in response to stressors such as invasive procedures, pain, and uncertainty. She also identified an increasing focus on the future for children in late childhood and early adolescence. Ritchie (2001) found that although age was not correlated with hopefulness in a sample of adolescents with cancer, when the adolescents were divided into three age groups the younger adolescents (12 to 14 years old) scored significantly higher in hopefulness than middle or later adolescents. Grey et al. (1991) found that adolescents were more likely than younger children to report using coping strategies characterized as negative. It is difficult to draw any conclusions from these few studies with heterogeneous samples, different methodologies, and inconsistent conceptualizations of coping, and therefore it must be said that very little is known about the developmental trajectory of children's coping with chronic illness.

An interesting and promising exception is a study by Thies and Walsh (1999) that systematically analyzed children's responses to illness-related stressors within an explicitly cognitive developmental framework. The primary goal of the study was to determine if chronically ill children's appraisal of and responses to stressors reflected a developmentally predictable sequence of cognitive maturation across middle childhood and adolescence. Combined qualitative and quantitative methods were employed to elicit children's appraisals of what was stressful and what they could do about it, which were then scored for the highest level of maturity reflected. The authors' findings supported a developmentally predictable trajectory in the types of stressors, behavioral and cognitive responses, and levels of emotional distress expressed by the three groups. In general, children's appraisals moved from a focus on external factors toward an internalized representation of stressors as assaults on their personal context and coping strategies as personal standards for behavior. The authors concluded that children's cognitive appraisal of stress and coping represent a developmental phenomenon that changes across childhood in an hierarchical, rather than strictly stagelike, progression that reflects an increasingly complex organizational structure. They suggest that by understanding the developmentally hierarchical nature of children's stress and coping processes, future studies can better address important clinical issues such as who is at greatest risk for negative psychological outcomes and how best to intervene with children at different maturational levels.

In summary, findings from the reviewed studies support the idea that children and adolescents display an impressive array of strategies for coping with the demands of chronic illness. These strategies can be categorized broadly as accessing supportive social resources; solving problems in response to illness and social demands; using cognitive, behavioral, and emotional strategies for ameliorating the aversive consequences of stressors that cannot be controlled or avoided; and relying on spirituality and faith in a positive future. The few studies that explicitly addressed developmental differences suggest that maturation does influence how children of different ages cope with chronic illness, but there is currently not enough evidence to support a comprehensive understanding of the developmental nature of children's responses to chronic illness.

Consequences of Illness Demands and Coping Responses: Child Outcomes

Nearly all of the reviewed studies employed the concept of adjustment in addressing the consequences of chronic illness for children. How children's adjustment was characterized in the various studies, however, depended in large part on the methodological approach used: quantitative studies tended to measure adjustment with established indices that varied along a continuum, whereas qualitative studies uncovered intrapersonal qualities or processes evolving over time that represented adjustment as a state of being. Taken together, these two approaches yielded a largely cohesive picture of how children's lives may be affected by chronic illness.

Traditional indices of children's adjustment were well represented in the reviewed studies. The variables most commonly employed in the quantitative studies included mood state, particularly measured as anxiety, depression, and/or global psychological distress (Grey, Cameron, Lipman, & Thurber, 1994, 1995; Hains et al., 2000; Neville, 1998; Thies & Walsh, 1999); indices of social adaptation such as self-perception and social role performance (Grey et al., 1991; Grey et al., 1995; McNelis et al., 2000; Ritchie, 2001; Yoos & McMullen, 1996); and a sense of personal achievement measured as self-efficacy or mastery (Amer, 1999a, 1999b; Kieckhefer & Spitzer, 1995; Magyary & Brandt, 1996). Similar constructs also emerged as central themes from several qualitative studies, including emotional distress (Instone, 2000), worry (Yoos & McMullen, 1996), mastery and self-esteem (Horner, 1999; Rydstrom et al., 1999), and social and emotional well-being (Rehm & Franck, 2000). In addition to these global indices of adjustment, several researchers employed illness-specific markers of adjustment, such as metabolic control in diabetes, symptom frequency and utilization of emergency services, adherence to medical regimens, and positive attitudes toward illness. These outcome variables were used to describe levels of adjustment associated with particular stressors and/or coping strategies, compared across age, illness, and/or peer groups, and tested in intervention studies. As in the broader children's chronic illness literature, the findings from comparative studies were mixed, demonstrating some differences but mostly similarities between ill children and their non-ill peers (Grey et al., 1994, 1995) as well as across age groups (Grey et al., 1991; Hinds et al., 1999; Thies & Walsh, 1999).

There was remarkable congruence in the characterization of normalcy as the primary adjustment outcome across illness contexts and age groups in the reviewed qualitative studies. The predominant theme in most of the studies was children maintaining a sense of normalcy despite their illness (Haase & Rostad, 1994; Horner, 1999; Rehm & Franck, 2000; Weekes & Kagan, 1994; Yeh, 2001). Several different markers of normalcy were identified in the various studies, including school participation (Rehm & Franck, 2000), defining the self as an ordinary person (Admi, 1996; Amer,

1999a), a reduced sense of difference from non-ill peers (Christian & D'Auria, 1997), shifting the illness to the background and focusing on the routine and ordinary (Horner, 1998, 1999; Stewart, 2003), and accepting increasing responsibility for illness self-care (Horner, 1998). Stewart (in press) suggests that this return to normalcy is indicative of the formation of a sufficient cognitive schema within which children can interpret their illness-related experiences as familiar and nonthreatening.

Intervention Studies

Only eight of the reviewed studies presented findings from nursing intervention studies aimed at improving outcomes for children with chronic illnesses. Six represented interventions designed for and implemented with children themselves; the other two studies were included in the review because they represented alternative intervention approaches. Five of the six child-focused interventions utilized a small group format to deliver the intervention to individual children. These groups were conducted in treatment centers (Grey et al., 1998; Grey, Boland, Davidson, Li, & Tamborlane, 2000; Hains et al., 2000; Hinds et al., 2000), at school (Magyary & Brandt, 1996), and at an illness-specific camping program (Sawin, Lannon, & Austin, 2001). The sixth study utilized an individual intervention delivered by the nurse researcher to children in the treatment setting (Amer, 1999a). The most common intervention format was instruction in the use of cognitive and behavioral coping strategies aimed at improving control over illness-related stressors.

The findings from the studies by Grey et al. (1998, 2000) and by Hinds et al. (2000) will be presented in detail in the discussion of these two nurse researchers' programs of research (see below). Of the remaining four child-focused interventions, only two (Hains et al., 2000; Magyary & Brandt, 1996) approximated a traditional experimental design. Magyary and Brandt (1996) utilized a quasi-experimental, delayed-intervention control group design to test a 12-week cognitive coping/self-management intervention conducted with 65 children aged 7 to 13 with various chronic medical conditions. They used small groups in an after-school setting and found that the intervention was effective in increasing therapeutic adherence, self-responsibility, and illness-related knowledge, and in decreasing the frequency and severity of reported health problems. The intervention study by Hains et al. (2000) tested a traditional cognitive-behavioral training intervention delivered in six weekly sessions to 12 to 15 year old children with diabetes. The study was grossly underpowered with a sample of only 14 children, and indeed no between-group differences were found post intervention. The researchers compared pre- and postintervention scores for the 8 intervention subjects and found that there were significant decreases in self-reported anxiety, stress, and use of negative coping strategies.

Two individual-level intervention studies are nonexperimental but are included here to suggest the types of intervention approaches that could be systematically tested and if effective adapted into nursing practice. Sawin et al. (2001) evaluated 20 children aged 8 to 16 years with seizure disorders before and after a recreational camping experience. There was no significant difference in children's attitudes toward their illness four weeks after camp, and there was a trend toward more positive attitudes for the subgroup of children with more frequent seizures ($p = .06$). Amer (1999a) engaged 27 children aged 7 to 16 years with endocrine conditions in discussions about works of fiction that portrayed children with similar conditions managing the medical and social demands of illness. Through analysis of open-ended interviews during which the children discussed their reactions to reading the book, related similar experiences to those portrayed in the book, and freely talked about their feelings, the author concluded that bibliotherapy can be effective in stimulating open and therapeutic discussions with children about their illness-related experiences. .

The remaining two intervention studies represent alternative types of studies that may be employed by nurse scientists in intervention research. Thies and McAllister (2001) describe their process evaluation of a community-level nursing intervention delivered to school principals who participated in a nurse-led workshop focusing on strategies to minimize the social and academic impact of chronic illness. Participating principals reported an increased understanding of the effect of chronic illness on academic and social achievement and improvements in school procedures to address special needs and involve parents in planning and evaluating individualized educational programs. Wesseldine, McCarthy, and Silverman (1999) conducted a randomized controlled clinical trial to test a brief educational intervention delivered at discharge to parents of 160 children admitted with asthma symptoms. Children in the experimental group had fewer readmissions and outpatient visits for asthma exacerbation as well as fewer daytime and nighttime symptoms managed at home. Unfortunately, the study provided little insight into how the intervention worked, and therefore missed the opportunity to evaluate mediating processes as well as additional outcomes that might be related to the medical outcomes, such as children's quality of life or social functioning.

Taken together, the findings from these few intervention studies suggest that a variety of traditional as well as innovative nursing approaches may be effective in helping children manage the demands of chronic illness. However, they may be most noteworthy in illuminating some of the methodological problems common to intervention research with clinical samples, particularly small sample sizes, uncontrolled conditions, and incompletely conceptualized models of how and with whom interventions work.

Two Exemplars of Systematic Programs of Research

By far the individual studies included in this review represent nonsystematic approaches to specific questions about children's experiences with chronic illness, and as such contribute valuable descriptive, associative, and comparative information about children's stressors, coping responses, and adjustment outcomes. However, they offer limited insight into relationships among these important constructs and the processes by which favorable outcomes arise or can be supported for children with chronic illness. Two notable exceptions are the programs of nursing research conducted by Margaret Grey and her colleagues on adjustment in children and adolescents with diabetes, and by Pamela Hinds and her colleagues on hopefulness in adolescents. (A similarly systematic program of research by Christian, D'Auria, and their colleagues with children with cystic fibrosis is not included here because it is presented in a separate chapter in this volume.) These two programs of research illustrate the value of systematically questioning and refining the empirical and conceptual findings from earlier studies in order to support the development and testing of interventions to improve chronically ill children's lives.

The program of research by Grey and her colleagues began with an investigation of the relationships between age, coping, and adaptation in children aged 8 to 18 years with insulin-dependent diabetes (Grey et al., 1991), which demonstrated maturation-related differences in children's choice of coping strategies, their mood states, self-perceptions, and metabolic control, with younger children (preadolescents) faring better across all adaptation outcomes. Coping behaviors characterized as negative, such as avoidance and blaming others, were associated both with older adolescents and more negative outcomes, and the interaction between age and coping contributed significantly to the explanation of variance in metabolic control. Their next two studies (Grey et al., 1994, 1995) included a non-ill comparison group and examined adaptation over time; they identified two periods of vulnerability for children with diabetes. Immediately following diagnosis, children with diabetes were more withdrawn, reported higher levels of trait anxiety, and had lower ratings of general health status than their non-ill peers. Then, although children with diabetes were comparable in all outcomes to their non-ill peers at 1 year post diagnosis, by 2 years post diagnosis the children with diabetes were again more withdrawn, reported more problems with dependency and hostility, manifested more depressive symptoms, and had lower ratings of health status than their non-ill peers. The authors conclude that children with diabetes adjust rapidly to the initial stress of diagnosis, but by 2 years post diagnosis are manifesting some negative consequences of living with diabetes. They characterize children's normal developmental trajectory of adjustment, represented by non-ill children's outcomes over time, as being vulnerable to the impact of illness at initial diagnosis and once the chronicity of the illness is well established.

Next the research team returned to an examination of the relationship between children's choice of coping strategies and their adjustment outcomes. In a sample of 43 children with diabetes aged 8 to 12 years, Boland and Grey (1996) found that younger age and more frequent use of cognitive coping strategies were associated with better metabolic control. In a separate analysis of the data from the previously described longitudinal study, Grey, Lipman, Cameron, and Thurber (1997) tested the relationship of coping choices at diagnosis and adjustment outcomes 1 year later, and found that younger age, higher levels of self-care, more frequent endorsement of humor as a coping strategy, and less frequent use of avoidant coping strategies at diagnosis predicted better psychological adjustment 1 year post diagnosis. Male gender and greater use of avoidant coping strategies at diagnosis predicted poorer metabolic control 1 year post diagnosis. The authors conclude that the adoption of self-care and coping behaviors at diagnosis has significant implications for psychological and medical adjustment to diabetes over time, especially for older children and boys.

Grey and her colleagues' most recently published reports present the short-term (Grey et al., 1998) and 1-year (Grey et al., 2000) findings from a randomized clinical trial of a coping intervention for adolescents with diabetes. Analysis of the baseline data demonstrated that negative impact on quality of life was predicted by higher levels of depressive symptoms, lower ratings of self-efficacy, greater use of rebellious coping, and finding diabetes more upsetting. Metabolic control over diabetes was positively associated with adolescents' perceptions of their families as providing guidance and control. The goal of the intervention study was to determine if a coping intervention would improve medical outcomes over a control condition of intensive diabetes management (Diabetes Control and Complications Trial Research Group, 1994), as well as lessen the impact of diabetes on adolescents' broader adjustment. Intervention subjects participated in small group training sessions over 6 weeks and then individual monthly visits with their nurse-trainer for the 12-month follow-up period. Both intervention subjects and those receiving the control condition of intensive diabetes management showed steady improvements in their metabolic control and psychological adjustment; however, intervention subjects improved more quickly and to a greater extent, with group differences being significant by 6 months and sustained over the follow-up period. By providing training in cognitive and behavioral coping skills in the context of an intensified diabetes management regimen, both medical outcomes and adolescents' overall quality of life were improved.

Hinds (2000) recently reviewed the program of research conducted by herself and her colleagues focusing on hopefulness as an important outcome for adolescents coping with cancer. That review is repeated here to highlight the steps that led from her early descriptive work to the development of measurement and conceptual models and then to the recent implementation and testing of a coping intervention. Hinds's initial qualitative studies of hopefulness with non-ill adolescents as well as those with substance abuse problems and cancer provided the conceptual definition of hopefulness as a comforting, reality-based belief in a positive future for oneself and others, and the characterization of hopefulness as an internal, dynamic experience that varies by individual, context, and time frame (Hinds, 1988). Based on this conceptual definition, Hinds developed and tested (Hinds & Gattuso, 1991) the Hopefulness Scale for Adolescents, which has demonstrated strong internal consistencies and has theoretically predicted relationships to self-esteem and hopelessness in samples of adolescents with substance abuse problems (Hinds, 1988) and cancer (Hinds et al., 1990, 1999, 2000). Additional qualitative work with 58 adolescents undergoing cancer treatment (Hinds & Martin, 1988; Hinds, Martin, &

Vogel, 1987) yielded a conceptualization of how ill adolescents become hopeful, a process the researchers labeled the "adolescent self-sustaining model." The ultimate goal of the self-sustaining process for adolescents is to achieve self-comfort and competence in managing health threats. Within this process the researchers uncovered coping strategies that adolescents employed to achieve these goals, including stopping and reframing negative thoughts and replacing them with positive thoughts and cognitive distraction. In addition, adolescents identified nursing behaviors that promoted their effective use of these cognitive strategies, including caring involvement and use of humor.

The adolescent self-sustaining model was then tested within a randomized, controlled clinical trial of a brief coping intervention in 78 adolescents with cancer (Hinds et al., 2000). The intervention consisted of information on self-care coping as well as modeling and rehearsal of the coping strategies. There were no significant differences in outcome measures between the intervention and control groups during the 6-month follow-up period; a process evaluation revealed that adolescents found the coping strategies helpful but that the intervention should be reinforced over time with additional opportunities for recall and rehearsal. In addition, the coping strategies most frequently used by the adolescents placed them into two contrasting groups who used either monitoring/information seeking or blunting/information avoiding, suggesting the influence of preexisting coping style preferences on adolescents' response to the intervention. Based on this test of the conceptual model, Hinds and her colleagues have proposed testing a revised intervention that is strengthened with repeated opportunities for rehearsal and matched to adolescents' baseline coping style preferences (Hinds, 2000).

Both Grey's and Hinds's programs of research illustrate the systematic process by which knowledge is built as constructs are identified and defined, measurement approaches are developed and refined, and conceptual models are derived and tested. Intervention studies based on the accumulated body of knowledge provide critical information about how best to improve the lives of children living with chronic illness. While the populations studied in these programs of research were both limited to a single illness, their theoretical, measurement, and intervention principles could easily be applied to other illness groups or to noncategorical samples. As such these programs of research make valuable contributions to nursing science that extend beyond the understanding of, and the benefits conveyed to, children with specific illnesses.

CRITIQUE AND DISCUSSION

Theoretical and Methodological Issues

As noted previously, the primary limitation of the collective body of reviewed studies is the lack of explicitly employed developmental models or other theoretical perspectives. This limitation is typical of clinical studies that employ isolated empirical approaches to generating findings rather than building on previous studies to build both conceptual and empirical validity. The primary consequence is that very little is still known about the processes by which individual characteristics, stressors, coping strategies, and outcomes relate. Stronger theoretical frameworks would provide the conceptual links between these constructs that could be tested in mediator and moderator analyses without necessarily requiring larger samples than are apparently currently available to many researchers. Such analyses would yield much more useful information than that which is generated by the comparative studies still common to the field.

The inclusion criteria that reviewed studies must focus on children's perspectives and use children as primary informants limited the information yielded about the influence of family characteristics, family functioning, or parental involvement on children's responses to chronic illness. As noted previously, research that utilizes parental perspectives to examine the impact of chronic illness on children and families seldom includes findings from children's perspectives. Given that the collective studies successfully employed a variety of reliable and valid quantitative and qualitative methodologies to represent children' perspectives, future studies should employ methodologies for combining children's and adults' perspectives to better understand the family as the context within which children's coping with chronic illness takes place.

With the notable exception of Thies and Walsh's (1999) systematically developmental evaluation of a maturational trajectory in children's responses to illness, most of the reviewed studies addressed children's development only as the context within which their illness experiences take place or as differences in understanding about illness, stressors appraised, coping strategies employed, and outcomes manifested by children in various age categories. The resulting findings provide rich detail about what stress, coping, and adjustment might look like in school-age children and adolescents with chronic illness, but they do not constitute a developmental science of children's responses to illness. Perhaps the most important developmental contribution that these studies do make, particularly those conducted within the qualitative research paradigm, is an appreciation for how illness-related stressors and the developmental tasks of childhood and adolescence intersect to intensify the impact of illness on children's lives, particularly in the social domain of peer relationships.

The primary methodological issue to be addressed in any study of children is the challenge of generating valid data with young informants. The majority of findings in the current review come from studies of school-age children and adolescents, as age sets real limits on the validity of the verbal self-report mechanisms typically employed for data generation. As such, very little is known about children's responses to chronic illness prior to their achieving the cognitive maturity to engage in our established methods for generating knowledge. Some researchers are attempting to push the age envelope by employing creative strategies such as projective drawing techniques (Instone, 2000; Sartain et al., 2000) and bibliotherapy (Amer, 1999a) to enhance narrative findings from children as young as 6 years. These techniques, as well as observational methods for deriving reliable findings from children's observable behaviors, deserve further attention as tools for broadening the age range possible for learning directly from children. In the meantime, the quantity and richness of findings from the reviewed studies support the idea that children and adolescents are exceptionally valuable informants about their experiences with chronic illness.

SUMMARY AND RECOMMENDATIONS
FOR FUTURE RESEARCH

An understanding of the psychological, social, and functional consequences of chronic illness is essential for nursing research to meet the important goal of improving the lives of ill children and their families. In her review of the state of knowledge about families of children with chronic illness, Hayes (1997) described the collective research as "at once prolific and dissipated" (p. 260), such that there were no comprehensive or organized models that provided direction for knowledge development in the field. The current review suggests that the related body of research about children's own responses to chronic illness reflects a similar tradition of individual studies that contribute valuable information about specific situations but fall short of constituting an organized body of knowledge.

The study of children's coping with chronic illness represents a unique opportunity for cross-disciplinary collaboration with real potential to generate a truly developmental science for studying the impact of chronic illness during childhood. Nursing researchers can provide their expertise in studying children within the chronic illness context, and developmental psychologists can provide their theoretical and methodological expertise in studying changing developmental trajectories and the processes that influence them. The reviewed study by Thies and Walsh (1999) represents such a collaboration and makes a valuable contribution to our understanding of how children's maturing cognitive abilities affect their appraisal of stress and utilization of coping strategies in response to the demands of chronic illness. Nurses should actively seek opportunities to collaborate with their developmental science colleagues to uncover the mechanisms by which development and illness interact to affect children's present and future lives.

Given these persistent challenges and limitations, the current review finds that we have considerable knowledge about what chronically ill children cope with, how they respond to illness-related demands, and what constitutes adjustment to chronic illness. The mandate for future research is that we develop and test conceptual models that will promote our understanding of how these factors, along with individual, family, and environmental characteristics, affect children's medical, psychosocial, and developmental outcomes. Only by doing so will nursing derive the knowledge with which to support the development of effective interventions for improving the lives of children facing chronic illness.

ACKNOWLEDGMENTS

The author wishes to acknowledge the following sources of support for her doctoral study, during which this chapter was prepared: predoctoral fellowships from the National Cancer Institute (NCI R25 CA57726-07) and the National Institute of Nursing Research (NIH 1 T32 NR07091-01), and the American Cancer Society's Doctoral Scholarship in Cancer Nursing.

REFERENCES

Admi, H. (1996). Growing up with a chronic health condition: A model of an ordinary lifestyle. *Qualitative Health Research, 6,* 163–183.

Amer, K. (1999a). Bibliotherapy: Using fiction to help children in two populations discuss feelings. *Pediatric Nursing, 25,* 91–95.

Amer, K. S. (1999b). A conceptual framework for studying child adaptation to Type I diabetes. *Issues in Comprehensive Pediatric Nursing, 22,* 13–25.

Bennett, D. S. (1994). Depression among children with chronic medical problems: A meta-analysis. *Journal of Pediatric Psychology, 19,* 149–169.

Bibace, R., & Walsh, M. E. (1980). Development of children's concepts of illness. *Pediatrics, 66,* 912–917.

Boland, E. A., & Grey, M. (1996). Coping strategies of school-age children with diabetes mellitus. *Diabetes Educator, 22,* 592–597.

Boland, E. A., Grey, M., Mezger, J., & Tamborlane, W. V. (1999). A summer vacation from diabetes: Evidence from a clinical trial. *Diabetes Educator, 25,* 31–38.

Chi, M. T. H., & Ceci, S. J. (1987). Content knowledge: Its role, representation, and restructuring in memory development. In H. W. Reese (Eds.), *Advances in child behavior and development* (pp. 91–142). New York: Academic Press.

Christian, B. J., & D'Auria, J. P. (1997). The child's eye: Memories of growing up with cystic fibrosis. *Journal of Pediatric Nursing, 12,* 3–12.

Crisp, J., Ungerer, J. A., & Goodnow, J. J. (1996). The impact of experience on children's understanding of illness. *Journal of Pediatric Psychology, 21,* 57–72.

D'Auria, J. P., Christian, B. J., & Richardson, L. F. (1997). Through the looking glass: Children's perceptions of growing up with cystic fibrosis. *Canadian Journal of Nursing Research, 29,* 99–112.

Diabetes Control and Complications Trial (DCCT) Research Group (1994). Effect of intensive insulin treatment on the development and progression of long-term complications in adolescents with insulin-dependent diabetes mellitus. *Journal of Pediatrics, 125,* 177–188.

Eisenberg, N., Fabes, R. A., & Guthrie, I. K. (1997). Coping with stress: The roles of regulation and development. In S. A. Wolchik & I. N. Sandler (Eds.), *Handbook of children's coping: Linking theory and intervention* (pp. 41–70). New York: Plenum Press.

Ellerton, M., Stewart, M. J., Ritchie, J. A., & Hirth, A. M. (1996). Social support in children with a chronic condition. *Canadian Journal of Nursing Research, 28*(4), 15–36.

Grey, M., Boland, E. A., Davidson, M., Li, J., & Tamborlane, W. (2000). Coping skills training for youth with diabetes mellitus has long-lasting effects on metabolic control and quality of life. *Journal of Pediatrics, 137,* 107–113.

Grey, M., Boland, E. A., Davidson, M., Yu, C., Sullivan-Bolyai, S., & Tamborlane, W. V. (1998). Short-term effects of coping skills training as adjunct to intensive therapy in adolescents. *Diabetes Care, 21,* 902–908.

Grey, M., Cameron, M. E., Lipman, T. H., & Thurber, F. W. (1994). Initial adaptation in children with newly diagnosed diabetes and healthy children. *Pediatric Nursing, 20,* 17–22.

Grey, M., Cameron, M. E., Lipman, T. H., & Thurber, F. W. (1995). Psychosocial status of children with diabetes in the first 2 years after diagnosis. *Diabetes Care, 18,* 1330–1336.

Grey, M., Cameron, M. E., & Thurber, F. W. (1991). Coping and adaptation in children with diabetes. *Nursing Research, 40,* 144–149.

Grey, M., Lipman, T., Cameron, M. E., & Thurber, F. W. (1997). Coping behaviors at diagnosis and in adjustment one year later in children with diabetes. *Nursing Research, 46,* 312–317.

Haase, J. E., & Rostad, M. (1994). Experiences of completing cancer therapy: Children's perspectives. *Oncology Nursing Forum, 21,* 1483–1492.

Hains, A. A., Davies, W. H., Parton, E., Tatka, J., & Amoroso-Camarata, J. (2000). A stress management intervention for adolescents with Type 1 diabetes. *Diabetes Educator, 26,* 417–424.

Hayes, V. E. (1997). Families and children's chronic conditions: Knowledge development and methodological considerations. *Scholarly Inquiry for Nursing Practice, 11,* 259–298.

Hinds, P. (1988). Adolescent hopefulness in health and illness. *Advances in Nursing Science, 10,* 79–88.

Hinds, P. S. (2000). Fostering coping by adolescents with newly diagnosed cancer. *Seminars in Oncology Nursing, 16,* 317–327.

Hinds, P., & Gattuso, J. (1991). Measuring hopefulness in adolescence. *Journal of Pediatric Oncology Nursing, 8,* 92–94.

Hinds, P. S., & Martin, J. (1988). Hopefulness and the self-sustaining process in adolescents with cancer. *Nursing Research, 37,* 336–340.

Hinds, P. S., Martin, J., & Vogel, R. (1987). Nursing strategies to influence adolescent hopefulness during oncologic illness. *Journal of Pediatric Oncology Nursing, 4,* 14–22.

Hinds, P. S., Quargnenti, A., Bush, A. J., Pratt, C., Fairclough, D., Rissmiller, G., et al. (2000). An evaluation of the impact of a self-care coping intervention on psychological and clinical outcomes in adolescents with newly diagnosed cancer. *European Journal of Oncology Nursing, 4,* 6–19.

Hinds, P., Quargnenti, A., Fairclough, D., Bush, A. J., Betcher, D., Rissmiller, G., et al. (1999). Hopefulness and its characteristics in adolescents with cancer. *Western Journal of Nursing Research, 21,* 600–620.

Hinds, P., Scholes, S., Gattuso, J., Riggins, M., & Heffner, B. (1990). Adaptation to illness in adolescents with cancer. *Journal of Pediatric Oncology Nursing, 7,* 54–55.

Horner, S. D. (1998). Catching the asthma: Family care for school-aged children with asthma. *Journal of Pediatric Nursing, 13,* 356–366.

Horner, S. D. (1999). Asthma self-care: Just another piece of school work. *Pediatric Nursing, 25,* 597, 600–604.

Instone, S. L. (2000). Perceptions of children with HIV infection when not told for so long: Implications for diagnosis disclosure. *Journal of Pediatric Health Care, 14,* 235–243.

Kieckhefer, G. M., & Spitzer, A. (1995). School-aged children's understanding of the relations between their behavior and their asthma management. *Clinical Nursing Research, 4,* 149–168.

Kliewer, W. (1997). Children's coping with chronic illness. In S. Wolchik & I. Sandler (Eds.), *Handbook of children's coping: Linking theory and intervention* (pp. 275–300). New York: Plenum Press.

Lavigne, J. V., & Faier-Routman, J. (1992). Correlates of psychological adjustment to pediatric physical disorders: A meta-analytic review and comparison with existing models. *Journal of Developmental and Behavioral Pediatrics, 14,* 117–123.

Lazarus, R. S., & Folkman, S. (1984). *Stress, appraisal, and coping.* New York: Springer Publishing.

Magyary, D., & Brandt, P. (1996). A school-based self-management program for youth with chronic health conditions and their parents. *Canadian Journal of Nursing Research, 28*(4), 57–77.

McNelis, A. M., Huster, G. A., Michel, M., Hollingsworth, J., Eigen, H., & Austin, J. K. (2000). Factors associated with self-concept in children with asthma. *Journal of Child and Adolescent Psychiatric Nursing, 13,* 55–68.

Neville, K. (1998). The relationships among uncertainty, social support, and psychological distress in adolescents recently diagnosed with cancer. *Journal of Pediatric Oncology Nursing, 15,* 37–46.

Rehm, R. S., & Franck, L. S. (2000). Long-term goals and normalization strategies of children and families affected by HIV/AIDS. *Advances in Nursing Science, 23,* 69–82.

Ritchie, M. A. (2000). Sources of emotional support for adolescents with cancer. *Journal of Pediatric Oncology Nursing, 18,* 105–110.

Ritchie, M. A. (2001). Self-esteem and hopefulness in adolescents with cancer. *Journal of Pediatric Nursing, 16,* 35–42.

Ryan-Wenger, N. M. (1992). A taxonomy of children's coping strategies. *American Journal of Orthopsychiatry, 62,* 256–263.

Ryan-Wenger, N. M., & Walsh, M. (1994). Children's perspectives on coping with asthma. *Pediatric Nursing, 20,* 224–228.

Rydstrom, I., Englund, A. D., & Sandman, P. (1999). Being a child with asthma. *Pediatric Nursing, 25,* 589–596.

Sandler, I. N., Wolchik, S. A., MacKinnon, D., Ayers, T. S., & Roosa, M. W. (1997). Developing linkages between theory and intervention in stress and coping processes. In S. A. Wolchik & I. N. Sandler (Eds.), *Handbook of children's coping: Linking theory and intervention* (pp. 3–40). New York: Plenum Press.

Sartain, S. A., Clarke, C. L., & Heyman, R. (2000). Hearing the voices of children with chronic illness. *Journal of Advanced Nursing, 32,* 913–992.

Sawin, K. J., Lannon, S. L., & Austin, J. K. (2001). Camp experiences and attitudes toward epilepsy: A pilot study. *Journal of Neuroscience Nursing, 33,* 57–64.

Stewart, J. L. (2003). "Getting used to it": Children finding the ordinary and routine in the uncertain context of cancer. *Qualitative Health Research, 13,* 394–407.

Stewart, J. L., & Mishel, M. H. (2000). Uncertainty in childhood illness: A synthesis of the parent and child literature. *Scholarly Inquiry for Nursing Practice, 14,* 299–319.

Thies, K. M., & McAllister, J. W. (2001). The Health and Education Leadership Project: A school initiative for children and adolescents with chronic health conditions. *Journal of School Health, 71,* 167–172.

Thies, K. M., & Walsh, M. E. (1999). A developmental analysis of cognitive appraisal of stress in children and adolescents with chronic illness. *Children's Health Care, 28,* 15–32.

Thomas, R. B. (1987). Introduction and conceptual framework. In M. H. Rose & R. B. Thomas (Eds.), *Children with chronic conditions: Nursing in a family and community context* (pp. 3–12). Orlando, FL: Grune & Stratton.

Thompson, R. J., Jr., & Gustafson, K. E. (1996). *Adaptation to chronic childhood illness.* Washington, DC: American Psychological Association.

Wallander, J. L., & Marullo, D. S. (1993). Chronic medical illness. In C. G. Last & M. Hensen (Eds.), *Handbook of prescriptive treatments for children and adolescents* (pp. 402–416). Boston: Allyn & Bacon.

Wallander, J. L., & Thompson, R. J., Jr. (1995). Psychosocial adjustment of children with chronic physical conditions. In M. C. Roberts (Eds.), *Handbook of pediatric psychology* (2nd ed.) (pp. 124–141). New York: Guilford Press.

Weekes, D. P. (1995). Adolescents growing up chronically ill: A life-span developmental view. *Family and Community Health, 17*(4), 22–34.

Weekes, D. P., & Kagan, S. H. (1994). Adolescents completing cancer therapy: Meaning, perception, and coping. *Oncology Nursing Forum, 21,* 663–670.

Weisz, J. R. (1990). Development of control-related beliefs, goals, and styles in childhood and adolescence: A clinical perspective. In J. Rodin, C. Schooler, & K. W. Schaie (Eds.), *Self-directedness: Cause and effects throughout the life course* (pp. 147–154). Hillsdale, NJ: Lawrence Erlbaum Associates.

Wesseldine, L. J., McCarthy, P., & Silverman, M. (1999). Structured discharge procedure for children admitted to hospital with acute asthma: A randomised controlled trial of nursing practice. *Archives of Diseases in Childhood, 80,* 110–114.

Yeh, C. (2001). Adaptation in children with cancer: Research with Roy's model. *Nursing Science Quarterly, 14,* 141–148.

Yoos, H. L., & McMullen, A. (1996). Illness narrative of children with asthma. *Pediatric Nursing, 22,* 285–290.

PART III

Parents and Families

Chapter 9

Parents of Children With Chronic Health Problems: Programs of Nursing Research and Their Relationship to Developmental Science

MARGARET SHANDOR MILES

ABSTRACT

This review identified nurse researchers and research teams that have current programs of research focused on parents and parenting of children with chronic health problems. Researchers were included if they had at least five publications since 1990, with at least three of these articles first-authored. These programs of research were critiqued from a developmental science perspective. Multiple methods were used for the search, including examination of previous review articles, hand search of journals, online computer searches, and review of the curriculum vitae of authors. Seven programs of research were identified. Two programs of research focused on childhood cancer—Ida M. Martinson et al. and Marsha H. Cohen. Three programs of research used a noncategorical approach encompassing a variety of childhood chronic conditions—Katherine A. Knafl and Janet A. Deatrick, Sharon O. Burke, and Ann Garwick. One program focused primarily on parents of children with Down syndrome and disabilities—Marsha Van Riper—and another on parents of infants with a variety of chronic health problems—Margaret S. Miles and Diane Holditch-Davis. Diverse theories and conceptual frameworks were used, and most had some focus on ecological systems that might affect parents and parenting. Many used a family perspective and included fathers. Still broader aspects of the family and community ecology and the health care were not generally included. Few examined the bidirectionality of the relationship between the child and aspects of the child's illness and parental responses. There was variability in the extent to which ethnicity and socioeconomic status were considered. Studies provide important insight into the responses of parents and their parenting of children with chronic health problems. The studies provide a sound base for continuing to build a developmentally sensitive body of knowledge related to parents and parenting of the child with chronic health problems.

Chronic health problems in children include a wide array of chronic conditions that are the result of birth defects, genetic disorders, chronic illness, sequelae of prematurity or acute illness or injury, and developmental disabilities. Many children have more than one disorder. These chronic health problems generally require special treatments or medications, necessitate ongoing health supervision, and may involve repeated hospitalizations. Some involve dependence on medical technology temporarily or for a lifetime (Faux, 1998). Others necessitate developmental interventions and special education. The prevalence of children with chronic health problems has increased over the past decades because of advances in medical science and health care (Thompson & Gustafson, 1996). Preterm and term infants with serious health problems at birth, the so-called medically fragile, are surviving their acute hospitalization but often have one or more chronic health problems as sequelae of their illness. Children with birth defects, genetic disorders, and chronic illnesses such as cancer, who would have died decades ago, are now living because of advances in diagnosis and treatment. In addition, children are now diagnosed with new illnesses such as HIV (Faux, 1998). Parents of these children must cope with the meaning of a health problem in their child and with increased responsibility in caring for their child's special needs. Many parents are called upon to care for children with serious and unstable chronic health problems at home, such as children who are technology dependent (e.g., ventilator-dependent children) and children who are seriously ill as a result of their treatments (e.g., bone marrow transplant).

Because of the pivotal role of parents in the care of their child as well as their role in managing family life around the child's illness, nurse researchers have for decades focused on the needs and responses of parents or have conducted interventions with parents. Previous reviews in the *Annual Review of Nursing Research* done by Barnard and Denyes in the first issue in 1984 and by Austin in 1991 included a focus on parents. A chapter on parenting the prematurely born child was written by Holditch-Davis and Miles in 1997. In a 1998 edited book, Austin and Sims (1998) reviewed assessment models and Deatrick (1998) reviewed intervention research on children with chronic conditions and their families, while Faux (1998) reviewed this literature historically. These publications clearly indicate the substantial advances as well as continued weaknesses in the conceptualization and design of research focused on parents and parenting of infants, children, and adolescents with chronic health problems. It is obvious from these reviews that synthesizing the nursing research on parenting is challenging because there are so many researchers who focus on so many different areas. In addition, these authors show the increasing numbers of nurse researchers who have built on their own work over a decade. It is timely to identify the nurse researchers with programs of research and to synthesize their work because they have especially important contributions to make in this domain of research. Thus the purpose of this review was to identify nurse researchers and research teams with current programs of research focused on parents and parenting of children with chronic health problems. Researchers were included if they had at least five publications since 1990, with at least three of these articles first-authored. The year 1990 was chosen to ensure that the individual had a current program of research.

Over the past several decades, another influence on research with parents in psychology, sociology, and other disciplines is the increasing sophistication of developmental science (see Miles & Holditch-Davis in Chapter 1 of this issue). Developmental science is important in the conceptualization and design of studies of parents because it places the parent and parenting within an ecological, systems, and intergenerational perspective, views parenting as a developmental process, encompasses child outcomes, and views the parent-child relationship as having reciprocal influences. This review, then, is unique in that the programs of research were critiqued from a developmental science perspective. It is hoped that the synthesis of these bodies of research will provide direction for future research as well as help researchers and clinicians together to design and test appropriate intervention studies that reduce the distress of parents, strengthen the parent-child relationship, improve parenting, and, since parents have a pivotal role in the family's response, reduce the distress of the family.

METHOD

Criteria for Inclusion

Criteria used to identify researchers and research teams with a "current program of research" related to parents and parenting of children with chronic health problems include the following: (a) the research had to focus on parents or parenting of children with a chronic health problem, including chronic conditions that are the result of birth defects, genetic disorders, chronic illness, sequelae of prematurity or acute illness or injury, and developmental disabilities; (b) only data-based research articles or related theoretical papers written in English were included; (c) papers that focused on parents, parental experiences or responses, and parenting a child with a serious health problem were included; and (d) the chronically ill children could be any age through adolescence. Programs of research on parents of and parenting the prematurely born child were not included unless there was an ongoing focus on chronic health problems related to prematurity. The researcher or research team had to include a nurse or be a researcher who has conducted research with a nursing perspective. An investigator was considered to have an ongoing program of research related to parents or parenting the child with a chronic health problem if he or she had at least five publications since 1990, with at least three of these articles first-authored. If two authors published extensively together, they were considered as one combined program of research.

Search Method

Multiple methods were used for the search. Searches were done for authors with programs of research known to the author to determine if they met the criteria. Previous review articles were examined to identify multiple publications by an author. CINAHL, MEDLINE, and PsycINFO were used to search the nursing literature since 1990 that focused on parents or parenting children with chronic health problems. Google was also used to search. Keywords included *parent, parenting, mother, father, chronic illness,* and *chronically ill child,* and words that focused on concepts of interest, such as *technology dependent, normalization,* and *parental uncertainty,* were also used.

Once a potential author was identified, an attempt was made to obtain the curriculum vitae (CV) of the author to provide an accurate and up-to-date list of all relevant publications. If the CV was not obtainable, an additional search was done to ensure that all publications were located. A number of important nurse researchers with strong programs of research in the past were not included in this review because they did not have sufficient publications in the 1990s. Additionally, several authors had new ongoing programs of research that had not yet met the criteria for number of publications.

Analytic Strategies

An iterative process was used to summarize, synthesize, and critique the programs of research. The first step was to ascertain which articles of a researcher or research team focused on parents and parenting of children with chronic health problems; studies that focused on other areas were not included. The next step was to review the research in order to write a descriptive summary of the studies. A critique of the body of research focused on the extent to which the study (a) used a developmental systems, ecological, and sociocultural perspective in the conceptual model; (b) allowed for and recognized the complex nature of parenting; (c) used a design that allowed for the study of processes over time, such as longitudinal methods, considered developmental transitions of the child and their impact on parenting, made some linkage between parents' responses and parenting and the chronically ill child, and recognized the bidirectional nature of these influences; (d) had a sample that was adequate in terms of sample size, the age span of the children, and inclusion of parents with different ethnic backgrounds and socioeconomic status; and (e) used data analytic methods that enhanced our understanding of ecological influences, processes and change over time, and the bidirectionality of influences. The final step was to summarize key findings across programs of research in order to identify what is known about parenting infants and children with chronic health problems. Areas for further research were identified.

FINDINGS

Seven programs of research were identified. Two were collaborative efforts, but almost all of the programs of research involved multiple authors in various publications. Two programs focused on childhood cancer—Ida M. Martinson et al. and Marsha H. Cohen. Three programs of research used a noncategorical approach (Stein & Jessop, 1982) by encompassing a variety of childhood chronic conditions—Katherine A. Knafl and Janet A. Deatrick, Sharon O. Burke, and Ann Garwick. One program focused primarily on parents of children with Down syndrome and disabilities—

Marsha Van Riper—and another on parents of infants with a variety of chronic health problems—Margaret S. Miles and Diane Holditch-Davis.

Ida M. Martinson and Colleagues

Ida M. Martinson, RN, PhD, has an extensive program of research from 1976 to the present focused primarily on children with cancer and their families. Martinson's program of research includes cohorts of children and families from the United States, Taiwan, China, Hong Kong, and South Korea. Most studies included both quantitative and qualitative data and were longitudinal, allowing opportunities for continued analysis by Martinson, her students, and colleagues.

Martinson's research program started in 1976 with a study from the National Cancer Institute that examined whether it was feasible and desirable for a family to care for a dying child at home, if necessary health care support were provided. Fifty-eight Caucasion families from urban and rural hospitals across Minnesota were enrolled. Families were followed from the time the child was known to be dying to 7 to 9 years post death. Early papers are a description and evaluation of the program and thus provide little insight into the experience or processes of parenting the children (Martinson et al., 1978, 1986; Martinson, 1986–1987). Most families (79%) were able to keep their child at home until the child's death. Parents adequately provided comfort measures and pain control at home with nursing support. A majority of families viewed the experience positively; only two were uncertain whether they would choose to bring the child home to die again. The costs of home care for parents were substantially lower than for hospital care (Moldow, Armstrong, Henry, & Martinson, 1982).

Later analyses of longitudinal data from this study provided a rich description of how parents and families coped. In interviews 2 years after the child's death, parents showed significant distress (Moore, Gilliss, & Martinson, 1988), and depressive symptoms were particularly salient (Martinson, Davies, & McClowry, 1991). Seven to 9 years after death, families still considered the child's death a significant event, suggesting that the death of a child creates an "empty space" in the family (McClowry, Davies, May, Kulenkamp, & Martinson, 1987). Three patterns of response were identified: "getting over it," "filling the emptiness," and "keeping the connection." Some parents recognized life as fleeting and fragile and so had a greater appreciation for life, while others had a sense of impending doom and vulnerability (Martinson, McClowry, Davies, & Kuhlenkamp, 1994). Publications from this project resulted in nationwide attention toward the development of hospice programs for the care of dying children at home (Martinson, 1995).

Martinson and her colleagues then asked further questions about the impact of childhood cancer on the well-being of the family. Another cohort of 40 mostly lower-middle-class, Caucasion families whose child had been newly diagnosed with cancer were enrolled, and 16 were followed annually for 5 years. In a qualitative descriptive analysis focused on parental responses, 17 themes were identified. The three most salient were being unprepared for the diagnosis, normalizing family life as quickly as possible, and fearing that the cancer would recur or that a sibling would develop the disease (Martinson & Cohen, 1988). Further analysis examined how chronic uncertainty related to parental understanding of their child's health as well as its impact on family life (Cohen & Martinson, 1988).

Opportunities to conduct related studies with families coping with childhood cancer in Taiwan, China, and Korea allowed Martinson and colleagues to explore parental responses in different cultures. A descriptive study was conducted with 75 Chinese families living in Taiwan whose children had been newly diagnosed, had relapsed, or had died of cancer (Chen, Chao, & Martinson, 1987; Martinson et al., 1982). The most salient issues were secrecy with the child, family, and community and lack of understanding about the causes and treatments of childhood cancer. Families also experienced many work-related and financial burdens. The primary source of support was the family. This study was pivotal in forming the Childhood Cancer Foundation, which improved the care of children with cancer in Taiwan (Martinson, 1989).

Subsequently, 50 families of children with cancer in the People's Republic of China were enrolled in another descriptive study (Martinson, Chong, & Liang, 1997; Martinson, Yin, & Liang, 1993; Martinson, Zhong, & Liang, 1994). Again issues related to disclosure with the child and extended family were identified, the understanding of cancer was limited and frightening, and costs associated with care were high. Distress symptoms reported by parents, especially mothers, included loss of appetite, weight loss, sleeping difficulty, headaches, dizziness, and colds. A subsequent Chinese study focused on a mother's reactions to home care of a child with a chronic illness (Martinson, Davis, et al., 1995; Martinson et al., 1997). Mothers reported that caregiving had financial, social, emotional, and physical impacts on their lives.

A similar descriptive study was conducted with 74 children with cancer and their families in Korea (Martinson, Kim, et al., 1995). As with the Chinese families, there was a lack of understanding about the causes of cancer, and the illness caused a financial burden on the family since fathers often changed jobs to live near Seoul, where treatment was available. More of the Korean children knew they had cancer. Family perspectives varied from hopeless to confidant. Parents got support from each other, from physicians and nurses, and from family and neighbors.

Having studied families of children with cancer across several cultures, the researchers had questions regarding how family responses and needs were similar or different based on cultural beliefs, values, and resources of the country. Thus, a small exploratory longitudinal design was used to compare the caregiving experience of United States (US) immigrant Chinese families from the People's Republic of China and Taiwan ($n = 10$) and US Caucasion ($n = 8$) families of children newly diagnosed with cancer (Leavitt et al., 1999; Martinson et al., 1999). Data were collected at three key points over the course of the first year after diagnosis using a semistructured interview guide and questionnaires assessing functional status of the child, family impact, health status of parents, and caregiving patterns. No differences between the groups were reported; however, details about how data were analyzed were not given, and it is not clear how the longitudinal data are considered in analysis. Chinese families used alternative therapies such as herbs, nutritional remedies, and therapeutic touch, had fewer resources, and were more isolated. Caucasion families emphasized emotional care. All families reported emotional and physical fatigue at the end of the first year as emotional demands, concerns about siblings, and marital conflict increased. Another cross-cultural analysis examined family responses to the death of a child among parents of children from Taiwan, Korea, and America (Martinson, Lee, & Kim, 2000). Death of a child in all three cultures was viewed as highly unusual and difficult. All parents experienced physical and psychological manifestations, but they were expressed in different ways. External expression of grief was discouraged in Korea and Taiwan. Feelings of stigma and expressions of guilt, blame, and regret were high in Korean families.

An important contribution of this body of descriptive research is the clinically relevant information about the experiences of parents of children with cancer in the United States and Asia. Findings would have been strengthened by linking them to broader research about cultural perspectives of illness and parenting in these cultures. In general, these studies were not guided by a conceptual framework, and the complex nature of parenting was not considered. An ecological, systems framework might have paid more specific attention to socioecological factors affecting parental responses and the interplay between their responses and various family and community systems. Furthermore, findings from these extensive studies were not used to develop a conceptual framework. Given the rich data collected over the years, moving toward a conceptual model about parental response to childhood cancer would have been helpful in guiding practice as well as future research. Another weakness is the lack of specificity about the analysis strategies used with both qualitative and quantitative data. Most of the qualitative papers did not cluster findings conceptually. A strength of this research is that many of the studies included longitudinal data that followed families for many years, some even after the death of the child. Attempts are made to look at processes over time, and insight previously unavailable was gained about the experiences of families over time. However, analysis of the longitudinal data would have been strengthened if longitudinal statistical analyses had been used and if clearer analysis of the qualitative data had more systematically shown patterns and changes over time. The age range of children in the study was very broad, as would be expected in a population that is relatively small. However, the studies would be strengthened by a more developmental perspective, such as examining how the age of the child at diagnosis and developmental transitions affected parents and the family.

To her credit, Martinson's research and especially her mentoring of students, clinicians, and faculty have had a lasting impact on the care of children across the world, thus showing the importance of descriptive research in uncovering needs and changing practice. Her work has resulted in concrete applications to the development of nurse-directed systems of care. According to Martinson (2001), the three most important applications are (a) development of systems of hospice care for dying children nationally and internationally; (b) establishment of the Childhood Cancer Foundation in Taiwan, which provided free chemotherapy to all newly diagnosed children with cancer until national health insurance covered the cost; and (c) development of a Childhood Cancer project in China, which improved care to these children and their families.

Marsha H. Cohen

Marsha H. Cohen, RN, DNS, had a program of research focused on parents of children with a variety of chronic illnesses, including cancer.

Dr. Cohen's contributions to nursing were cut short in 2000 when she was diagnosed with a terminal illness (Martinson, 2001).

Two publications were written as a doctoral student with her mentor Dr. Ida Martinson. These involved secondary analyses with data from 10 families in Martinson's longitudinal study of parents of children with cancer (Martinson & Cohen, 1988; Cohen & Martinson, 1988). The authors identified uncertainty to be a multidimensional concept that affects parents' ability to appraise the health status of their child and also many aspects of family life. Four subsequent articles are based on her dissertation. Data included the 10 parents of children from Martinson's longitudinal study and interviews with a cross-sectional sample of parents of 21 children with a variety of chronic, life-threatening illnesses. She also used biographical accounts written by parents of chronically ill children. One paper, which focused on identifying the dimensions of uncertainty, resulted in a conceptual model depicting how diagnosis of a chronic illness ended diagnostic uncertainty but led to many other types of uncertainty (Cohen, 1993a). A related paper described how living under conditions of sustained uncertainty transformed their world, necessitated management strategies at many levels, and affected the fabric of their family life (Cohen, 1993b). Building on these analyses, Cohen identified a perceptual-interpretive-behavior process that is linked to the emergence and intensification of uncertainty during the prediagnostic phase of a child's illness (Cohen, 1995a). Three stages were identified: the lay explanatory stage, the legitimating stage, and the medical diagnostic stage. Evidence also emerged that sustained uncertainty is a source of family stress and a greater threat to family life than the diagnosis of a serious illness. Further analyses identified that each family had a unique illness trajectory that sustained their uncertainty. Certain triggers, such as medical appointments, changes in the medical regime, and new developmental demands, heightened the level of awareness of their uncertainty (Cohen, 1995b).

Building on these grounded theory analyses, Cohen then conducted a grounded theory longitudinal study of parents' experiences in the transition of technology-dependent children to home and community-based care (Cohen, 1999). Families were followed for 2 years, and multiple sources of data were collected. Family social status accounted for significant variation in the moral distress of families.

Cohen's body of research provides rich insight into the experiences of parents surrounding the diagnosis and management of a child's chronic illness. While her first paper was conceptualized using stress and coping theory, subsequent studies used grounded theory methods to derive a theory about family behavior under conditions of sustained uncertainty brought about by the diagnosis of a chronic, life-threatening illness of a child. Imbedded in her analysis is an appreciation for the complex nature of parenting, and noteworthy is the fact that, unlike many who study parents of chronically ill children, she recognized the impact of the illness on the developmental course of the parents. Cohen's methods for qualitative analysis are clearly described in the articles and are sound. She had a longitudinal perspective, and several papers involved analysis of longitudinal data collected over 5 years. Aspects of the child's illness course as well as developmental demands as the children matured were considered. However, there is limited focus in her work on the link between parental responses and child responses or outcomes. Likewise, limited attention was paid to the ecology of the family.

Kathleen A. Knafl and Janet Deatrick

Kathleen A. Knafl, PhD, has both her undergraduate and graduate degrees in sociology. She is included in this review because she has spent her entire academic career in schools of nursing, has incorporated a nursing perspective in her research, and has worked in very close collaboration with other nursing scholars. Her most notable collaborator, Janet Deatrick, RN, PhD, is included in this review.

Knafl's early program of research was a study on how mothers and fathers managed a child's hospitalization (Knafl, Cavallari, & Dixon, 1988). Different patterns of parental participation were identified, ranging from very active to passive. Aspects of the organizational context of nursing care that influenced parent participation were also examined. Another focus brought attention to how parents manage family life and jobs during a child's hospitalization (Knafl, 1985; Knafl, Deatrick, & Kodadek, 1982). Some fathers maintained their usual role with emphasis on providing comfort and routine care, while others expanded their role to also monitor the child's care and interact with the health care team (Knafl & Dixon, 1984).

Knafl, Deatrick, and colleagues then focused their attention on how families define and manage a child's chronic illness. Using methods of concept analysis, they reviewed the literature on families managing childhood chronic illness (Knafl & Deatrick, 1986). The researchers then conducted an exploratory study based on their findings about family management (Deatrick, Knafl, & Walsh, 1988) and on another concept analysis (Deatrick & Knafl, 1990; Knafl & Deatrick, 1990). This resulted in their framework of Family Management Styles (FMS). In the FMS framework, family responses to illness are thought to be the configuration of each individual family member's definition of the situation, their management behaviors, and also the sociocultural context (Knafl & Deatrick, 1990). *Definition of the situation* is the subjective meaning of the illness for a family member. *Management behaviors* are the changes family members use to manage the illness on a daily basis. Meaning and management behavior are thought to be interrelated (Knafl, Gallo, Zoeller, & Breitmayer, 1993).

The research team then conducted a naturalistic, qualitative study grounded in this working model of FMS. A purposive sample of 63 families with a school-age child with a chronic illness that required daily monitoring and management, such as diabetes, asthma, and juvenile rheumatoid arthritis, were enrolled. Most were Caucasion, although 10 were African American and 2 were Asian. There was a broad range of incomes and levels of education. Data were collected from both mothers and fathers, where possible, the child with chronic illness, and siblings, interviewed separately. Data were collected at two time points 1 year apart and included semistructured interviews on how family members defined and managed their situation, as well as questionnaires measuring family functioning and mood states (Knafl & Zoeller, 2000). A number of papers resulted from this study. While siblings and the child with chronic illness were interviewed, most of the paper focused on the data from the parents, thus elucidating primarily their perspective on family responses to childhood chronic illness.

Data from the interviews were analyzed using methods of content analysis (Knafl, Gallo, Zoeller, Breitmayer, & Ayres, 1993). There was a diversity of perspectives. Most parents viewed the child as normal. While most families viewed the chronic illness as manageable and incorporated management into their everyday existence, some families experienced it as an enduring burden or tragedy that made their family different. The parenting philosophy of most parents was accommodative, but some used restrictive and other approaches. Again, while most families were confident in their ability to manage the treatment regimen, some, particularly mothers, saw this as a burden. Parents' view of the child related to their view of the illness and treatment regimen and their parenting philosophy: Parents who viewed their child as normal more often saw the illness as manageable, used accommodative parenting, and routinized the treatment regimen. If neither parent viewed the child as normal, there was a more negative view of the illness, a more negative parenting philosophy, and a view of treatment as a burden. Mothers and fathers generally had a shared view of the experience and its impact on their lives (Knafl, Breitmayer, et al., 1996; Knafl & Zoeller, 2000). Parents who disagreed on views of the illness also tended to disagree on other themes. In the minority of cases where parents held discrepant views, mothers reported more negative aspects of the chronic illness.

Three approaches to illness management were identified in another analysis (Gallo & Knafl, 1998). These were strict adherence (38% of families), flexible adherence (36%), and selective adherence (22%). Mothers more often had flexible adherence approaches. There were no differences by illness, child gender, or number of other children. Considering all of the themes, fire overall FMS styles were identified (Knafl, Breitmayer, Gallo, & Zoeller, 1996). The "thriving FMS" family had a normalcy view with the illness seen as manageable and had a "life goes on" in-spite-of-it attitude. "Accommodative FMS" also included a normalcy theme, but one or more subthemes were negative or showed difficulty managing in some area. "Enduring FMS" encompassed difficulty as the overriding theme, with negative views of the situation and much effort in management. In "struggling FMS" families there was parental conflict, and in "floundering FMS" families there was confusion and negative defining themes. There were few differences in FMS patterns by child gender and none by socioeconomic status (SES) or ethnicity. "Floundering FMS" families more often had older children, were less educated, and had children with diabetes. There was some evidence that changes in style over time were more likely if there was evidence of difficulty in managing.

Narrative analysis was used to identify pathways to diagnosis (Knafl, Ayres, Gallo, Zoeller, & Breitmayer, 1995). These pathways were direct, delay, detour, quest, and ordeal and were influenced by the parental role and by parent-provider relationships. Pathways differed by diagnosis based on the presenting symptoms but not by gender or child age. Most parents were satisfied with the working relationship they had with their child's health care providers (Knafl, Breitmayer, Gallo, & Zoeller, 1992). They preferred providers who interacted effectively and enhanced parental sense of competence. In a comparison of families in which a child had diabetes or a life-threatening illness, variance in patterns of decision making—

dependent, independent, and collaborative—was related to the amount of reliance on health care professionals, expectations of professionals, trust, and information exchange (Kirschbaum & Knafl, 1996).

One family management strategy identified in the earlier concept analysis was normalization (Knafl & Deatrick, 1986). Four processes were identified in normalization. More recently, the authors refined the concept of normalization based on additional content analysis of related literature (Deatrick, Knafl, & Murphy-Moore, 1999). Normalization attributes now include (a) acknowledging the chronic condition and its potential to threaten lifestyle; (b) adopting a "normalcy lens" for defining the child and the family; and (c) engaging in parenting behaviors and family routines and interacting with others based on the view of the child and family as normal. Fifteen parents of children with osteogenesis imperfecta described normalization as a constant process of active accommodation to the physical and emotional needs of the child or adolescent (Deatrick, Knafl, & Walsh, 1988). Subsequent analysis was conducted to explore families whose response to the illness was not characterized by normalization (Knafl & Deatrick, 2001). Of 59 families, 24 (41%) never normalized. Instead, they emphasized how the child was different from other children and how their parenting style had changed to accommodate these differences. The illness was a major focus of family life and source of conflict, and the treatment regimen a significant burden affecting family life. Another 14 (25%) described changing experiences of normalization during the year between the two data collection periods. Sustaining normalization was closely linked to the status of the illness: normalization worked when in remission but did not always work when there was a health crisis. Other barriers to normalization include cultural differences in normalization goals, including different views between parents leading to conflict.

Overall, this body of research has elucidated many aspects of how families, particularly parents, manage childhood chronic illness. Of particular importance is the focus on important phenomena such as family management strategies and normalization as a family process. A strength of this body of research is the framework—Family Management Styles—which was inductively derived from content analyses of empirical literature focused on childhood chronic illness and on pilot research. The design of the studies was guided by a strong family perspective in which the family's management style was thought to be a configuration formed by individual family members' views of the situation, their management behaviors, and the sociocultural context of the family (Knafl, Gallo, Zoeller, Breitmayer, &

Ayres, 1993). Thus, data were collected from all members of the family and comparisons were made across individual family members to identify family unit responses. Still, in reviewing papers, it appears that most of the analyses focused on parental interviews, and it is not clear how the data from the child with chronic illness or from siblings informed analysis. Another strength of this body of research is the identification of the many aspects involved in managing and parenting a child with chronic illness and the examination of how mothers and fathers differed in their perspectives, as well as the implications of these differences for FMS. Still, the complex nature of parenting, including differences in maternal and paternal roles with chronically ill children and developmental aspects of the parents, is not clearly conceptualized in the FMS model or in most analyses. In addition, there is no clear conceptualization of the family based on family theory. For example, an ecological, systems theory perspective might have added additional views about the phenomena and especially about interfamilial and ecological factors affecting family management. While sociocultural aspects of the family are a construct in their model, limited attention is placed in analysis on culture and socioeconomic status.

The developmental age and gender of the child with chronic illness were considered. The study was limited to chronically ill school-aged children, and a number of analyses examined whether there were differences based on the age and gender of the child. The investigators chose to use a noncategorical approach (Stein & Jessop, 1982) and including a wide range of chronic conditions, which strengthens the generalizability of findings. The impact of different FMS on the child with chronic illness is not addressed. This would be an important direction for future research.

The rich description of normalization as a process in these families is important. However, an assumption is made that normalization is positive, but it is not clear when normalization is a positive outcome and when it can be problematic to the family. Another strength is the triangulation of data collection methods using interviews and some questionnaires, and the repeated measures design in which families were interviewed twice a year apart, allowing for exploration of processes over time. Of note is the fact that the investigators attempted to use a more "person-oriented" approach by using cases to illustrate the model and to describe differences in family responses (Gallo, 1990; McCarthy & Gallo, 1992; Obrecht, Gallo, & Knafl, 1992). This approach could be further strengthened by more sophisticated use of multiple case study design or person-centered analysis.

Sharon O. Burke and Colleagues

Sharon O. Burke, RN, PhD, and colleagues have an ongoing program of research focused on the stressors of families with chronically ill and handicapped children both in the hospital and at home. For a comprehensive and detailed description of their program of research, readers are referred to their own review article (Burke, Kauffmann, Harrison, & Wiskin, 1999). These authors conducted both quantitative and qualitative descriptive studies of the experiences and perceptions of parents (Burke, Costello, & Handley-Derry, 1989; Burke, Kauffmann, Costello, & Dillon, 1991; Burke, Kauffmann, LaSalle, Harrison, & Wong, 2000). Based on their research, they developed the Burke Stressors and Tasks Framework for Families with a Child with a Chronic Condition (Burke, Kauffmann, Costello, Wiskin, & Harrison, 1998). This framework was then validated based on a synthesis of the available qualitative research focused on these parents. The authors used this framework to develop a family-focused, stress-point nursing intervention for parents to reduce distress and improve child and family functioning related to hospitalization (Kauffmann, Harrison, Burke, & Wong, 1998). The Stress-Point Intervention by Nurses (SPIN) identified the family concerns, provided preparatory information, and helped parents develop strategies for coping with the upcoming hospitalization. In a hospital-based randomized clinical trial of SPIN, intervention parents had better coping and family functioning than those in the usual care group (Burke, Handley-Derry, Costello, Kauffmann, & Dillon, 1997). In turn, their children showed reduced short-term developmental regression and improved developmental gains. A subsequent three-site randomized study was conducted in an ambulatory care setting. Families of chronically ill children who were expected to be hospitalized were randomly assigned to SPIN or a control group (Burke, Harrison, Kauffmann, & Wong, 2001). SPIN parents were more satisfied with family functioning and had better parental coping after hospitalization than control parents. Secondary analysis of data from these studies revealed that distance to hospital had a negative effect on family functioning (Yantzi, Rosenberg, Burke, & Harrison, 2001).

Burke and colleagues focused much of their program of research in a neglected area of practice, namely, the impact of repeated hospitalization of a child with a chronic illness or disability on parents and the family. Their program of research is an excellent example of building on descriptive studies to design an intervention. The Burke Stressors and Tasks

Framework for Families with a Child with a Chronic Condition, which guided their intervention, is ecological in that many aspects of personal and family life as well as of the child's illness are included (Burke et al., 1999). This model did acknowledge the complex nature of parenting chronically ill children. The model included financial strains and family values and beliefs, but limited attention was placed in analysis on culture and ethnicity or on socioeconomic status of families. In testing their intervention, the authors included parent, family, and child outcomes. Burke et al. used a noncategorical approach to their study and thus included children with a wide variety of chronic conditions. Given their focus on the stresses of hospitalization as the common experience of parents, this was appropriate. However, it would have added to our body of knowledge had there been some analysis based on experiences during hospitalization such as critical care, invasive surgery, or diagnosis of relapse of a serious chronic illness. Another limitation was the lack of attention to child age in the design and analysis; children ranged in age from 1 to 17 (Burke et al., 1997). Family stresses are likely affected by the developmental level of the child. The descriptive studies used cross-sectional or qualitative methods. While none of them were longitudinal, one study did ask parents about their perceptions of the past, present, and future course of their child's health problem (Burke et al., 2000). Longitudinal descriptive studies would provide a more process-oriented view of the stressors of these parents. The intervention studies used a short-term longitudinal design, measuring outcomes to 3 months post discharge.

Ann Garwick and Colleagues

Ann Garwick, PhD, RN, along with an interdisciplinary group of colleagues, has a program of research that evolves from Project Resilience, a multisite longitudinal research project with families of children with a variety of chronic health problems. In a well-designed qualitative analysis, Garwick and colleagues identified factors that influence the reactions of families to the diagnosis of Down syndrome or congenital heart disease (Garwick, Patterson, Bennett, & Blum, 1995). The differing characteristics of the two conditions that affected reactions were identified, as well as predisposing family factors that crossed the diagnostic category. Of most importance is the finding that emotional reactions to the diagnosis were related to the quality of the information as well as to the manner in which they were told.

Ethnocultural aspects of caring for a child with a chronic condition were analyzed in two papers. One explored variations in families' explanations of childhood chronic conditions across different ethnic groups (Garwick, Kohrman, Titus, Wolman, & Blum, 1999). Another analysis explored recommendations for improving the care of children with chronic conditions from the perspective of three ethnocultural groups: African American, Hispanic, and European American families (Garwick, Kohrman, Wolman, & Blum, 1998). No differences in recommendations were found by ethnicity. All families focused on the need to improve the quality of health care services; to decrease barriers to services and programs; to improve the training of health care professionals, families, and the public about chronic conditions and their management; and to improve the quality and availability of community-based services.

Parents' perceptions of support in managing the care was explored in two papers. Both helpful and unhelpful support were identified (Patterson, Garwick, Bennett, & Blum, 1997). Perceptions of support for parents of preadolescents with chronic conditions was examined with data from 124 parents (Garwick, Patterson, Bennett, & Blum, 1998). Family members were the primary source of emotional and tangible support for both mothers and fathers, while health care providers were the primary source of informational support. Unsupportive behaviors were attributed primarily to health professionals and extended family.

Differences in the perspectives of mothers and fathers were examined using a large sample of parents of young children with chronic health problems (Dodgson et al., 2000). No differences were found between mothers' and fathers' report of family distress about the degree of uncertainty in the child's life expectancy and the unpredictability of the child's symptoms. Parents of children with intermittently unpredictable symptoms reported significantly more family distress than parents of children with more predictable symptoms.

The research of Garwick and her research team was built on a family systems perspective. As such, they included a focus on the ecology of the family as well as some focus on the health care resources. Both fathers and mothers were included, and the unique perspective of the father was examined in at least one paper. In addition, the sample was ethnically diverse, and at least one analysis explored ethnic differences. Furthermore, the sample enrolled a cohort of families with young children and followed them longitudinally. Developmental age of the child was considered in several analyses, including uncertainty and family stress in families with young children and support in managing preadolescents with chronic health problems. The influence of the child's illness, such as life expectancy and unpredictability of symptoms, was considered in the analysis. The samples were generally large, strengthening the quantitative analyses and allowing for subanalyses of select groups.

Marcia Van Riper

Marcia Van Riper, RN, PhD, has a program of research focused on parent and family responses to the birth and care of a child with Down syndrome and other disabilities. As a master's student, Van Riper interviewed 16 parents using life transition theory to explore their responses to becoming parents of a child with Down syndrome (Van Riper & Selder, 1989). Uncertainty was a major characteristic of such transitions. Sources included the unexpected diagnosis, concern about the future, apprehensions regarding their ability to parent the child, and the initial responses of health care professionals. Ongoing uncertainties revolved around the child's education and future health and developmental status. While parents described the impact of having a child with Down syndrome as profound, they also identified positive outcomes.

In her doctoral studies, Van Riper broadened her focus to examine the effects of Down syndrome on family, marital, and individual functioning. A unique aspect of this and future work was her inclusion of positive outcomes using a multidimensional conception of psychological well-being derived from life-span developmental, personal growth, and mental health literature (Van Riper, Ryff, & Pridham, 1992; Van Riper, 2000). The design incorporated a control group, and criteria for enrollment considered both the age of the child and the level of functioning. No differences were found between parents who had a child with Down syndrome and parents with normal children, suggesting a competence model for parents with Down syndrome.

Another study using symbolic interaction as a framework found that health care providers "set the tone" for parental response to the diagnosis (Van Riper, 1992). Building on this research, Van Riper's doctoral dissertation described parental perception of family-provider relationships and the linkages to family well-being (Van Riper, 1999). The study was based on the "parental working model of family-provider relationships," a synthesis of theoretical perspectives that explain how families appraise and respond to their relationships with health care providers. When mothers viewed their relationships with health care providers as positive and family-centered, they were more satisfied with care and had higher levels of individual and family well-being. Using a similar framework and design, Van Riper (2001) examined family-provider relationships in mothers of preterm infants hospitalized in a neonatal intensive care unit. Again, mothers who depicted their family's relationship as positive and family-centered reported more satisfaction with the care received and higher levels of well-being.

Several important phenomena are explored by Van Riper—uncertainty, family-provider relationships, and family well-being. A particular strength is the positive focus, which moves research with families who have a child with a disability such as Down syndrome from a negative bias in which signs of distress and dysfunction are sought, to more positive designs. Van Riper's studies are based on well-thought-out conceptual models that fit the design. These models, however, have some limitations from a developmental perspective. The Parental Working Model of Family-Provider Relationships includes a perspective on the complex nature of parenting. While the studies revolve around children with health problems (Down syndrome and prematures), the children themselves are not included in the conceptual model or design. Van Riper paid attention to the age range of children in one study, but more recent studies included a wide age range of children and no attention was placed on age or level of disability. However, it must be noted that Van Riper's research is with a population that is not easy to access. Another limitation of the designs from a developmental perspective is the lack of focus on the ecology and sociocultural aspects of the health care environment and the family that may affect relationships with staff and well-being.

Margaret Shandor Miles and Diane Holditch-Davis

Margaret Shandor Miles, RN, PhD, and Diane Holditch-Davis, RN, PhD, have a current ongoing program of research focused on parents of prematurely born and medically fragile infants that is primarily reviewed here. Previous research of Miles that is focused on parenting of children with chronic health problems is also included. Holditch-Davis has a program of research on the behavior and development of prematurely born children (see Chapter 2 in this volume) and on parent-infant interaction with mothers and prematurely born children (Holditch-Davis & Miles, 1997); these studies are not included.

Building on her extensive program of research on the stressors experienced by parents when a child was admitted to a pediatric (Miles, Carter, Riddle, Hennessey, & Eberly, 1989; Miles, Carter, Eberly, Hennessey, & Riddle, 1989) or neonatal (Miles, Funk, & Kasper, 1991) intensive care unit (ICU), Miles focused on what it was like to parent a chronically ill child. Several small studies were conducted with graduate students. One identified problems mothers faced in managing children with diabetes (Banion, Miles, & Carter, 1983). Another identified alterations in the parental role, such as enhanced feeling of responsibility to protect the child and to advocate on behalf of the child, that resulted when a child had a chronic illness (Miles, D'Auria, Hart, Sedlack, & Watral, 1993). Parents of children diagnosed with serious oncology or hematology disorders had high levels of depression (Nelson, Miles, Reed, Poprawa, & Cooper, 1994).

Miles and Holditch-Davis collaborated to focus on the long-term impact of premature birth on parenting. Mothers in Holditch-Davis's longitudinal study of prematurely born children were interviewed about their parenting when the children were 3 years old; many had developmental delays and other chronic health problems (Huber, Holditch-Davis, & Brandon, 1993). A compensatory parenting process was identified in which the child who survived the neonatal ICU experience was treated as special but also vulnerable (Miles & Holditch-Davis, 1995). As a result, the mothers provided extra stimulation and had difficulty setting limits and disciplining the children (Miles, Holditch-Davis, & Shepherd, 1998).

This led to a focus on parents of medically fragile infants—term and preterm infants with serious health problems that necessitated dependence on technology and long hospitalizations and that resulted in chronic health problems. Interviews with parents during hospitalization revealed their struggle to assume their parental role with the nursing staff member who was responsible for the care of the infant (Miles & Frauman, 1993). A longitudinal study of parental role attainment with medically fragile infants using a developmental, ecological parental role attainment framework was conducted to examine how maternal identity, presence, and competence developed over time, how ecological factors influenced these constructs, and how level of maternal role attainment affected the quality of parenting in the second year of life. Personal, family, and infant health characteristics influenced the development of parental role attainment (Miles, Holditch-

Davis, & Burchinal, 2001). Further, parental role attainment influenced many parenting outcomes including parental competence, sensitivity, and involvement at 16 months (Holditch-Davis, Miles, & Burchinal, 2001). Mothers experienced moderately high depressive symptoms at both time points, but there was also evidence of growth, especially at 16 months (Miles, Holditch-Davis, Burchinal, & Nelson, 1999). Distress was influenced by maternal characteristics, hospital environmental stress, and worry about the child's health. Growth was influenced by characteristics of the child's illness, hospital environmental stress, worry, and level of maternal role attainment. Maternal worry about the child's health was not related to the diagnosis of the child but rather to maternal educational level (Docherty, Miles, & Holditch-Davis, 2002). There were few differences between Caucasion and African American mothers in stress or support during hospitalization, but again mothers with a lower educational level reported more stress (Miles, Holditch-Davis, Brunssen, Burchinal, & Wilson, 2002). In a small adjunct study, African American mothers indicated that they were stressed by separation and worried about when they could take their baby home (Miles, Wilson, & Docherty, 1999). Fathers reported high distress associated with seeing their sick child, and African American fathers were especially distressed (Miles & Docherty, 2001). Fathers of infants with severe congenital heart disease described conflicting responses as they coped with the child's diagnosis and early treatment (Clark & Miles, 1999). A comparison of parent-child interactions with infants with and without an abnormal neurological finding indicated that neurological status had little impact on the early interactions of these medically fragile infants and their mothers (Holditch-Davis, Tesh, Burchinal, & Miles, 1999). No differences were found in mother-infant interactions between infants with bronchopulmonary dysplasia and other infants (Holditch-Davis, Docherty, Miles, & Burchinal, 2001).

This body of research provides some insights into the processes and complexities of parenting a child with chronic health problems. Of particular note is the focus on becoming a parent while coping with an infant's serious illness and hospitalization. Many of the early studies were atheoretical, descriptive studies with small samples. Later studies were strengthened by larger and more diverse samples and by the use of longitudinal designs. A strength of the study of medically fragile infants was the ecological, developmental systems model and the use of appropriate longitudinal statistical analyses for the longitudinal data. Attention was paid to examining responses of African American mothers and fathers, although the sample sizes were relatively small.

DISCUSSION

A number of common themes related to the responses of parents to and parenting of children with chronic health problems can be identified across studies. The period surrounding the diagnosis of a child's chronic condition is a critical period for parental adaptation. Parents experience a myriad of feelings while coping with the diagnosis. Parents of infants also struggle to attain their normal parental role (Miles et al., 1998). The response of the health care team is an important factor in parental responses (Garwick et al., 1995, 1998; Knafl et al., 1992, 1995; Miles & Frauman, 1993; Van Riper, 1999, 2001). Parents who perceive parent-provider relationships more positively are more satisfied with care and show better adaptation. Uncertainty surrounding the diagnosis and the dimensions of uncertainty involved in managing a child's chronic illness over time were identified (Cohen, 1995b; Dodgson et al., 2000; Van Riper & Selder, 1989). Unpredictable symptoms caused more parental distress (Dodgson et al., 2000). Physical and emotional distress of parents and stressors affecting family life were described in many studies. There was a beginning attempt to look at the positive outcomes as well as the negative (Knafl et al., 1993; Miles et al., 1999; Van Riper, 2000).

Another important theme revolved around family support. Many studies, including cross-cultural studies of Asian parents, identified family as an important source of support (Patterson et al., 1997; Martinson et al., 1982). However, findings also indicate difficulties related to disclosure of diagnosis, especially in Asian families (Martinson et al., 1993). In addition, unsupportive behaviors of families were described (Patterson et al., 1997). More research is needed that explores the processes involved in getting and sustaining support.

An important strategy used by families to manage their child's illness was normalization (Knafl & Deatrick, 1986; Deatrick et al., 1999). There is some evidence of a compensatory parenting approach with previously acutely ill prematurely born children in which parents balanced their desire to have a normal child with their concerns about developmental and health problems (Miles & Holditch-Davis, 1995). Further work is needed to examine how parents and families normalize the child with a chronic illness and the extent to which they treat the child as different and special.

The theories and frameworks used for this body of research are so diverse that it is difficult to synthesize the findings. Garwick used a family systems perspective (Garwick et al., 1998). Knafl and colleagues inductively derived a family management model (Knafl & Deatrick, 1990). Cohen's work involved a grounded theory method in developing theory (Cohen, 1993a). Martinson's studies were atheoretical. Van Riper used symbolic interaction and a multidimensional conception of psychological well-being in her studies (Van Riper et al., 1992; Van Riper, 1999). Miles and Holditch-Davis (Miles et al., 2001) used developmental systems theory and theories of maternal role attainment. Many of the theories and frameworks had some aspects of a developmental perspective. Still, the ecology of the broader family and community and of the health care system was not adequately included in most designs. Few studies used a perspective on parenting that acknowledged the complex nature of parenting. There was some focus on how the child's chronic illness affected parenting and the parent-child relationship (Cohen, 1995a, 1995b; Knafl et al., 1993; Miles et al., 2001; Holditch-Davis et al., 2001), but few studies examined how parental responses and parenting influenced child responses and outcomes. An important developmental premise that needs exploration is the bidirectional interaction of influences. Clearly, to move this field of research along, there is a need for scholars to develop a comprehensive, developmentally based family and parenting framework for future research.

Many studies used a family perspective, and several included data from all family members (Knafl et al., 1993). Of particular interest here is the use of fathers in many studies, including an exploration of their differing experiences (Dodgson et al., 2000; Knafl & Dixon, 1984; Knafl & Zoeller, 2000) and their unique experiences (Clark & Miles, 1999; Miles & Docherty, 2001). There was wide variability across studies in the extent to which ethnicity was considered. Many studies had samples that were primarily Caucasion. On the other hand, some investigators explored parental responses by ethnicity (Garwick et al., 1999; Knafl, Breitmayer, et al., 1983; Miles et al., 2001, 2002). Martinson's program of research (Martinson et al., 1999, 2000) is particularly unique in focusing on US Caucasion and US Asian families as well as Asian families internationally. It is essential that ethnically diverse samples be recruited and that we explore the impact of ethnicity on parental responses and parenting. Socioeconomic status was rarely considered in an analysis, although educational level, which might be considered a proxy for SES, was considered by some (Docherty et al., 2002; Knafl, Breitmayer, et al., 1996; Miles et al., 2002).

Many of the studies involved small cross-sectional samples of children of diverse ages and differing length of time with the chronic condition. Combining samples with widely diverse ages creates confusion about the meaning of the findings, as parenting is likely vastly different for an infant than for an adolescent. In order to increase the sample size needed for such analyses, more collaborative, multisite studies are needed. The qualitative designs used in many studies provided an in-depth perception of parental experiences, and triangulation of both qualitative and quantitative methods was another strength. Longitudinal or repeated measures designs were used by many investigators; however, many studies with longitudinal data did not analyze them using methods of longitudinal analysis. More longitudinal studies are needed, and new, evolving methods of longitudinal analysis should be used as appropriate.

In general, this rich body of research provides important information that has relevance for clinical practice in a variety of settings. The studies provide a sound base for continuing to build a developmentally sensitive body of knowledge related to parents and parenting of the child with chronic health problems. Of utmost importance are longitudinal designs and the inclusion of child outcomes.

ACKNOWLEDGMENTS

The author wishes to acknowledge partial support from Grants NR02868 and NRO5263, National Institute of Nursing Research, National Institutes of Health. The assistance of Andrea Blickman in identifying and procuring references is gratefully acknowledged.

REFERENCES

Austin, J. K. (1991). Family adaptation to a child's chronic illness. In H. H. Werley & J. J. Fitzpatrick (Eds.), *Annual review of nursing research* (Vol. 9, pp. 103–120). New York: Springer.

Austin, J. K., & Sims, S. L. (1998). Integrative review of assessment models for examining children's and families' responses to chronic illness. In M. E. Broome, K. Knafl, K. Pridham, & S. Feetham (Eds.), *Children and families in health and illness* (pp. 196–220). Thousand Oaks, CA: Sage Publications.

Banlon, C., Miles, M. S., & Carter, M. C. (1983). Problems of mothers in management of children with diabetes. *Diabetes Care, 6,* 548–551.

Barnard, K. E. (1984). Nursing research related to infants and young children. In H. H. Werley & J. J. Fitzpatrick (Eds.), *Annual review of nursing research* (Vol. 1, pp. 3–26). New York: Springer.

Burke, S. O., Costello, E., & Handley-Derry, M. (1989). Maternal stress and repeated hospitalizations of children who are physically disabled. *Children's Health Care, 18,* 82–90.

Burke, S. O., Handley-Derry, M. H., Costello, E. A., Kauffmann, E. A., & Dillon, M. C. (1997). Stress-point intervention for parents of repeatedly hospitalized children with chronic conditions. *Research in Nursing & Health, 20,* 475–485.

Burke, S. O., Harrison, M. B., Kauffmann, E., & Wong, C. (2001). Effects of stress-point intervention with families of repeatedly hospitalized children. *Journal of Family Nursing, 7,* 128–158.

Burke, S. O., Kauffmann, E., Costello, E. A., & Dillon, M. C. (1991). Hazardous secrets and reluctantly taking charge: Parenting a child with repeated hospitalizations. *Image: Journal of Nursing Scholarship, 23,* 39–45.

Burke, S. O., Kaufmann, E., Costello, E. A., Wiskin, N., & Harrison, M. B. (1998). Stressors in families with a child with a chronic condition: An analysis of qualitative studies and a framework. *Canadian Journal of Nursing Research, 30,* 71–95.

Burke, S. O., Kauffmann, E., Harrison, M. B., & Wiskin, N. (1999). Assessment of stressors in families with a child who has a chronic condition. *MSN: American Journal of Maternal-Child Nursing, 24,* 98–106.

Burke, S. O., Kauffmann, E., LaSalle, J., Harrison, M. B., & Wong, C. (2000). Parents' perceptions of chronic illness trajectories. *Canadian Journal of Nursing Research, 32,* 19–36.

Chen, Y. C., Chao, Y. Y., & Martinson, I. (1987). Parents' reactions to childhood cancer in the family in Taiwan. *Recent Advances in Nursing, 16,* 61–84.

Clark, S., & Miles, M. S. (1999). Conflicting responses: The experiences of fathers of infants diagnosed with severe congenital heart disease. *Journal of the Society of Pediatric Nurses, 4,* 1, 714.

Cohen, M. H. (1993a). Diagnostic closure and the spread of uncertainty. *Issues in Comprehensive Pediatric Nursing, 16,* 135–146.

Cohen, M. H. (1993b). The unknown and the unknowable: Managing sustained uncertainty. *Western Journal of Nursing Research, 15,* 77–96.

Cohen, M. H. (1995a). The stages of the prediagnostic period in chronic, life-threatening childhood illness: A process analysis. *Research in Nursing & Health, 18,* 39–48.

Cohen, M. H. (1995b). The triggers of heightened parental uncertainty in chronic, life-threatening childhood illness. *Qualitative Health Research, 5,* 63–77.

Cohen, M. H. (1999). The technology-dependent child and the socially marginalized family: A provisional framework. *Qualitative Health Research, 9,* 654–668.

Cohen, M. H., & Martinson, I. M. (1988). Chronic uncertainty: Its effect on parental appraisal of a child's health. *Journal of Pediatric Nursing, 3,* 89–96.

Deatrick, J. A. (1998). Integrative review of intervention research with children who have chronic conditions and their families. In M.E. Broome, K. Knafl, K. Pridham, & S. Feetham (Eds.), *Children and families in health and illness* (pp. 221–235). Thousand Oaks, CA: Sage Publications.

Deatrick, J. A., & Knafl, K. A. (1990). Management behaviors: Day-to-day adjustments to childhood chronic conditions. *Journal of Pediatric Nursing, 5,* 15–22.

Deatrick, J. A., Knafl, K. A., & Murphy-Moore, C. (1999). Clarifying the concept of normalization. *Image: Journal of Nursing Scholarship, 31,* 209–214.

Deatrick, J. A., Knafl, K. A., & Walsh, M. (1988). The process of parenting a child with a disability: Normalization through accommodations. *Journal of Advanced Nursing, 13,* 15–21.

Denyes, M. J. (1984). Nursing research related to school-age children and adolescents. In H. H. Werley & J. J. Fitzpatrick (Eds.), *Annual review of nursing research* (Vol. 1, pp. 27–54). New York: Springer.

Docherty, S., Miles, M. S., & Holditch-Davis, D. (2002). Perception of illness severity and worry about infant health in mothers of hospitalized medically fragile infants. *Advances in Neonatal Care, 2,* 84–92.

Dodgson, J., Garwick, A., Blozis, S., Patterson, J., Bennett, F., & Blum, R. (2000). Uncertainty in childhood chronic conditions and distress in families of young children. *Journal of Family Nursing, 6,* 252–266.

Faux, S. A. (1998). Historical overview of responses of children and their families to chronic illness. In M. E. Broome, K. Knafl, K. Pridham, & S. Feetham (Eds.), *Children and families in health and illness* (pp. 179–195). Thousand Oaks, CA: Sage Publications.

Gallo, A. (1990). Family management style in juvenile diabetes: A case illustration. *Journal of Pediatric Nursing, 5,* 23–32.

Gallo, A. M., & Knafl, K. A. (1998). Parents' reports of "tricks of the trade" for managing childhood chronic illness. *Journal of the Society of Pediatric Nurses, 3,* 93–102.

Garwick, A., Kohrman, C., Titus, J., Wolman, C., & Blum, R. W. (1999). Variations in families' explanations of childhood chronic conditions: A cross-cultural perspective. In H. I. McCubbin & A. Thompson (Eds.), *The dynamics of resilient families* (pp. 165–202). Thousand Oaks, CA: Sage Publications.

Garwick, A., Kohrman, C., Wolman, C., & Blum, R. W. (1998). Families' recommendations for improving services for children with chronic conditions. *Archives of Pediatrics and Adolescent Medicine, 152,* 440–448.

Garwick, A., Patterson, J., Bennett, C. F., & Blum, R. W. (1995). Breaking the news: How families first learn about their child's chronic condition. *Archives of Pediatrics and Adolescent Medicine, 149,* 991–997.

Garwick, A., Patterson, J., Bennett, C. F., & Blum, R. W. (1998). Parents' perceptions of helpful versus unhelpful types of support in managing the care of pre-adolescents with chronic conditions. *Archives of Pediatrics and Adolescent Medicine, 152,* 665–671.

Holditch-Davis, D., Docherty, S., Miles, M. S., & Burchinal, M. (2001). Developmental outcomes of infants with bronchopulmonary dysplasia: Comparison with other medically fragile infants. *Research in Nursing and Health, 24,* 181–193.

Holditch-Davis, D., & Miles, M. S. (1997). Parenting the prematurely born child. In J. J. Fitzpatrick & J. Norbeck (Eds.), *Annual review of nursing research* (Vol. 15, pp. 3–34). New York: Springer.

Holditch-Davis, D., Miles, M. S., & Burchinal, P. (2001, February). *The impact of parental role attainment with parents of medically fragile infants on the parent-*

child relationship at 16 months. Paper presented at the Southern Nursing Research Society, Baltimore, Maryland.

Holditch-Davis, D., Tesh, E. M., Burchinal, M., & Miles, M. S. (1999). Early interactions between mothers and their medically fragile infants. *Applied Developmental Science, 3,* 155–167.

Huber, C., Holditch-Davis, D., & Brandon, D. (1993). High-risk preterms at three years of age: Parental response to the presence of developmental problems. *Children's Health Care, 22,* 107–122.

Kauffmann, E., Harrison, M. B., Burke, S. O., & Wong, C. (1998). Family matters: Stress-point intervention for parents of children hospitalized with chronic conditions. *Pediatric Nursing, 24,* 362–366.

Kirschbaum, M. S., & Knafl, K. A. (1996). Major themes in parent-provider relationships: A comparison of life-threatening and chronic illness experiences. *Journal of Family Nursing, 2,* 195–216.

Knafl, K. A. (1985). How families manage a pediatric hospitalization. *Western Journal of Nursing Research, 7,* 174–176.

Knafl, K. A., Ayres, L., Gallo, A. M., Zoeller, L. H., & Brietmayer, B. J. (1995). Learning from stories: Parents' accounts of the pathway to diagnosis. *Pediatric Nursing, 21,* 411–415.

Knafl, K., Breitmayer, B., Gallo, A., & Zoeller, L. (1992). Parents' views of health care providers: An exploration of the components of a positive working relationship. *Children's Health Care, 21,* 90–95.

Knafl, K., Breitmayer, B., Gallo, A., & Zoller, L. (1996). Family response to childhood chronic illness: Description of management styles. *Journal of Pediatric Nursing, 11,* 315–326.

Knafl, K. A., Cavallari, K. A., & Dixon, D. M. (1988). *Pediatric hospitalization: Family and nurse perspectives.* Glenview, IL: Scott, Foresman, and Company.

Knafl, K. A., & Deatrick, J. A. (1986). How families manage chronic conditions: An analysis of the concept of normalization. *Research in Nursing & Health, 9,* 215–222.

Knafl, K. A., & Deatrick, J. A. (1990). Family management style: Concept analysis and development. *Journal of Pediatric Nursing, 5,* 4–14.

Knafl, K. A., & Deatrick, J. A. (2001). *The challenge of normalization for families of children with chronic conditions.* Unpublished paper.

Knafl, K. A., Deatrick, J. A., & Kodadek, S. (1982). How parents manage jobs and a child's hospitalization. *MCN: American Journal of Maternal-Child Nursing, 7,* 125–127.

Knafl, K. A., & Dixon, D. M. (1984). The participation of fathers in their children's hospitalization. *Issues in Comprehensive Pediatric Nursing, 7,* 269–281.

Knafl, K. A., Gallo, A. M., Zoeller, L., & Breitmayer, B. (1993). Family response to a child's chronic illness: A description of major defining themes. In S. G. Funk (Ed.), *Key aspects of caring for the chronically ill: Hospital and home* (pp. 290–303). New York: Springer.

Knafl, K. A., Gallo, A. M., Zoeller, L. H., Breitmayer, B. J., & Ayres, L. (1993). One approach to conceptualizing family response to illness. In S. L. Feetham, S. B.

Meister, J. M. Bell, & C. L. Gillis (Eds.), *The nursing of families: Theory, research, education, practice* (pp. 70–78). Newbury Park, CA: Sage.

Knafl, K., & Zoeller, L. (2000). Childhood chronic illness: A comparison of mothers' and fathers' experiences. *Journal of Family Nursing, 6,* 287–302.

Leavitt, M., Martinson, I. M., Liu, C. Y., Armstrong, V., Hornberger, L., Zhang, J. Q., & Han, X. P. (1999). Common themes and ethnic differences in family caregiving the first year after diagnosis of childhood cancer. Part II. *Journal of Pediatric Nursing, 14,* 110–122.

Martinson, I. M. (1986–1987). Home care for the dying child with cancer: Feasibility and desirability. *Loss, Grief & Care, 1,* 97–114.

Martinson, I. M. (1989). Impact of childhood cancer on family care in Taiwan. *Pediatric Nursing, 15,* 636–637.

Martinson, I. (1995). Pediatric hospice nursing. In J. Fitzpatrick & J. Stevenson (Eds.), *Annual review of nursing research* (pp. 195–214). New York: Springer.

Martinson, I. (2001). In tribute to Marsha Cohen: Once my doctoral student and always a friend. *Journal of Family Nursing, 7,* 227–229.

Martinson, I. M., Armstrong, G., Geis, D., Anglim, M., Gronseth, E., MacInnis, H., Kersey, J., & Nesbit, M. (1978). Home care for children dying of cancer. *Pediatrics, 62,* 106–113.

Martinson, I. M., Chen, Y. C., Liu, B. Y., Lo, L. H., Ou, J. C., Wang, R. H., & Chao, Y. M. (1982). Impact of childhood cancer on the Chinese families. *Medical Science, 4,* 1395–1415.

Martinson, I., Chong, Y. L., & Liang, Y. H. (1997). Distress symptoms and support systems of Chinese parents of children with cancer. *Cancer Nursing, 20,* 94–99.

Martinson, I. M., & Cohen, M. (1988). Themes from a longitudinal study of family reaction to childhood cancer. *Journal of Psychosocial Oncology, 6,* 81–98.

Martinson, I. M., Davies, B., & McClowry, S. (1991). Parental depression following the death of a child. *Death Studies, 15,* 259–267.

Martinson, I., Davis, A., Armstrong, V., Gan, I., Jin, Q., Liang, Y., & Lin, J. (1997). The experience of the family of children with chronic illness at home in China. *Pediatric Nursing, 23,* 371–376.

Martinson, I., Davis, A., Liu, C. Y., Gan, I., Jin, C., Liang, Y., & Lin, J. (1995). Chinese mothers' reactions to their child's chronic illness. *International Healthcare for Women, 16,* 365–375.

Martinson, I. M., Kim, S., Yang, S. O., Young, S. C., Lee, J. S., & Young, H. L. (1995). Impact of childhood cancer on Korean families. *Journal of Pediatric Oncology Nursing, 12,* 11–17.

Martinson, I. M., Leavitt, M., Liu, C., Armstrong, V., Hornberger, L., Ziang, J. Q., & Han, X. (1999). Common themes and ethnic differences in family caregiving the first year after diagnosis of childhood cancer. Part I. *Journal of Pediatric Nursing, 14,* 99–109.

Martinson, I. M., Lee, H. O., & Kim, S. (2000). Culturally based interventions for families whose child dies. *Illness, Crisis & Loss, 8,* 17–31.

Martinson, I. M., McClowry, S. G., Davies, B., & Kuhlenkamp, E. J. (1994). Changes over time: Family bereavement following childhood cancer. *Palliative Care, 10,* 19–25.

Martinson, I. M., Moldow, D. G., Armstrong, G. D., Henry, W. F., Nesbit, M. E., & Kersey, J. H. (1986). Home care for children dying of cancer. *Research in Nursing and Health, 9,* 11–16.

Martinson, I. M., Yin, S. X., & Liang, Y. H. (1993). The impact of childhood cancer on fifty Chinese families. *Journal of Pediatric Oncology Nursing, 10,* 13–18.

Martinson, I. M., Zhong, B. H., & Liang, Y. H. (1994). The reaction of Chinese parents to terminally ill children with cancer. *Cancer Nursing, 17,* 72–76.

McCarthy, S. M., & Gallo, A. M. (1992). A case illustration of Family Management Style. *Journal of Pediatric Nursing, 17,* 395–402.

McClowry, S. G., Davies, E. B., May, K. A., Kulenkamp, E. J., & Martinson, I. M. (1987). The empty space phenomenon: The process of grief in the bereaved family. *Death Studies, 11,* 361–374.

Miles, M. S., Carter, M. C., Eberly, T. W., Hennessey, J., & Riddle, I. I. (1989). Toward an understanding of parent stress in the pediatric intensive care unit: Overview of a program of research. *Maternal-Child Nursing Journal, 18,* 181–185.

Miles, M. S., Carter, M. C., Riddle, I., Hennessey, J., & Eberly, T. W. (1989). The pediatric intensive care unit environment as a source of stress for parents. *Maternal-Child Nursing Journal, 18,* 199–206.

Miles, M. S., D'Auria, J., Hart, E. M., Sedlack, D. A., & Watral, M. A. (1993). Parental role alterations experienced by mothers of children with a life-threatening chronic illness. In S. Funk, E. M. Tornquist, M. T. Champagne, & R. A. Wiese (Eds.), *Key aspects of chronic illness care: Home and hospital* (pp. 281–289). New York: Springer.

Miles, M. S., & Docherty, S. (2001). *The response of African American and Caucasion fathers to hospitalization of a medically fragile infant.* Unpublished paper submitted for publication.

Miles, M. S., & Frauman, A. (1993). Barriers and bridges: Nurses' and parents' negotiation of caregiving roles with medically fragile infants. In S. Funk, E. M. Tornquist, M. T. Champagne, & R. A. Wiese (Eds.), *Key aspects of chronic illness care: Home and hospital* (pp. 239–250). New York: Springer.

Miles, M. S., Funk, S. G., & Kasper, M. A. (1991). The neonatal intensive care unit environment: Sources of stress for parents. *AACN Clinical Issues in Critical Care Nursing, 2,* 346–354.

Miles, M. S., & Holditch-Davis, D. (1995). Compensatory parenting: How mothers describe parenting their 3-year-old prematurely born children. *Journal of Pediatric Nursing, 10,* 243–253.

Miles, M. S., Holditch-Davis, D., Brunssen, S., Burchinal, P., & Wilson, S. (2002). Perceptions of stress, worry, and support in Black and White mothers of hospitalized medically fragile infants. *Journal of Pediatric Nursing, 17,* 82–88.

Miles, M. S., Holditch-Davis, D., & Burchinal, P. (2001, February). *Parental role attainment with medically fragile infants.* Paper presented at the Southern Nursing Research Society, Baltimore, MD.

Miles, M. S., Holditch-Davis, D., Burchinal, P., & Nelson, D. (1999). Distress and growth outcomes in mothers of medically fragile infants. *Nursing Research, 48,* 129–140.

Miles, M. S., Holditch-Davis, D., & Shepherd, H. (1998). Concerns of mothers in parenting three-year-old prematurely born children. *Journal of Maternal-Child Nursing, 23*(2), 70–75.

Miles, M. S., Wilson, S., & Docherty, S. (1999). African American mothers' response to hospitalization of a seriously ill infant. *Neonatal Networks, 18,* 17–25.

Moldow, D. G., Armstrong, G. D., Henry, W. F., & Martinson, I. M. (1982). The cost of home care for dying children. *Medical Care, 20,* 1114–1160.

Moore, I. M., Gilliss, C. L., & Martinson, I. M. (1988). Psychosomatic manifestations of bereavement in parents two years after the death of a child with cancer. *Nursing Research, 37,* 104–107.

Nelson, A., Miles, M. S., Reed, S. B., Poprawa, C., & Cooper, H. (1994). Depressive symptomatology in parents of children with life-threatening oncologic and hematology disorders. *Journal of Psychosocial Oncology, 12,* 61–75.

Obrecht, J. A., Gallo, A. M., & Knafl, K. A. (1992). A case illustration of Family Management Style in childhood end stage renal disease. *American Nephrology Nurses Association Journal, 19,* 255–259.

Patterson, J. M., Garwick, A. W., Bennett, F. C., & Blum, R. W. (1997). Social support in families of children with chronic conditions: Supportive and nonsupportive behaviors. *Journal of Developmental and Behavioral Pediatrics, 18,* 383–391.

Stein, R. E. K., & Jessop, D. J. (1982). A noncategorical approach to chronic childhood illness. *Public Health Reports, 97,* 354–362.

Thompson, R. J., & Gustafson, K. E. (1996). *Adaptation to chronic childhood illness.* Washington, DC: American Psychological Association.

Van Riper, M. (1992). Symbolic interactionism: A perspective for understanding parent-nurse interactions following the birth of a child with Down syndrome. *Maternal-Child Nursing Journal, 20,* 21–40.

Van Riper, M. (1999). Maternal perceptions of family-provider relationships and well-being in families of children with Down syndrome. *Research in Nursing & Health, 22,* 357–368.

Van Riper, M. (2000). Family variables associated with well-being in families of children with Down syndrome. *Journal of Family Nursing, 6,* 267–286.

Van Riper, M. (2001). Family-provider relationships and well-being in families of preterm infants. *Heart and Lung, 30,* 74–84.

Van Riper, M., Ryff, C., & Pridham, K. (1992). Parental and family well-being in families of children with Down syndrome: A comparative study. *Research in Nursing & Health, 15,* 227–235.

Van Riper, M., & Selder, F. E. (1989). Parental responses to the birth of a child with Down syndrome. In J. Rainer, S. Rubin, M. Bartalas, et al. (Eds.), *Genetic disease: The unwanted inheritance* (pp. 59–76). New York: Haworth.

Yantzi, N., Rosenberg, M. W., Burke, S. O., & Harrison, M. B. (2001). The impacts of distance to hospital on families with a child with a chronic condition. *Social Science & Medicine, 52,* 1777–1991.

Chapter 10

The Sibling Experience of Living With Childhood Chronic Illness and Disability

MARCIA VAN RIPER

ABSTRACT

The main purpose of this integrative review is to summarize existing nursing research on the sibling experience of living in a family that includes a child with a chronic illness or disability, specifically highlighting nurse researchers who have conducted more than two studies concerning the sibling experience. A secondary purpose is to determine to what extent nurse researchers interested in the sibling experience have used or been informed by a developmental science perspective. A final purpose is to discuss future research needed to further develop the existing knowledge base concerning the sibling experience of living with childhood chronic illness and disability. Forty of 86 published research articles were authored or coauthored by nurses. There were four nurse researchers with programs of research. Most studies used a categorical approach and were descriptive, cross-sectional designs; there were few longitudinal studies. Multiple factors were identified that affect how siblings respond to childhood chronic illness and disability. Future research needs to focus on siblings and families from diverse cultural and socioeconomic backgrounds, and outcomes need to be assessed at multiple levels. Furthermore, intervention studies building on the descriptive research are needed.

During the past three decades, the amount of research on the sibling experience of living with childhood chronic illness and disability has increased dramatically. This increase reflects a growing awareness that chronic illness and disability are relatively common features of childhood (McDaniel, Hepworth, & Doherty, 1992), and the effects of these chronic conditions are not limited to the individual who has the illness or disability (Rolland, 1994). Family members are interconnected and dependent upon one another. When there is a change in the health of one member, all family members are affected in some way and the family unit as a whole is altered (McCubbin & McCubbin, 1993; McDaniel, Hepworth, & Doherty, 1992; Rolland, 1994; Wright & Leahey, 2000; Wright, Watson, & Bell, 1996).

Approximately 18% to 31% of all children in the United States have a chronic health condition (Newacheck, 1994; Newacheck et al., 1998), and a large percentage of these children have one or more siblings. Siblings spend more time with each other than with other family members (Bank, 1982; Bank & Kahn, 1975). Because of their time together, siblings exert a powerful influence on each other. When one sibling has a chronic condition, this influence may be even stronger, especially if the typically developing sibling takes on additional caretaking responsibilities (Gallo, 1988; Gath, 1974; McHale & Gamble, 1989; Siemon, 1984). Given that advances in science continue to increase the life expectancy for children with chronic conditions, there will most likely continue to be a large number of siblings who take on long-term caretaking challenges and burdens. Therefore, it is critical that nurses be able to make sense of and use the existing research in this area.

Nursing has made significant contributions to the existing knowledge base concerning the sibling experience of living with childhood chronic illness and disability. Notably, four nurse researchers have conducted more than two studies concerning the sibling experience (Craft, Gallo, Murray, Williams). In addition, at least 25 other published reports of nursing research concern the sibling experience of childhood chronic illness and disability. Nurses have been the authors or coauthors for literature reviews on siblings of hospitalized children (Craft, 1993); siblings and childhood cancer (Kramer, 1981; Murray, 1999a; Ross-Alaolmolki, Heinzer, Howard, & Marszal, 1995); siblings and childhood chronic illness (Brett, 1988; Drotar & Crawford, 1985; Gallo & Knafl, 1993; McKeever, 1983; Williams, 1997); and siblings of children with disabilities (Faux, 1993).

To date, none of the existing reviews concerning the sibling experience of living with childhood chronic illness and disability have focused specifically on nursing research, nor have these reviews explored the extent to which the researchers used or were informed by a developmental science perspective. Therefore, the main purpose of this integrative review is to summarize existing nursing research on the sibling experience of living in a family that includes a child with a chronic illness or disability, specifically highlighting nurse researchers who have conducted more than two studies concerning the sibling experience. A secondary purpose is to determine to what extent nurse researchers interested in the sibling experience have used or been informed by a developmental science perspective. A final purpose is to discuss future research needed to further develop the existing knowledge base concerning the sibling experience of living with childhood chronic illness and disability.

METHODS

This chapter is an integrative review of 40 studies concerning the sibling experience of living in a family that includes a child with a chronic illness or disability. All of the studies were conducted by nurse researchers and published after 1972. For the purpose of this chapter, children with a chronic illness or disability are defined as children who (a) have a chronic physical, developmental, behavioral, or emotional condition and (b) require health and related services of a type or amount beyond that required by children in general. Studies that focus on the sibling response to the death of a child were excluded from this review, as were studies concerning siblings of individuals who develop chronic illnesses or disabilities in adulthood. No limitation was placed on the age of the sibling.

Several strategies were used to obtain the sample of studies. First, computer-based searches (i.e., CINAHL, MEDLINE, PUBMED, and PSYCHLIT) were conducted using the following keywords: *siblings, chronic illness, chronic conditions, disability, mental retardation, mental illness,* and *childhood cancer*. Next, reference lists from the identified studies, as well as those from review articles, were searched for additional studies. Then, specific journals were searched, including *Children's Health Care, Journal of Pediatric Nursing: Nursing Care of Children and Families, Issues in Comprehensive Pediatric Nursing, Journal of Family Nursing*, and *Pediatric Nursing*. Finally, work by nurse researchers known to be interested in the sibling experience (e.g., Craft, Faux, Gallo, Murray, and Williams) was searched.

Questions addressed in this review include: How has nursing research concerning the sibling experience of living with chronic illness and disability changed during the past three decades in terms of areas of focus, theoretical approaches, methods, and findings? To what extent have nurse researchers interested in the sibling experience of chronic illness and disability incorporated key aspects of the developmental science perspective (e.g., holistic approach, use of developmentally appropriate measures and constructs, longitudinal designs, person-oriented analysis) into their research? What research is needed to further develop the nursing research base concerning the sibling experience of chronic illness and disability?

FINDINGS

Eighty-six published research articles concerning the sibling experience of chronic illness and disability were identified. Of these, 40 were authored or coauthored by nurses. The articles reviewed in this chapter have been organized into three groups: early research (1972–1992), recent research (1992–present), and the four programs of research.

Early Research

The initial stimulus for nursing research on siblings of children with chronic conditions appears to have come from clinical nurse specialists and other nurses who noted that some children have difficulty adjusting to their sibling's chronic illness or disability (Craft, 1979; Everson, 1977; Thibodeau, 1988). In early publications, siblings of children with chronic conditions were referred to as "the family's neglected 'other' child" (Craft, 1979, p. 297), "the neglected group" (Menke, 1987, p. 132), and "the forgotten group" (Brett, 1988, p. 43). Sibling counseling was identified as "a forgotten part of family-centered care in pediatrics" (Everson, 1977, p. 644). Signs of poor sibling adjustment described by nurses include fatigue, weakness, poor appetite, overeating, enuresis, nightmares, irritability, impatience, restlessness, overactivity, lack of initiative, social withdrawal, poor school performance, school phobia, increased sibling rivalry, self-blame, and preoccupation with thoughts of the affected child (Craft, 1979; Everson, 1977; Thibodeau, 1988).

Prior to 1992, most nursing studies concerning the sibling experience of chronic illness and disability were descriptive studies that used a qualitative approach (Faux, 1991; Gallo, 1990; Harder & Bowditch, 1982; Iles, 1979; Kramer, 1984; Martinson, Gilliss, Colaizzo, Freeman, & Bossert, 1990; Menke, 1987; Pinyerd, 1983; Taylor, 1980; Walker, 1988). Typically, semi-structured interviews were conducted with the siblings and, for some studies, both the siblings and their parents (e.g., Faux, 1991; Menke, 1987; Pinyerd, 1983; Walker, 1988). A number of the early nurse researchers interested in the sibling experience used additional data collection techniques. For example, Walker (1988) used puppet play, drawings, cartoon storytelling, and a sentence-completion test to enhance sibling communication during the interviews. In addition to interviewing mothers of children with developmental disabilities, Scheiber (1989) did in-home observations of interactions between these mothers and their children (children with developmental disabilities and their typically developing siblings). While interviewing siblings was very common in early nursing research concerning the sibling experience, it was not that common in other disciplines. Sibling researchers in other disciplines were more likely to interview parents, most often mothers, about the sibling experience. They seldom interviewed the siblings.

Most of the early nursing research on the sibling experience of chronic illness and disability used a categorical or disease entity approach (Gallo & Knafl, 1993). That is, the focus was limited to siblings of children with specific diseases, rather than siblings of children who have diseases with similar illness characteristics (e.g., onset, visibility, incapacitation, disease course, treatment demands, and outcome). In seven of the early sibling studies conducted by nurses, the sample was limited to siblings of children with a single condition or disease entity. For example, in four of the studies the specific condition or disease entity was childhood cancer (Iles, 1979; Kramer, 1984; Martinson et al., 1990; Walker, 1988). In the study conducted by Harder and Bowditch (1982), all of the siblings who were interviewed were living in a family that included a child with cystic fibrosis. Pinyerd (1983) limited her sample to siblings of children with myelomeningocele. The family presented in the case study by Gallo (1990) included a child with juvenile diabetes and two healthy siblings.

Three nurse researchers included siblings of children with two or more chronic conditions in their sample. Taylor (1980) interviewed 25 school-age siblings of children with three different chronic conditions (asthma, congenital heart disease, and cystic fibrosis). In the study by Faux (1991), the sample not only included siblings of children with two chronic conditions (craniofacial anomalies and cardiac anomalies), but it also included a comparison group of siblings of typically developing, healthy children. Menke (1987) interviewed 72 siblings of school-age children with five conditions (cancer, cystic fibrosis, congenital heart disease, burns, and myelomeningocele) and their parents. Menke's (1987) study is one of earliest sibling studies in which the researcher clearly identified the noncategorical illness characteristics used to select the sample. As noted by Gallo and Knafl (1993), Menke selected her sample in a specific way to obtain divergent experiences based on disease trajectory as reflected in the degree of incapacitation and prognosis.

In general, findings from early nursing research on the sibling experience of chronic illness and disability provided support for the belief that siblings of children affected by chronic illness and disability experience ongoing stressors and challenges. In the study by Walker (1988), content analysis of sibling data revealed major stressor themes of loss, fear of death, and change. The majority of siblings in the study by Menke (1987) expressed worries about their affected family member. In addition, they noted changes in their parents, such as being more worried and tired, having more fights, and spending more time with the ill child. For siblings in the study by Harder and Bowditch (1982), the most frequently reported unresolved problem was parents spending too much time with the child with cystic fibrosis. In a study concerning siblings of children with childhood cancer, dominant themes for siblings were the need for information, feelings of being displaced and unimportant, and the need for involvement in the life of the affected child (Martinson et al., 1990).

Findings from early nursing research on the sibling experience did not provide support for the common assumption that chronic childhood conditions invariably have a deleterious effect on family members. In fact, most researchers reported both positive and negative effects. For example, Taylor (1980) noted that while two thirds of the siblings of children with chronic illnesses expressed feelings of isolation, egocentricity, deprivation, inferiority, or inadequate knowledge, one third of them reported positive effects, such as increased self-esteem, empathy, cognitive mastery, cooperation, and rewards. In Pinyerd's (1983) study of siblings of children with myelomeningocele, some of the siblings did not share their worries and concerns with their parents, but none expressed overwhelming concerns, and the majority had an accurate understanding of their sibling's condition. Themes of loss, change, and growth in human relations and self-concept were revealed in a small study concerning five school-age siblings of children with cancer (Iles, 1979). Three major sources of stress (emotional realignment within the family, separation from family members, and family disruptions and changes brought on by the ill child's therapeutic regiment) were noted in a study about siblings living with childhood cancer (Kramer,

1984), but positive consequences were also noted (increased sensitivity and empathy for the ill child, enhanced personal maturation, and greater family cohesion). In the study by Harder and Bowditch (1982), 12 of the 19 siblings reported that their families were closer together because of the cystic fibrosis.

Findings from these early nursing studies concerning the sibling experience of chronic illness and disability are somewhat contradictory and inconclusive, and their generalizability is limited because most were based on data from small, convenience samples, without control groups. However, these early studies did lay the groundwork for future sibling studies. Findings from them sensitized nurse researchers to the unique issues and concerns experienced by siblings of children with chronic conditions. In addition, they helped to elucidate factors that may influence sibling adjustment (e.g., sibling age and gender, family size, family definition or meaning of the chronic illness or disability, patterns of communication in the family, sibling understanding of the chronic condition, family resources, sibling involvement in decision making and caretaking). Nurse researchers who conducted these early studies on the sibling experience of living with chronic illness and disability consistently emphasized the need for longitudinal studies with age-matched control groups of typically developing, healthy children.

Crisis theory, stress and coping frameworks, and family systems theory were the most common theoretical perspectives employed in early nursing research concerning the sibling experience of living in a family that includes a child with a chronic condition (Brett, 1988). The child's chronic condition was typically conceptualized as a stressor that affected the behavioral, psychological, and cognitive development of other family members (Gallo & Knafl, 1993). Areas of focus in these early sibling studies included (a) fears, worries, and concerns of the siblings; (b) sibling awareness and understanding of the chronic condition; (c) losses experienced by the siblings; (d) changes and disruptions in peer and family relationships; (e) changes in the sibling's environment; and (f) indicators of sibling maladjustment (anxiety, behavior problems, feelings of isolation, egocentricity, deprivation, and stigma). Despite their interest in understanding the negative aspects of this rather unique sibling experience, early nurse researchers in this area were open to the possibility that there might be positive aspects. This openness to the possibility of positive aspects was not true of early sibling researchers from other disciplines, who focused almost exclusively on the negative aspects of the sibling experience of chronic illness and disability.

Recent Research

The most commonly used theoretical perspectives in recent nursing studies concerning the sibling experience of chronic illness and disability include Orem's Self-Care Deficit Theory (Orem, 1991); Lazarus and Folkman's (1984) Framework of Stress and Coping; the Resiliency Model of Stress, Adjustment, and Adaptation (McCubbin & McCubbin, 1993); the Family Management Style Model (Knafl & Deatrick, 1990); and House's (1981) conceptualization of social support. While the assumption that a child's chronic condition will invariably have a negative impact on other family members is less common than it was in early sibling research, the child's chronic condition is still conceptualized as a stressor that affects the behavioral, psychological, and cognitive development of other family members.

Recent nursing studies concerning the sibling experience continue to focus on many of the areas examined in earlier studies (e.g., fears, worries, and concerns of the siblings; sibling awareness and understanding of the chronic condition; losses experienced by the siblings; changes and disruptions in peer and family relationships; changes in the sibling's environment; and indicators of sibling maladjustment, such as anxiety, behavior problems, and feelings of isolation, depression, and stigma), but there has been a greater emphasis on indicators of psychological well-being (e.g., self-esteem, self-concept, and social competence) in recent research. In addition, there is growing interest in the broader etiology that influences sibling adjustment, especially factors that are modifiable. For example, Van Riper (2000) examined the relationship between family demands, family resources, family problem-solving communication, family coping, and sibling well-being.

While the primary method of data collection in sibling studies conducted by nurses prior to 1992 was semistructured interviews, the primary method of data collection in recent sibling studies has been self-report questionnaires (Davies, 1993; Heffernan & Zanelli, 1997; Lee, Phoenix, Brown, & Jackson, 1997; Mandleco, Olsen, Dyches, & Marshall, in press; Murray, 1995, 2001b; Phuphaibul & Muensa, 1999; Williams et al., 1997; Williams et al., 1999; Van Riper, 2000) or a combination of interviews and self-report questionnaires (e.g., Gallo, Breitmayer, Knafl, & Zoeller, 1992, 1993; Gallo & Szychlinksi, in press; Kiburz, 1994; Mims, 1997; Wang & Martinson, 1996). Interviews were the sole source of data in only five of the recent sibling studies (Faulkner, 1996; Kendall, 1998; Lehna, 1998; Smith, 1998; Williams, Lorenzo, & Borja, 1993).

In the majority of studies, data were collected from both the siblings and their parents (Gallo & Szychlinski, in press; Heffernan & Zanelli, 1997; Kiburz, 1994; Mims, 1997; Murray, 2001a; Van Riper, 2000; Wang & Martinson, 1996; Williams et al., 1997; Williams et al., 1999). In two studies, data were collected from the child with the chronic condition, the sibling, and one or both parents (Faulkner, 1996; Kendall, 1998). Lee and colleagues collected data from 14 children with sickle cell disease and their 14 siblings. Mandleco and colleagues (in press) collected data from siblings, parents, and the sibling's teacher. Five studies collected data from siblings only (Lee et al., 1997; Lehna, 1998; Murray, 1998, 2001b; Smith, 1998), and four collected data from mothers only (Davies, 1993; Gallo et al., 1993; Phuphaibul & Muensa, 1999; Williams et al., 1993). Murray (1995) was the only nurse researcher to collect data about siblings from nurses.

Unlike the earlier sibling research conducted by nurse researchers, a number of the more recent sibling studies included a control or comparison group (Davies, 1993; Gallo & Szychlinski, in press; Mims, 1997; Mandleco et al., in press). The sample in the study by Gallo and Szychlinski (in press) included 45 siblings of children with diabetes, 45 siblings of children with asthma, and 45 healthy siblings. The sample in the study by Mims (1997) included 10 siblings of children with frequent seizures, 10 siblings of children with infrequent seizures, and 11 siblings of children with no chronic illness.

Much of the recent sibling research conducted by nurse researchers continues to use a categorical approach. However, a number of the recent studies have used a noncategorical approach. The study conducted by Gallo and colleagues (Gallo et al., 1992, 1993) is a good example of a sibling study that used a noncategorical approach. The sample for this study included 28 siblings of children with a wide variety of conditions (e.g., diabetes, renal failure, juvenile rheumatoid arthritis, Crohn's disease, systemic lupus, scleroderma, ankylosing spondylitis, and asthma) differing in terms of onset, visibility, incapacitation, disease course, treatment demands, and outcome.

Despite growing recognition of the need for longitudinal studies of the sibling experience of chronic illness and disability, they remain the exception rather than the norm. One of the few longitudinal sibling studies conducted by nurses is the examination by Gallo and colleagues (1992) of the psychological adjustment of well siblings of chronically ill children. Another is the study by Wang and Martinson (1996) that explored the behavioral responses of healthy Chinese siblings to the stress of childhood cancer in the family. A third longitudinal study conducted by nurses was the intervention study by Williams et al. (1997), which is also one of the only sibling intervention studies that has been conducted in nursing.

As with the findings from the early sibling studies, findings from the recent nursing research concerning the sibling experience of living with chronic illness and disability are inconclusive and often contradictory. While some researchers (Heffernan & Zanelli, 1997; Kendall, 1998; Lee et al., 1997; Mims, 1997; Phuphaibul & Muensa, 1999; Smith, 1998; Williams et al., 1993, 1997, 2000) have reported that siblings living with chronic illness and disability are at increased risk for negative consequences (e.g., behavior problems, increased stress, depression, and isolation), others have suggested that siblings living with chronic illness and disability are not necessarily at greater risk for negative consequences (Faulkner, 1996; Gallo et al., 1992; Kiburz, 1994; Mandleco et al., in press; Murray, 1998; Van Riper, 2000) and may, in fact, experience positive consequences, such as increased empathy, cooperation, and patience, higher self-concept, and increased family cohesion.

Studies conducted to identify factors that influence sibling response to living with chronic illness (e.g., Gallo et al., 1993; Gallo & Szychlinski, in press; Mandleco et al., in press; Murray, 2001b; Van Riper, 2000) have identified the following factors: age and gender of the sibling; perceived controllability of the chronic condition; prognosis for the child with the chronic condition; social support; family demands; family resources; family problem-solving communication; and family coping. An important finding for nurses and other clinicians working with families who are dealing with childhood chronic illness and disability is that most of these factors are modifiable.

Programs of Research

There were four nurse researchers with programs of research on the sibling response to illness and disability. These included M. J. Craft and colleagues, A. Gallo and colleagues, J. S. Murray, and P. D. Williams and colleagues.

M. J. CRAFT AND COLLEAGUES

Craft is one of the first nurse researchers to focus on the sibling experience. To date, she has published a clinical article on siblings of hospitalized children (Craft, 1979), five data-based articles on siblings of hospitalized children (Craft, 1986; Craft & Craft, 1989; Craft, Lakin, Oppliger, Clancy, & Vanderlinden, 1990; Craft & Wyatt, 1986; Craft, Wyatt, & Sandell, 1985), and a literature review on siblings of hospitalized children (Craft, 1993).

Craft's first study (Craft et al., 1985; Craft & Craft, 1989) was a descriptive study designed to assess changes in feelings and behaviors experienced by 123 siblings (5 to 17 years of age) of children hospitalized for acute, chronic, and progressive illness. Her second study (Craft, 1986) involved validation of the Perceived Changes Scale. This scale was used in Craft's first study, and it has two versions (an interview using projective techniques for siblings between 5 and 10 years and a questionnaire for siblings 11 years and older). For her third study, Craft joined Wyatt (Craft & Wyatt, 1986) and used a quasi-experimental design to explore the impact of sibling visitation on 32 siblings of hospitalized children. In the fourth study (Craft et al., 1990), Craft and colleagues examined the effectiveness of a 4-month intervention program in which 31 siblings of children with cerebral palsy were taught about cerebral palsy and what they could do to encourage their sibling with cerebral palsy to be more independent.

An important finding from Craft's program of research is that parents of hospitalized children may not be aware of all the changes in feelings and behavior experienced by their other children. Another important finding is that certain factors (e.g., sibling age, relationship of the sibling with the hospitalized child, fear of getting the disease, residence of the sibling during the hospitalization of the sick child, and perceived changes in parenting) may influence the number and kind of changes experienced by siblings of hospitalized children. An exciting finding from Craft's program of research is that siblings can be important teachers, role models, and agents of change in families that include a child with a chronic condition.

Craft's program of research concerning siblings of hospitalized children is notable for a number of reasons. First, her work is grounded in her experience as a pediatric nurse. Next, she has built each study on findings from her prior work. Another strength is that over time her studies have become more methodologically sophisticated. Her first study was descriptive, her next involved validation of an instrument, her third was a comparison study that included a quasi-experimental design, and her fourth was an intervention study. A final reason why Craft's program of research is notable it that she has consistently taken into account the developmental level of the siblings. She has designed, tested, and validated a measure of perceived change so that it is developmentally appropriate for siblings of different ages. For researchers and clinicians interested in the sibling experience of chronic illness and disability, it would have been helpful if Craft had explored how the three groups of siblings compare on the type and number of changes that they experience.

A. GALLO AND COLLEAGUES

Gallo has a program of research on well siblings of children with chronic illness. To date, she has published a clinical article on the special sibling relationship in chronic illness and disability (Gallo, 1988), a case study on a family that includes a child with juvenile diabetes (Gallo, 1990), three data-based articles on siblings of children with chronic illness (Gallo et al., 1992, 1993; Gallo & Szychlinski, in press), and a literature review on siblings of chronically ill children (Gallo & Knafl, 1993).

In Gallo's first study (Gallo et al., 1992; Knafl, Breitmeyer, Gallo, & Zoeller, 1987), she used parental ratings on the Child Behavior Checklist to examine the psychological adjustment of 28 well siblings (age 6 to 16 years) of children with different types of chronic illnesses at two time points, 12 months apart. In a subsequent publication (Gallo et al., 1993), Gallo used data from the sample in her first study to examine variations in sibling behavioral adjustment in relation to mothers' perceptions of the illness experience and family life. Based on mothers' ratings on the behavior problem scale of the Child Behavior Checklist, five siblings considered to be very well adjusted and five siblings considered to be poorly adjusted were compared with respect to mothers' reports of individual family members' response to illness, illness management, parenting philosophy, presence of other stressors, availability of social supports, and impact of the illness on family members and family life. The recently completed study by Gallo and Szychlinski (in press) was a comparative study of 135 healthy siblings of children with diabetes, asthma, or healthy children. Siblings completed the Family APGAR for Children (Austin & Huberty, 1989) and Harter's Self Perception Profile for Children (Harter, 1985a).

Findings from Gallo's program of research suggest that siblings of children with chronic illness may not be uniformly at risk for behavior and social competence problems. Two major differences were noted between mothers who rated their healthy siblings as either very well adjusted or poorly adjusted: (a) the effects of the illness on the healthy sibling, the ill child, and the marital relationship and (b) perceived controllability of the chronic illness. In Gallo's recent study, female sibling pairs in the diabetic group had lower family functioning scores than female pairs in the asthma or healthy group, whereas male sibling pairs had lower self-concept scores than male pairs in the asthma group. Healthy siblings of children with diabetes were most at risk for self-concept difficulties. They exhibited difficulties in the following areas: scholastic competence, social acceptance, and global self-worth. In addition, siblings in the diabetic group were less satisfied with how their parents talked about and shared problems than siblings in the healthy group. For the siblings in the diabetic group, physical appearance, behavioral conduct, athletic competence, scholastic competence, and global self-worth were associated with satisfaction in family functioning.

Gallo's work has added significantly to our understanding of the sibling experience of chronic illness. She has conducted a longitudinal study concerning the sibling experience of chronic illness, as well as a cross-sectional study with a comparison group of siblings of healthy children. Her research is conceptually grounded in the Family Management Style Model (Knafl & Deatrick, 1990). She has used both a categorical and a noncategorical approach in her work. She has collected data concerning the sibling experience from multiple sources (i.e., siblings, mothers, and fathers) using a mixed-method approach. The measures that she has used have been valid and reliable, as well as developmentally appropriate. Findings from her work have helped sibling researchers to identify factors that may influence whether or not siblings living in a family that includes a child who has a chronic condition will be resilient and thrive, or suffer negative consequences.

J. S. MURRAY

The focus of Murray's program of research is siblings of children with cancer. He has published three conceptual papers concerning how different theoretical perspectives (i.e., attachment theory, developmental theory, and House's conceptualization of social support) can help to understand the sibling experience of cancer (Murray, 2000a, 2000b, 2000e), three methodological papers (Murray, 1999b, 2000c, 2000d), a literature review (Murray, 1999a), and four data-based papers (Murray 1995, 1998, 2001a, 2001b).

In his first study, which was guided by House's conceptualization of social support, Murray (1995) used an instrument that he had developed, the Sibling Support Questionnaire, to identify nursing interventions used by 134 pediatric oncology nurses to provide social support to siblings of children with cancer. Murray's next study (1988) was a phenomenological study designed to gain a better understanding of the lived experience of a 14-year-old who had a sibling with childhood cancer. In his third study, a descriptive, exploratory study guided by House's conceptualization of social support, Murray (2001b) investigated the social support interventions received by school-age siblings of children with cancer. He also examined which of these interventions siblings and parents perceived as helpful. He collected data from 50 school-age siblings and their parents using either the sibling or parent version of the Nurse-Sibling Support Questionnaire. For his fourth study, Murray used the Personal Attribute Inventory for Children (PAIC) with the sample of 50 school-age children described above to examine self-concept in school-age siblings of children with cancer who attended summer camp.

According to Murray's findings, the two interventions that nurses use most to support siblings of children with cancer are (1) encouraging parents to spend time with their other children and (2) encouraging parents to provide honest responses to questions asked by siblings. Themes that emerged from Murray's phenomenological study of one sibling's experience with childhood cancer include emotional intensity, increased empathy for others, need for support, personal growth, and a desire to help others. Siblings in Murray's third study indicated that interventions aimed at providing emotional and instrumental support were the most helpful. Parents perceived interventions aimed at meeting the siblings' need for emotional and informational support as the most helpful. Parents reported a higher frequency of emotional, informational, and appraisal support for their children than their children reported. Siblings who attended summer camp scored higher on the PAIC than siblings who did not. According to Murray, this finding suggests that a camp experience may play an important role in how siblings cope with having a brother or sister with childhood cancer.

Murray's work has made significant contributions to our knowledge base concerning the sibling experience of cancer. In his conceptual papers, he has shown how researchers and clinicians can use different theoretical perspectives to better understand how siblings respond to the experience of living in a family that includes a child with cancer. His methodological papers provide support for the increased use of mixed-method designs in studies concerning the sibling experience of cancer. The measure that he has developed to assess social support interventions received by siblings of children with cancer may prove very useful to researchers and clinicians interested in the sibling experience of cancer and other chronic conditions. Findings from Murray's program of research highlight the need for nurses and other clinicians to realize that healthy siblings' perceptions of their own need for social support may not be congruent with those of their parents or clinicians.

P. D. WILLIAMS AND COLLEAGUES

Williams and her colleagues have conducted three studies concerning siblings of chronically ill children (Williams et al., 1997; Williams, Lorenzo, & Borja, 1993; Williams et al., 1999). In addition, Williams (1997) has published a review of the literature on siblings and pediatric chronic illness.

In the first study, Williams, Lorenzo, and Borja (1993) used structured interviews to collect information about sibling and maternal activities from 100 Filipino mothers of children with chronic conditions (57 with cardiac conditions and 43 with neurological conditions). The items included in the interviews were based on Duvall's (1977) concept of family developmental tasks and a review of the literature. The second study (Williams et al., 1997) was a one-group, pretest-post-test pilot study to evaluate the outcomes of a structured educational and support group nursing intervention for 22 siblings of children with four chronic illnesses (cancer, cystic fibrosis, diabetes, and spina bifida). An additional purpose of the study was to describe sibling and parent perceptions of sibling experiences at home. The third study (Williams et al., 1999) was based on data collected from the families that participated in study two. Siblings completed Harter's Social Support Scale for Children (Harter, 1985b), Harter's Self-Perception Profile for Children (Harter, 1985a), and the Mood Scale developed by Sahler and Carpenter (1989). Mothers completed the Family Adaptability and Cohesion Scales (FACES II) developed by Olson and colleagues (1985) and the Profile of Mood States—Short Form (McNair, Lorr, & Droppleman, 1992).

Findings from the first study by Williams and colleagues (1993) suggest that having a child with a chronic illness in the family significantly increased sibling household activities and decreased sibling social and school activities, especially for girls. Parents' average evaluation rating of the sibling intervention used in study two was 9 on a 10-point scale (Williams et al., 1997). Positive comments by the parents supported their positive ratings of the intervention. Sibling and parent perceptions of sibling experiences at home were congruent. The most common consequences for siblings were feelings of isolation and resentment.

In the third study by Williams and colleagues (1999), an exploratory path analysis was done to generate a causal model for further testing. Results showed significant path coefficients, indicating that positive maternal mood was associated with sibling perception of higher social support, which in turn was related to higher self-esteem and more positive sibling mood. In addition, positive maternal mood was related to higher family functioning, which in turn was related to positive sibling mood. Considering the small sample size ($n = 22$), these results must be viewed with extreme caution.

The work by Williams and colleagues has broadened our understanding of sibling activities in families that include a child with a chronic condition. In addition, their work has provided an example of a nursing intervention that may prove helpful with siblings of children with a broad range of chronic conditions. However, one should use caution when interpreting the findings from these studies. Findings from the first study may not accurately reflect the current situation because the study was conducted in 1981. The sample size for the second study may have been too small for the analyses that were conducted.

USE OF THE DEVELOPMENTAL SCIENCE PERSPECTIVE IN SIBLING RESEARCH BY NURSES

The developmental science perspective is a holistic, interdisciplinary framework that transcends the constructs, methods, and subject matter of developmental psychology and other fields of psychology (Cairns, 2000). In the developmental science perspective, a child's development is viewed as a reflection of the dynamic interactions in which the child is involved— interactions between internal biological states as well as interactions between the child's biology and external systems (e.g., families, social networks, communities, and cultures). Researchers informed by the developmental science perspective advocate for a holistic approach that acknowledges the complexity of development by using longitudinal designs as well as comparative, cross-cultural, and intergenerational research strategies. In addition, they encourage the use of both person-oriented and variable-oriented analyses.

Because of its holistic, interdisciplinary nature and its emphasis on the development of the child within the context of the child's family, culture, and society, the developmental science perspective is ideally suited to be a guiding framework for the study of the sibling experience of chronic illness and disease. While none of the nurse researchers cited in this review have explicitly stated that they have used the developmental science perspective, several have used theories compatible with developmental science, such as Erickson's theory of psychosocial development (Kiburz, 1994), family systems theory (Loebig, 1990; Taylor, 1980), the Resiliency Model of Stress, Adjustment, and Adaptation (Mandleco et al., in press; Van Riper, 2000), and the Family Management Style Model (Gallo et al., 1992, 1993; Gallo & Szychlinski, in press). In addition, many of the nurse researchers have incorporated key aspects of the developmental perspective in their research. However, future research will be strengthened by using a more ecological, systems framework. Of particular interest is exploring systems aspects of parent-sibling and sibling-sibling relationships.

However, it is important to note that nurse researchers, consistent with developmental perspectives, acknowledged that age, gender, birth order, and developmental level play an important role in how siblings respond to the experience of living with chronic illness and disability. Because of this, many researchers have limited their sample to siblings of a certain age, and they have tried to recruit similar numbers of boys and girls. By far, the most commonly studied age group has been siblings 6 to 12 years old (e.g., Faux, 1991; Iles, 1979; Kiburz, 1994; Martinson et al., 1990; Menke, 1987; Mims, 1997; Murray, 1998; Pinyerd, 1983; Phuphaibul & Muensa, 1999; Taylor, 1980; Walker, 1988; Wang & Martinson, 1996). Nurse researchers have not focused specifically on adolescent siblings. Typically, if adolescents were included in the sample, the age range of the sample was fairly wide (e.g., 6 to 18 years). Since adolescence is an important time for developmental change, studies should focus more on this age group.

Most of the sibling studies conducted by nurse researchers used a categorical approach, focusing on one illness or disability or comparing across several conditions. While there is an increasing interest in the noncategorical approach, the question remains as to whether and in what ways the sibling experience and ultimately sibling responses differ for different chronic conditions that have differing demands on the family. Principles of developmental science would suggest that studies need to include more about the chronically ill child's response to his illness and the ecology of the family system coping with the child's illness.

The majority of the early nursing studies concerning the sibling experience of chronic illness and disability were qualitative studies that emphasized the importance of using a holistic perspective to examine the sibling's response in the context of the child's family and other systems in which the child interacts (Faux, 1991; Gallo, 1990; Harder & Bowditch, 1982; Iles, 1979; Kramer, 1984; Menke, 1987; Pinyerd, 1983; Taylor, 1980; Walker, 1988). To date, most are cross-sectional, descriptive studies. There was limited use of longitudinal designs. Because of this, our understanding of how the experience of living with chronic illness and disability affects the sibling's development over time remains limited. Likewise, the vast majority of the studies used group analytic methods. The few researchers who did use a person-centered approach (e.g., Lehna, 1998; Murray, 1998) presented the individual data only descriptively. No examples were found of nurse researchers who conducted person-centered statistical analysis.

Nurses were some of the earliest researchers to conduct interviews with siblings. Recently, the use of self-report questionnaires has become more common in nursing studies of the sibling experience. The number of nurse researchers who have assessed both child and parent outcomes has increased (e.g., Gallo & Szychlinski, in press; Kendall, 1998; Mandleco et al., in press; Van Riper, 2000; Williams et al., 1999). In general, nurse researchers have used measures that are developmentally appropriate.

Limited emphasis has been placed on how culture, ethnicity, and socioeconomic status affect the sibling response. Most of the studies reviewed for this chapter provided information about sibling age and gender but little, if any, information concerning culture, ethnicity, and socioeconomic status. There have been at least two nursing studies concerning siblings in other countries (Wang & Martinson, 1996; Williams et al., 1993), but no cross-cultural nursing studies concerning the sibling experience.

RECOMMENDATIONS FOR FUTURE RESEARCH

There is now little doubt that no single factor determines how siblings respond to the experience of living in a family that includes a child with a chronic illness or disability. Factors that influence how siblings respond include but are not limited to: the age, gender, and developmental levels of the sibling and the child with the chronic condition; the birth order of siblings; the developmental stage of the family unit; the perceived controllability of the chronic condition; the prognosis for the child with the chronic condition; social support; family demands; family definitions of the chronic condition; family resources; family problem-solving communication; family coping; cultural beliefs about chronic illness and disability; and societal norms regarding the care and treatment of people with chronic illness and disability.

Future research concerning the sibling experience of chronic illness and disability should be guided by a holistic, interdisciplinary perspective that recognizes and more accurately captures the complexity of human development. Research methodologies and analyses need to include longitudinal designs, both person-oriented and variable-oriented analyses, and comparison groups. Study samples should include siblings and families from diverse cultural and socioeconomic backgrounds. Outcomes need to be assessed at multiple levels (e.g., child, parent, parent-child dyad, parent-parent dyad, and family level). There needs to be a greater emphasis on the identification of modifiable variables, so that interventions designed to promote healthy, adaptive functioning can be developed and implemented.

ACKNOWLEDGMENTS

The author wishes to acknowledge partial support from Grants NR 02868 and NR05263, National Institute of Nursing Research, NIH.

REFERENCES

Austin, J., & Huberty, T. (1989). Revision of the Family APGAR for use by 8-year-olds. *Family Systems Medicine, 7,* 323–327.

Bank, S. (1982). *Sibling bond.* New York: Basic Books.

Bank, S., & Kahn, M. (1975). Sisterhood-brotherhood is powerful: Sibling-subsystems in family therapy. *Family Process, 14,* 311–339.

Brett, K. M. (1988). Sibling response to chronic childhood disorders: Research perspectives and practice implications. *Issues in Comprehensive Pediatric Nursing, 11,* 43–57.

Cairns, R. B. (2000). Developmental science: Three audacious implications. In L. R. Bergman, R. B. Cairns, L. Nilsson, & L. Nystedt (Eds.), *Developmental science and the holistic approach* (pp. 49–72). Mahway, NJ: Lawrence Erlbaum.

Craft, M. J. (1979). Help for the family's neglected "other" child. *MCN: American Journal of Maternal-Child Nursing, 4,* 297–300.

Craft, M. J. (1986). Validation of responses by school-aged siblings of hospitalized children. *Children's Health Care, 15,* 6–13.

Craft, M. J. (1993). Siblings of hospitalized children: Assessment and intervention. *Journal of Pediatric Nursing: Nursing Care of Children and Families, 8,* 289–297.

Craft, M. J., & Craft, J. L. (1989). Perceived changes in siblings of hospitalized children: A comparison of sibling and parent reports. *Children's Health Care, 18,* 42–48.

Craft, M. J., Lakin, J. A., Oppliger, R. A., Clancy, G. M., & Vanderlinden, D. W. (1990). Siblings as change agents for promoting the functional status of children with cerebral palsy. *Developmental Medicine and Child Neurology, 32,* 1049–1057.

Craft, M. J., & Wyatt, N. (1986). Effect of visitation upon siblings of hospitalized children. *Maternal-Child Nursing Journal, 15,* 47–59.

Craft, M. J., Wyatt, N., & Sandell, B. (1985). Behavior and feeling changes in siblings of hospitalized children. *Clinical Pediatrics, 24,* 374–378.

Davies, L. K. (1993). Comparison of dependent-care activities for well siblings of children with cystic fibrosis and well siblings in families without children with chronic illness. *Issues in Comprehensive Pediatric Nursing, 16,* 91–98.

Drotar, D., & Crawford, P. (1985). Psychological adaptation of siblings of chronically ill children: Research and practice implications. *Journal of Developmental and Behavioral Pediatrics, 6,* 355–362.

Duvall, E. (1977). *Family development* (5th ed.). Philadelphia: Lippincott.

Everson, S. (1977). Sibling counseling: A forgotten part of family-centered care in pediatrics. *American Journal of Nursing, 77,* 644–646.

Faulkner, M. S. (1996). Family responses to children with diabetes and their influence on self-care. *Journal of Pediatric Nursing: Nursing Care of Children and Families, 11,* 82–93.

Faux, S. A. (1991). Sibling relationships in families with congenitally impaired children. *Journal of Pediatric Nursing: Nursing Care of Children and Families, 6,* 175–184.

Faux, S. A. (1993). Siblings of children with chronic physical and cognitive disabilities. *Journal of Pediatric Nursing: Nursing Care of Children and Families, 8,* 305–317.

Faux, S. A., & Seideman, R. Y. (1996). Health care professionals and their relationships with families who have members with developmental disabilities. *Journal of Family Nursing, 2,* 217–238.

Gallo, A. (1988). The special sibling relationship in chronic illness and disability: Parental communication with well siblings. *Holistic Nursing Practice, 2,* 28–37.

Gallo, A. (1990). Family management style in juvenile diabetes: A case illustration. *Journal of Pediatric Nursing: Nursing Care of Children and Families, 5,* 23–32.

Gallo, A., Breitmayer, B. J., Knafl, K., & Zoeller, L. H. (1991). Stigma in childhood chronic illness: A well sibling perspective. *Pediatric Nursing, 17,* 21–27.

Gallo, A., Breitmayer, B. J., Knafl, K., & Zoeller, L. H. (1992). Well siblings of children with chronic illness: Parents' reports of their psychologic adjustment. *Pediatric Nursing, 18,* 23–29.

Gallo, A., Breitmayer, B. J., Knafl, K., & Zoeller, L. H. (1993). Mothers' perceptions of sibling adjustment and family life in childhood chronic illness. *Journal of Pediatric Nursing: Nursing Care of Children and Families, 8,* 318–324.

Gallo, A., & Knafl, K. (1993). Siblings of children with chronic illnesses: A categorical and noncategorical look at selected literature. In Z. Stoneman & P. W. Bermann (Eds.), *The effects of mental retardation, disability, and illness on sibling relationships: Research issues and challenges* (pp. 215–234). Baltimore, MD: Paul H. Brookes.

Gallo, A., & Szychlinski, C. (in press). Self-concept and family functioning in healthy school-aged siblings of children with asthma, diabetes, and healthy children. *Journal of Family Nursing.*

Gath, A. (1974). Sibling reactions to mental handicap: A comparison of the brothers and sisters of mongol children. *Journal of Child Psychology and Psychiatry, 15,* 187–198.

Harder, L., & Bowditch, B. (1982). Siblings of children with cystic fibrosis: Perceptions of the impact of the disease. *Children's Health Care, 10,* 116–120.

Harter, S. (1985a). *Manual for the self-perception profile for children.* Denver: University of Denver.

Harter, S. (1985b). *Manual for the social support scale for children.* Denver: University of Denver.

Hefferman, S. M., & Zanelli, A. S. (1997). Behavior changes exhibited by siblings of pediatric oncology patients: A comparison between maternal and sibling descriptions. *Journal of Pediatric Oncology Nursing, 14,* 3–14.

House, J. S. (1981). *Work stress and social support.* Reading, MA: Addison-Wesley.

Iles, J. P. (1979). Children with cancer: Healthy siblings' perceptions during the illness experience. *Cancer Nursing, 2,* 371–377.

Kendall, J. (1998). Outlasting disruption: The process of reinvestment in families with ADHD children. *Qualitative Health Research, 8,* 839–857.

Kiburz, J. A. (1994). Perceptions and concerns of the school-age siblings of children with myelomeningocele. *Issues in Comprehensive Pediatric Nursing, 17,* 223–231.

Knafl, K. A., Breitmayer, B., Gallo, A., & Zoeller, L. (1987). How families define and manage a chronic illness (Grant #NR011594, funded by the National Center for Nursing Research). Washington, DC: National Center for Nursing Research.

Knafl, K. A., & Deatrick, J. A. (1990). Family management style: Concept analysis and development. *Journal of Pediatric Nursing, 5,* 4–14.

Kramer, R. F. (1981). Living with childhood cancer: Healthy siblings' perspective. *Issues in Comprehensive Pediatric Nursing, 5,* 155–165.

Kramer, R. F. (1984). Living with childhood cancer: Impact on the healthy siblings. *Oncology Nursing Forum, 11,* 44–51.

Lazarus, R. S., & Folkman, S. (1984). *Stress, appraisal, and coping.* New York: Springer.

Lee, E. J., Phoenix, D., Brown, W., & Jackson, B. S. (1997). A comparison study of children with sickle cell disease and their non-diseased siblings on hopelessness, depression, and perceived competence. *Journal of Advanced Nursing, 25,* 79–86.

Lehna, C. R. (1998). A childhood cancer sibling's oral history. *Journal of Pediatric Oncology Nursing, 15,* 163–171.

Loebig, M. (1990). Mothers' assessments of the impact of children with spina bifida on the family. *Maternal-Child Nursing Journal, 19,* 251–267.

Mandleco, B., Olsen, S. R., Dyches, T., & Marshall, E. (in press). The relationship between family and sibling functioning in families raising a child with a disability. *Journal of Family Nursing.*

Martinson, I. M., Gilliss, C., Colaizzo, D. C., Freeman, M., & Bossert, E. (1990). Impact of childhood cancer on healthy school-age siblings. *Cancer Nursing, 13,* 183–190.

McCubbin, M., & McCubbin, H. (1993). Families coping with illness: The resiliency model of family stress, adjustment, and adaptation. In C. Danielson, B. Hamel-Bissell, & P. Winstead-Fry (Eds.), *Families, health, and illness: Perspectives on coping and intervention* (pp. 21–63). St Louis: Mosby.

McDaniel, S. H., Hepworth, J., & Doherty, W. J. (1992). *Medical family therapy: A biopsychosocial approach to families with medical problems.* New York: Basic Books.

McHale, S. M., & Gamble, W. C. (1989). Sibling relationships of children with disabled and nondisabled brother and sisters. *Developmental Psychology, 25,* 421–429.

McKeever, P. (1983). Siblings of chronically ill children: A literature review with implications for research and practice. *American Journal of Orthopsychiatry, 53,* 209–218.

McNair, D., Lorr, M., & Droppleman, L. (1992). *POMS manual: Profile of mood states.* San Diego: EdiTS.

Menke, E. (1987). The impact of a child's chronic illness on school-age siblings. *Children's Health Care, 15,* 132–140.

Mims, J. (1997). Self-esteem, behavior, and concerns surrounding epilepsy in siblings of children with epilepsy. *Journal of Child Neurology, 12,* 187–192.

Murray, J. S. (1995). Social support for siblings of children with cancer. *Journal of Pediatric Oncology Nursing, 12,* 62–70.

Murray, J. S. (1998). The lived experience of childhood cancer: One sibling's perspective. *Issues in Comprehensive Pediatric Nursing, 21,* 217–227.

Murray, J. S. (1999a). Siblings of children with cancer: A review of the literature. *Journal of Pediatric Oncology Nursing, 16,* 25–34.

Murray, J. S. (1999b). Methodological triangulation in a study of social support for siblings of children with cancer. *Journal of Pediatric Oncology Nursing, 16,* 194–200.

Murray, J. S. (2000a). Attachment theory and adjustment difficulties in siblings of children with cancer. *Issues in Mental Health Nursing, 21,* 149–169.

Murray, J. S. (2000b). A concept analysis of social support as experienced by siblings of children with cancer. *Journal of Pediatric Nursing, 15,* 313–322.

Murray, J. S. (2000c). Clinical methods: Conducting psychosocial research with children and adolescents: A developmental perspective. *Applied Nursing Research, 13,* 151–156.

Murray, J. S. (2000d). Development of two instruments measuring social support for siblings of children with cancer. *Journal of Pediatric Oncology Nursing, 17,* 229–238.

Murray, J. S. (2000e). Understanding sibling adaptation to childhood cancer. *Issues in Comprehensive Pediatric Nursing, 23,* 39–47.

Murray, J. S. (2001a). Self-concept of siblings of children with cancer. *Issues in Comprehensive Pediatric Nursing, 24,* 85–94.

Murray, J. S. (2001b). Social support for school-aged siblings of children with cancer: A comparison between parents and sibling perceptions. *Journal of Pediatric Oncology Nursing, 18,* 90–104.

Newacheck, P. W. (1994). Poverty and childhood chronic illness. *Archives of Pediatric Adolescent Medicine, 148,* 1143–1149.

Newacheck, P. W., Strickland, B., Shonkoff, J. P., Perrin, J. M., McPherson, M., McManus, M., et al. (1998). An epidemiologic profile of children with special health care needs. *Pediatrics, 102,* 117–123.

Olson, D., Portner, J., & Lavee, Y. (1985). *Family adaptability and cohesion evaluation scales.* St Paul, MN: University of Minnesota.

Orem, D. E. (1991). *Nursing: Concepts of practice* (4th ed.). St. Louis: Mosby.

Phuphaibul, R., & Muensa, W. (1999). International pediatric nursing: Negative and positive adaptive behaviors of Thai school-aged children who have a sibling with cancer. *Journal of Pediatric Nursing: Nursing Care of Children and Families, 14,* 342–348.

Pinyerd, B. J. (1983). Siblings of children with myelomeningocele: Examining their perceptions. *Maternal-Children Nursing Journal, 12,* 61–70.

Rolland, J. S. (1994). *Families, illness, and disability: An integrative treatment model.* New York: Basic Books.

Rose, M. H., & Thomas, R. B. (1987). *Children with chronic conditions: Nursing in a family and community context.* Orlando: Grune Stratton.

Ross-Alaolmolki, K., Heinzer, M. M., Howard, R., & Marszal, S. (1995). Impact of childhood cancer on siblings and family: Family strategies for primary health care. *Holistic Nursing Practice, 9,* 66–75.

Sahler, O., & Carpenter, P. (1989). Evaluation of a camp program for siblings of children with cancer. *American Journal of Diseases of Children, 143,* 690–696.

Scheiber, K. K. (1989). Developmentally delayed children: Effects on the normal sibling. *Pediatric Nursing, 15,* 42–44.

Siemon, M. (1984). Siblings of the chronically ill or disabled child: Meeting their needs. *Nursing Clinics of North America, 19,* 295–307.

Smith, M. E. (1998). Protective shield: A thematic analysis of the experience of having an adult sibling with insulin-dependent diabetes mellitus. *Issues in Mental Health Nursing, 19,* 317–335.

Taylor, S. (1980). The effects of chronic childhood illnesses upon well siblings. *Maternal-Child Nursing Journal, 9,* 109–116.

Thibodeau, S. M. (1988). Sibling response to chronic illness: The role of the clinical nurse specialist. *Issues in Comprehensive Pediatric Nursing, 11,* 17–28.

Van Riper, M. (2000). Family variables associated with well-being in siblings of children with Down syndrome. *Journal of Family Nursing, 6,* 267–286.

Walker, C. L. (1988). Stress and coping in siblings of childhood cancer patients. *Nursing Research, 37,* 208–212.

Wang, R., & Martinson, I. M. (1996). Behavioral responses of healthy Chinese siblings to the stress of childhood cancer in the family: A longitudinal study. *Journal of Pediatric Nursing: Nursing Care of Children and Families, 11,* 383–391.

Williams, P. D. (1997). Siblings and pediatric chronic illness: A review of the literature. *International Journal of Nursing Studies, 34,* 312–323.

Williams, P. D., Hanson, S., Karlin, R., Ridder, L., Liebergen, A., Olson, J., et al. (1997). Outcomes of a nursing intervention for siblings of chronically ill children: A pilot study. *Journal of the Society of Pediatric Nurses, 2,* 127–137.

Williams, P. D., Lorenzo, F. D., & Borja, M. (1993). Pediatric chronic illness: Effects on siblings and mothers. *Maternal-Child Nursing Journal, 21,* 111–121.

Williams, P. D., Williams, A. R., Hanson, S., Graff, C., Ridder, L., Curry, H., et al. (1999). Maternal mood, family functioning, and perceptions of social support, self-esteem, and mood among siblings of chronically ill children. *Children's Health Care, 28,* 297–310.

Wright, L. M., & Leahey, M. (2000). *Nurses and families: A guide to family assessment and intervention* (3rd ed.). Philadelphia: F. A. Davis.

Wright, L. M., Watson, W. L., & Bell, J. M. (1996). *Beliefs: The heart of healing in families and illness*. New York: Basic Books.

Chapter 11

Maternal Mental Health and Parenting in Poverty

Linda S. Beeber and Margaret Shandor Miles

ABSTRACT

Maternal mental health is a key factor affecting the quality of parenting and, ultimately, a child's developmental outcomes. Thus, the persistence of mental health problems such as chronic depressive symptoms or addiction in low-income mother-child dyads may be the critical determinant of their collective future. This review examines the research conducted by nurses that focuses on maternal mental health, mothering, and child outcomes in the context of rearing children in poverty. Multiple methods were used for the search. Four programs showed evidence of sustained, related studies focused on the mental health of low-income mothers and their parenting. Two of these programs included intervention studies aimed at improving the mental health of mothers and developmental outcomes for their children. There were four newer programs of research in which the research teams had begun to focus on mothers rearing children in poverty and five other researchers who conducted single studies of maternal mental health. Additionally, two investigators focused on mothers who were prisoners, one team focused on homeless mothers, and another on mothers with HIV. Studies were critiqued using a developmental science framework. Studies varied widely in the degree to which they used developmentally based conceptual frameworks, designs, and measures. While nurse scientists have made progress in conducting research with mothers rearing children in poverty, there is an urgent need for more developmentally sensitive research aimed at strengthening maternal mental health and assisting mothers to be more effective parents in the midst of the challenges of poverty and welfare reform. By doing so, nursing interventions can improve the child's developmental outcomes.

Strong parenting can buffer or neutralize the assaults that poverty makes on the cognitive, emotional, and social development of children (Brody & Flor, 1998; Duncan & Brooks-Gunn, 2000; Furstenberg, 1993; Jarrett, 1995; Jarrett & Burton, 1999; Petterson & Albers, 2001; Wilson, 1997). One of the pathways through which parental protection occurs is the presence of a strong, mentally healthy mother who has logical thought processes, clear perception, appropriate emotional responses, adequate energy for action, and the developmental maturity required to maintain meaningful relationships, manage stressors, carry out life roles, and pursue personal growth and development (Beeber, 1998c). Nursing research with mothers rearing children in poverty builds on a long history of caring for the underserved, particularly mothers and their children (Backer, 1993; Buhler-Wilkerson, 1991). This review examines the research conducted by nurses that focuses on maternal mental health, mothering, and child outcomes in the context of rearing children in poverty.

MENTAL HEALTH OF MOTHERS AND THEIR CHILDREN: POVERTY AS A CONTEXT

Unfortunately, 25% of children in the United States (US) under the age of 6 years old are reared in poverty (US Department of the Census, 2001). Forty percent of families in poverty are headed by a single parent, most likely the mother (90%) (Ensminger, 1995; Olson & Banyard, 1993), who must manage severe stressors such as violence, poor housing, drug abuse, and illness. All of these factors threaten maternal mental health (Ensminger, 1995). For example, a low-income single mother of young children has four times the risk of other women to have severe depressive symptoms that persist for a year or longer (Brown & Moran, 1997). Other poverty-related threats, such as drug use, addiction, and incarceration, pose additional dangers to maternal mental health (Kearney, Murphy, Irwin, & Rosenbaum, 1995). Conversely, severe mental illnesses such as schizophrenia and bipolar disorder may predispose a mother to poverty (Beeber, Hendrix, Taylor, & Wykle, 1993). If a mother seeks help through public assistance, she will be required to work, a recent change that accompanied the Personal Responsibility and Work Opportunity Reconciliation Act of 1996, which ended welfare and began a program of time-limited benefits or Temporary Assistance for Needy Families (TANF). While introducing

additional stressors, this program stopped open-ended entitlement programs and provided limited cash assistance, education, and work-training
programs to help mothers achieve full-time employment. Mental health
has been a critical attribute of mothers who have permanently exited
welfare by using the opportunities for self-development that accompanied
these legislative changes (Duncan & Brooks-Gunn, 2000; Gennetian &
Miller, 2002).

Maternal mental health affects optimal development of the child,
as demonstrated in the case of maternal depressive symptoms. At all
socioeconomic levels, persistent depressive symptoms in the mother place
a child at risk for cognitive deficits, developmental delays, and long-term
speech and attention disorders (Brooks-Gunn, Kelbanov, & Duncan, 1996;
Field, 1998; Foss, Hirose, & Barnard, 1999; Goodman & Gotlib, 1999;
McLoyd, 1990; Petterson & Albers, 2001; Samaan, 1998). For the low-
income child, poor maternal mental health adds additional risk by compro-
mising the compensatory actions of parents that shield the child from the
damage of deficient housing, substandard schools, dangerous neighborhoods, and negative role models (Brooks-Gunn, 1995; Furstenberg, 1993;
Duncan, Brooks-Gunn, & Klebanov, 1994; Jackson, Brooks-Gunn, Huang, & Glassman, 2000; Jarrett, 1995; Wilson, 1997). Ultimately, it is a
diligent and sensitive mother who produces a resilient child who, despite
being reared in poverty, has realized his or her full potential (Brody &
Flor, 1998; Furstenberg, 1993; Jarrett, 1995; Jarrett & Burton, 1999).
Strong mothering protects the low-income child in three ways: through the
creation of a safe, nurturing home environment, provision of developmental
support for the child, and acquisition of compensatory enrichment resources (Brooks-Gunn et al., 1996; Duncan & Brooks-Gunn, 2000; Goodman & Gotlib, 1999; Harris, 1993; Mistry, Vanderwater, Huston, &
McLoyd, 2002; National Institute of Child and Human Development, 1999;
Petterson & Albers, 2001; Samaan, 1998).

In summary, mental health is a key factor affecting the quality of the
low-income mother's parenting and, ultimately, her child's developmental
outcomes. Maternal mental health is also critical in one of the most powerful changes a mother can make for herself and her child—permanently
transitioning out of poverty. Thus, the persistence of mental health problems such as chronic depressive symptoms or addiction in low-income
mothers may be the critical determinant of the collective future of the
mother-child dyad.

DEVELOPMENTAL SYSTEMS PERSPECTIVE ON MATERNAL MENTAL HEALTH AND PARENTING

Nursing research on maternal mental health, parenting, and child outcomes must be reviewed in the context of the broader literature on mental health of mothers in poverty and their children (Coll, 1990; Duncan & Brooks-Gunn, 2000; Halpern, 1990; Huston, McLoyd, & Coll, 1994). From a developmental systems perspective, mother and child are a dyad, with reciprocal interactions continuously determining the health and development of each member of the dyad (Barnard, Morisset, & Spieker, 1993; Magnusson & Cairns, 1996; Thelen & Smith, 1998; Thoman, Acebo, & Becker, 1983). Developmental systems theory also suggests that the context within which mother and child interact profoundly affects the dyad (Bronfenbrenner, 1989; Brooks-Gunn, 1995; Morisset, Barnard, Greenberg, Booth, & Spieker, 1990). Furthermore, intergenerational history and experiences have direct and indirect effects on mothers and their children (Chase-Landsdale, Brooks-Gunn, & Zamsky, 1994; Elder, 1998; Hammen, 1991; Lyons-Ruth & Zeanah, 1993). These contextual and intergenerational factors, particularly those associated with poverty, have a profound impact on the mental health of mothers and, hence, on the development of their children.

This review, which focuses on maternal mental health, mothering, and child outcomes in the context of poverty, identifies what nurse scientists have discovered about the mental health of mothers in poverty and critiques our theories and methods from the standpoint of developmental science. In addition, the review summarizes how maternal mental health protects the child, and it also identifies tested nursing interventions that strengthen the mental health of these mothers. The ultimate goal is to stimulate an increased interest in this research, explore how developmental science perspectives can strengthen this research, and, ultimately, develop theory-based interventions to improve maternal mental health. By assisting mothers to be more effective parents in the midst of the challenges of poverty and welfare reform, nursing interventions can improve the future of vulnerable children.

METHODS

Criteria for Inclusion

The main criterion for inclusion was that the research had to examine some aspect of the mental health of mothers who were rearing children in the context of poverty and the researcher or research team had to include a nurse or be a researcher who had conducted research with a nursing perspective. Specific criteria included (a) a clear focus on mothers and not on women in general; (b) inclusion of some measure of mental health, including psychiatric disorders, mental health symptoms of depression and anxiety, and drug addiction, as well as positive mental health outcomes such as maternal role development and parenting efficacy; and (c) clear evidence of low-income status as a variable. Excluded were (a) studies with low-income mothers that did not examine maternal mental health as a variable, (b) research about mental health of women that did not clearly focus on low-income mothers, (c) studies of battered and abused mothers (there are two excellent reviews already on this topic—Campbell & Parker, 1992, 2002), (d) research on postpartum depression, and (e) studies focused on the mental health or emotional distress of low-income mothers secondary to having an infant or child with special needs or complex health problems such as prematurity, chronic illness, or disabilities. Published articles, in-press publications, and abstracts of research in progress were included.

Search Method

Multiple methods were used for the search. CINAHL, Medline, and PubMed were used with the keywords *mother, parent, mental health, poverty, low-income, infants, toddlers, children, nursing research,* and *intervention,* along with additional formal mental illness descriptors such as *depression, substance abuse,* and *schizophrenia,* until repetitive searches yielded no new nursing studies. This was followed by searches of key authors until no new studies were found. When possible, the curriculum vitae of the researcher was requested or the web page was located to provide a complete and up-to-date list of publications. Researchers with ongoing research were contacted directly, and in several cases, they generously provided prepublication manuscripts. Unpublished researchers, located through abstracts of conference proceedings, were asked to provide reports on research in progress. Public search engines such as *Google.com* were used to locate researchers whose work appeared in government publications, technical reports, and lay magazines. Finally, two review papers that focused on general health issues in low-income women by Reutter, Neufeld, and Harrison (1998, 2000) were used to cross-validate the search.

Analytic Strategies

The critique of the research focused on the following points: (a) What theory, conceptual framework, or ecological perspective, if any, was used to guide the study? (b) Did the sample represent mothers currently living in poverty, was culture or ethnicity used in the design and analysis of the studies, and was the income of the study participants adequately reported, especially in relation to poverty threshold? (c) To what extent did the study designs capture the complex nature of parenting over time in the context of poverty? (d) What measures were used to assess mental health, and how valid, reliable, and appropriate were they for this population? (e) Did the research address maternal strengths as well as deficits, such as how mothers protect their children against the effects of poverty? (f) Did the study analyze the relationship of maternal development and mental health and the developmental outcomes of the child? Using these questions, the studies were critiqued in regard to the use of concepts and methods of developmental science. Finally, the critique identified areas for further research that are needed to develop the knowledge base about maternal mental health and parenting by low-income mothers.

RESULTS

Programs of research (a series of related, cumulative studies by a single researcher or team) as well as individual studies were reviewed. Several researchers focused on special populations such as prisoners, the homeless, and mothers with HIV.

Programs of Research on Mental Health in Mothers in Poverty

Four programs of research built bodies of evidence on the mental health of low-income mothers and their parenting. These include Barnard and her research team; Hall, Sachs, and Lutenberger and their colleagues; Kitzman and Olds; and Kearney and colleagues. Barnard and Kitzman and Olds conducted interventions aimed at improving the mental health of mothers.

One of the most influential teams studying low-income mothers and their parenting is that of Kathryn Barnard and her colleagues at the University of Washington. In the 1980s, they conducted an innovative intervention aimed at helping low-income pregnant women at high social risk and with low social support to improve their ability to initiate and maintain relationships supportive of their parenting role (Barnard et al., 1988; Barnard, Booth, Mitchell, & Telzrow, 1988; Morisset et al., 1990). Many papers were published from this longitudinal study. The earliest reported results of the intervention (Barnard et al., 1988). One group received an individualized mental health intervention built on a therapeutic relationship and using active problem solving toward better parenting; the other group received an information intervention. Mothers in the mental health group had less depression, perceived more support, increased their social competence, had a more positive view of the world, and showed higher parenting competencies. Although there were no differences in child outcomes for the entire sample, for women who began the intervention with low social skills, these changes in social skills related positively to the quality of mother-child interaction (Booth, Mitchell, Barnard, & Spieker, 1989). A longitudinal analysis also showed that mothers with low coping resources and social support who improved their social skills as a result of the intervention had children with higher IQ's and receptive language skills at 4 years (Bee, Hammond, Eyres, Barnard, & Snyder, 1986). Attrition was a limitation of this study. Hence, an analysis was conducted examining data from 28 intervention and 26 control mothers identified by the research team as "difficult to engage" (Spieker, Solchany, McKenna, DeKlyen, & Barnard, 2000). A higher proportion of these mothers were classified on the Adult Attachment Inventory as "unresolved" or "hard to classify," suggesting unresolved experiences of loss and trauma that might influence their ability to engage in a relationship. Indeed, further qualitative analysis revealed that these mothers experienced a profound sense of loss when they thought about their childhood.

Data from the entire sample were used to examine an ecological transactional model of the cognitive and linguistic skill development of the toddlers (Morisset et al., 1990). At 1 year of age, the impact of environmental risk on development was mediated more by the quality of early mother-child interaction than by family social status or maternal characteristics. At 30 months of age, quality of parenting was the only significant predictor of language utterance, and at 5 years of age, first-year parenting variables explained more variance in IQ than either social status or maternal risk over time (Barnard & Morisett, 1995). This demonstrates that mothering is of utmost importance in mediating the young child's environment.

This program of research contributed to the development of the Nursing Child Assessment Interaction Model and several related intervention programs—the Nursing Parent and Child Environment Program and the Nursing Systems Toward Effective Parenting–Preterm Program (Barnard et al., 1988, 1993; Barnard, Snyder, & Spietz, 1991). These programs have been adapted nationwide by public health nurses and others trained by Barnard and colleagues. Overall, this program of research was soundly based in developmental ecological theories of development. Longitudinal methods were used, and both mother-child interaction and child developmental outcomes were outcomes.

Another program of research by Hall, Sachs, and Lutenbacher consisted of a series of cross-sectional descriptive studies focused on stress, depressive symptoms, and parenting in low-income single mothers. Hall noted that most of the work on stressors had concerned general life events rather than the daily strains of poverty and had not linked stressors to the well-being of children. In the first study, 111 low-income mothers of young children were interviewed about social support, everyday stressors, and depressive symptoms (Hall, Williams, & Greenberg, 1985). Common problems, life events, quality of intimate relationships, social network, and income were associated with depressive symptoms in the unmarried mothers. Everyday stressors, combined with life events, were the strongest predictors of child behavior problems, but stress and child behavior problems were not mediated by maternal depressive symptoms (Hall & Farel, 1988). In another cross-sectional study of 196 low-income mothers, Hall (1990) found that demographic factors along with everyday stressors increased the risk for depressive symptoms. A pilot study showed that depressive symptoms were related to more unrealistic expectations of children, greater reports of behavior problems, and higher abuse potential (Sachs & Hall, 1991).

A subsequent study involved a three-panel longitudinal panel study of 225 low-income single-mother families. Analysis of the first panel found that parenting attitudes and avoidance coping were related to everyday stressors and depressive symptoms (Hall, Gurley, Sachs, & Kryscio, 1991). Low family support was associated with maternal depressive symptoms, while more stress, lower coping, and parenting attitudes predicted child behavior problems. In an analysis of the first and third panels, self-esteem along with childhood and partner sexual abuse and everyday stressors accounted for 58% of the variance in depressive symptoms (Lutenbacher & Hall, 1998). In the final panel, the presence rather than the severity of maternal childhood abuse (violence and sexual) was associated with maternal depressive symptoms; violent sexual abuse in childhood was the strongest predictor of severe depressive symptoms (Hall, Sachs, Rayens, & Lutenbacher, 1993). History of abuse and level of support resources emerged as important predictors of child abuse potential (Hall, Sachs, & Rayens, 1998). Interview data from nine mothers with high abuse potential revealed that idealistic expectations of family and children's functioning, high need for control, overwhelming familial responsibilities, poor support systems, absence of parenting strategies, and conscious halting of the mothers' personal development in order to care for their children were risk factors for abuse (Sachs, Pietrukowicz, & Hall, 1997). The authors also identified maternal strengths and coping capacities and found that the mothers showed strengths in their resolve not to repeat the mistakes of their own parents, willingness to sacrifice for their children, and skill in evaluation and use of community resources. Shifting the focus to the etiology of child maltreatment, Hall and colleagues studied 738 postpartum mothers (Hall, Kotch, Browne, & Rayens, 1996). Self-esteem was added to their conceptual model. Everyday stress and lower-quality intimate relationships were associated with lower self-esteem, which was a mediator between everyday stressors and depressive symptoms, and the effect of the primary intimate relationship on depressive symptoms.

Lutenbacher (2000, 2002) extended Hall's research using a transactional, ecological model in another three-panel study of 59 single mothers with young children. A high prevalence of abuse, depressive symptoms, and abusive parenting attitudes was found. Cross-sectional analysis found that abuse was related to higher daily stress and that stress, in turn, was associated with lower self-esteem. Childhood abuse and lower self-esteem were related to higher depressive symptoms, and partner abuse was correlated with abusive parenting attitudes and parent-child role reversal. Higher anger was associated with less parental empathy.

Hall and colleagues identified the sources of stress for mothers living in poverty and examined the link between these variables, other maternal characteristics, depressive symptoms, and parenting. Sample sizes were sufficient to examine important predictors of maternal depression and parenting. Mental health was measured consistently across each study using the Center for Epidemiological Studies—Depression scale (CES-D), a depressive symptom severity measure with stable reliability and validity in low-income populations (Radloff, 1977). The CES-D has standard risk cutpoints which permitted Hall and colleagues to validate that a high proportion of low-income mothers were significantly symptomatic. Their results suggest that intervention focused on reducing maternal stress and improving self-esteem and parenting attitudes may improve child outcomes. What is not clear, however, is how these factors interact over time. Unfortunately, although two repeated-measures panel studies were conducted, to date, there is no analysis of the data using longitudinal statistical methods. The framework for these studies was not always clearly articulated. The frameworks for the early studies appeared to be empirically based models, although those studies did consider some important aspects of the ecology of the mothers and children. Lutenbacher, however, clearly used a transactional framework (Lutenbacher, 2002; Lutenbacher & Hall, 1998). While the researchers included many ecological and intergenerational factors in their design, consideration of additional variables such as child gender and ethnicity in their analysis would strengthen the ecological perspective.

A program of experimental research by Kitzman, Olds, and colleagues has contributed longitudinal data about the impact of a nursing intervention directed at low-income, first-time mothers (Kitzman, 1999; Kitzman et al., 1997, 2000; Olds, Henderson, & Kitzman, 1994; Olds, Henderson, Kitzman, & Cole, 1995; Olds, Henderson, Phelps, Kitzman, & Hanes, 1993; Olds et al., 1997, 1998, 1999). Maternal mastery was the mental health outcome thought to mediate the impact of the intervention on parenting. Two randomized trials were conducted over a 20-year period involving home visits from a nurse that were initiated prenatally and continued for 2 years after delivery. Kitzman and Olds timed the intervention to occur during the mother's first pregnancy, which was proposed to be a pivotal developmental period during which the mother might make critical decisions about her own future and that of her child (Olds & Kitzman, 1990; Hanks, Kitzman, & Milligan, 1995). The intervention, a characteristical nursing model, was strength-focused, was culturally congruent, and used maternal choice, occupational skill development, and health habit change (smoking and drug cessation) (Hanks et al., 1995). Maternal role development was addressed through parenting skills and by helping the mother change her life course through control of her sexuality (Kitzman et al., 1997).

The intervention was initially tested in 400 white, rural mothers (Olds & Kitzman, 1990) and replicated with 1,139 African American urban mothers (Kitzman et al., 1997). The intervention led to positive changes in the maternal life course (deferral of pregnancies, work), reduction in psychological distress, and greater mastery (Kitzman et al., 2000; Olds et al., 1998, 1999). Children of intervention mothers had fewer injuries and antisocial behaviors and were less likely to smoke or use alcohol (Olds et al., 1994, 1998; Kitzman et al., 1997). The investigators also found that the reduction of stressors in the early developmental life of the child moderated the onset of problem behaviors and that the most positive results were in the mothers with the fewest resources (Olds et al., 1999; Eckenrode et al., 2000, 2001).

Strengths in the Kitzman and Olds studies were the well-designed preventive intervention study based on social support and human ecological models. The study design included a broad array of ecological environmental and personal factors, and extensive developmentally appropriate maternal and child measures were used. Cost analysis showed that in the low-income families, the intervention investment was recouped by the time the child was 4 years old (Olds et al., 1997). The longitudinal design allowed researchers to track the long-term impact of the intervention on factors in the mother and child's ecology, but the mediating effect of mastery was never analyzed. A stronger mental health measure would have provided more insight into the mental health impact of the intervention, and more specific linkage of the content and timing of the interventions to the outcomes also would have strengthened the analysis of findings.

The final program of research was that of Kearney and colleagues, who studied mothers with addictions—another mental health threat that shares high degrees of comorbidity with poverty. Kearney, Murphy, and Rosenbaum (1994a) conducted grounded theory research with 100 mostly low-income crack cocaine–addicted women residing in the San Francisco Bay area and found that the mothers' perception of being trapped and having narrowed life options preceded the use of crack cocaine. Further analysis of data from 68 of the women who were also mothers indicated that few planned their pregnancies but nonetheless embraced a strong sense of responsibility and pride in being mothers (Kearney, Murphy, & Rosenbaum, 1994b). Strategies of mothering included defensive compensation, shielding children from maternal drug use, and isolating them from drug cultures. Interestingly, these strategies were similar to those practiced by families to protect children from the dangers of living in low-income neighborhoods, such as avoidance, curfews, self-segregation from questionable neighbors, confinement, and chaperoning (Furstenberg, 1993; Jarrett, 1995). These researchers further studied the parallel developmental processes in mother and child and found that the developmental trajectory of the child required that the mother adjust her life-management strategies to fit the child's changing needs. Toddlerhood, the most demanding period for the mother because of the high need for nurturance and modeling, increased the temptation to use drugs. However, remaining in the drug culture was inherently dangerous because it sometimes resulted in losing their children. As a last resort, mothers surrendered their children to others when they perceived that they could not uphold their own standards of parenting. However, this thwarted their development as mothers.

Kearney and colleagues also reported on data from 60 of the mothers who used crack cocaine regularly during pregnancy (Kearney et al., 1995). Mothers were concerned about their babies, a departure from the previous stereotype about drug-addicted pregnant women. Threatened selfhood and the prospect of losing the baby or giving birth to a damaged infant led some mothers to "salvage self" and redirect their lives, while others resorted to deception. In a subsequent study of 14 mothers, Kearney (1996) found that mothers reconstructed their identity as they recovered from drug use and gained a new appreciation of their children and their mothering role. Based on this program of research, Kearney (1998) developed a grounded theory of women's addiction recovery. The basic process was truthful self-nurturing, which required recognition of addiction as a problem. Social and psychological change, abstinence, self-discovery, and connection were processes involved in the recovery. Of particular importance was that mothers made a gradual reconnection to society through the mothering role.

Kearney's program of research has strong developmental components, particularly the focus on the developmental processes of the mother against the backdrop of a severe mental health threat. Development of the child was considered in analysis, with the finding that risk for relapse may vary according to the changing demands of the child at different developmental stages. Limited attention was given to broader ecological factors, such as culture and ethnicity; societal attitudes, including threats of losing the child; relationship with family; and use of community resources that might affect responses to addiction, recovery, and parenting.

Emerging Programs of Research

There were four programs of research focused on mental health in middle-class women or mothers in which the research teams began to focus on mothers rearing children in poverty. This included the research teams of Walker, Webster-Stratton, Gross, and Beeber.

Building on Walker's earlier program of research on parenting of infants (Walker, 1989; Walker, Crain, & Thompson, 1986a, 1986b), Walker and Kim (in press) have begun the Austin New Mothers study, a longitudinal study that focuses on the relationship between depressive symptoms and stress in 305 African American, Hispanic, and white low-income mothers and their full-term newborns. Analysis of the first panel of data found that a large proportion of the sample had clinically significant depressive symptoms that were not associated with lower infant birthweight, as was found by others (Field, 1998; Hoffman & Hatch, 2000). This longitudinal study is ongoing and will provide data on maternal stress and the persistence, character, and influence of depressive symptoms over time. The use of a longitudinal design and a large, diverse sample of mothers is a strength, especially if ethnicity and culture are used in analysis. It is not clear how Walker and colleagues are building on their earlier conceptualizations of stress, depressive symptoms, and maternal role attainment, particularly maternal identity.

Webster-Stratton, although not a nurse, is director of a large parenting education center at the School of Nursing, University of Washington, where she developed a self-efficacy–based parent effectiveness training intervention—the Incredible Years Parenting Training Program (Webster-Stratton, 1982, 1987). The intervention, developed for parents of young children with severe behavior problems (Webster-Stratton, 1990; Webster-Stratton & Hammond, 1988), has now been tested with low-income Head Start children in an effort to prevent these problems (Webster-Stratton, Reid, & Hammond, 2001; Reid, Webster-Stratton, & Beauchaine, 2001). Head Start programs were randomized into experimental or control groups. The 12-session group training program was then offered to all parents of children enrolled in experimental centers (Webster-Stratton et al., 2001). Mothers in the experimental group showed lower negative and higher positive parenting scores and higher parent-teacher bonding and the children had fewer conduct problems at school than did control children. Intervention effects were maintained for parents who attended more than 6 sessions and for children with the most risk for behavior problems. Reid et al. (2001) found no differences in treatment responses across ethnic groups; parents from all ethnic groups reported high satisfaction. Webster-Stratton's work is built on a well-conceptualized, developmentally based, manualized intervention. The intervention and design have a strong ecological focus with a particular emphasis on the ecology of the school environment. Consistent with developmental science, the data collection used multiple methods, including parent self-report, teacher evaluations, and observation.

Gross, a nurse researcher, has used the Webster-Stratton training intervention with parents of toddlers with behavior problems (Gross, Fogg, & Tucker, 1995). This work builds on earlier longitudinal studies of maternal and child mental health in ethnically and socioeconomically diverse mothers (the level of poverty was unclear). In a longitudinal design, 126 mothers of 1-year-olds and 126 mothers of 2-year-olds were studied three times over a year. Depressed mothers were more likely to rate their toddler's temperament as difficult, and the more difficult the mother rated the child's temperament, the lower was her parenting self-efficacy. Lower self-efficacy, in turn, was related to greater depression. Further, mothers' depressive symptoms at enrollment were strong predictors of depressive symptoms 6 months later (Gross, Conrad, Fogg, & Wothke, 1994). In a follow-up at ages 3 and 4, maternal depression was significantly related to lower social competence and more behavior problems in the children, and boys with depressed mothers were more at risk (Gross, Conrad, Fogg, Willis, & Garvey, 1995).

Gross, Fogg, and Tucker (1995) then tested the Incredible Years Parenting Training Program with mothers and fathers of children with behavioral difficulties from a health maintenance organization. The training led to increases in maternal self-efficacy, lower maternal stress, and improvements in mother-toddler interactions. Gross and Grady (2002) are presently testing the intervention with parents and teachers of toddlers enrolled in day care centers. Gross's research used longitudinal design, linked maternal mental health to parenting skills and child behavior, and explored the influence of child gender on outcomes. No analyses were conducted examining the influence of culture and ethnicity. Broader ecological aspects such as family characteristics and intergenerational history, as well as the stresses of poverty, that might affect maternal mental health, parenting, and child behavior were not considered.

Building on a series of studies focused on depressive symptoms and interventions with college women (Beeber, 1998a, 1998b; Beeber & Caldwell, 1996; Beeber & Charlie, 1998), Beeber refocused her work on low-income mothers with infants and preschoolers in Early Head Start. An initial descriptive study in 26 Head Start and Early Head Start mothers, all of whom were in welfare-to-work programs, identified stressors and depressive symptoms (Beeber, 2000). Acute stressors were maternal and child health crises and economic hardship crises (e.g., loss of telephone, eviction). Chronic strains included time pressure, work tensions, lack of money, poor transportation and health care, and worry about having enough food. Uplifts included their children, family and home activities, and supportive relationships. Work in entry-level, minimum-wage jobs was not positive for these mothers. Depressed mothers confirmed that their symptoms severely hampered functioning. Stigma, dangerous environments, day-to-day survival, and child care were barriers to attending mental health clinics.

Based on these findings, Beeber and colleagues developed an intervention guided by Interpersonal Theory and Interpersonal Psychotherapy (Beeber, 1998c; Beeber & Caldwell, 1996) and by interventions conducted by Barnard (Barnard et al., 1993) and Kitzman (Hanks et al., 1995). The intervention was pilot-tested with 16 Early Head Start mothers of infants and toddlers in two sites in the Northeast and South (Beeber, Canuso, Holditch-Davis, Belyea, & Campbell, 2002). Fifty mothers were screened for depressive symptoms using the CES-D, and, of these, 50% scored over 16, indicating they were at risk. At-risk mothers were randomly assigned to an intervention or usual care group. Based on the findings of the previous study, the intervention addressed depressive symptoms, problematic life issues, access to social support, and parenting. There was a substantial drop in depressive symptom severity that was sustained over time (8 and 16 weeks post intervention), while depressive symptom severity in control mothers remained relatively stable. Maternal interactions with their child also improved in the intervention group. A strength of this research was the theory guiding the intervention and the focus on the significant relationships of the mother, maternal self-efficacy, and parenting skills. Ecological aspects were also considered. Developmentally sensitive observational methods were used as one outcome, but no other child outcomes were measured. Replication and study of the effects of culture and ethnicity are needed in future research.

Individual Studies

Five additional researchers studied the mental health of mothers. To identify the prevalence of severe psychiatric disorders, Flick and colleagues (2001b) assessed 528 low-income pregnant mothers for 19 psychiatric diagnoses using the Diagnostic Interview Schedule (DIS-IV). Most (54%) had at least one lifetime psychiatric disorder, and many (27%) had a current disorder. Post-traumatic stress disorders and nicotine dependence were the most prevalent diagnoses. Flick and colleagues (2001a) are also studying persistent tobacco use in pregnancy, as part of a longitudinal study of mothers from a Women, Infants and Children (WIC) Supplemental Nutrition program. Nineteen percent of mothers were tobacco dependent and had an elevated rate of psychiatric disorders, suggesting that smoking cessation is not likely to be successful unless underlying psychiatric disorders are addressed. These atheoretical descriptive studies did not include broader ecological aspects of the mother and child, and there were no assessments of parenting or child outcomes.

Murata (1995) studied family stress, social support, and depressive symptoms in 21 low-income single African American mothers and their sons. Family stress emerged as the major contributor to depressive symptoms. A strength was the use of an established model of family stress. However, no analysis was done of the interaction of family stress and the developmental stage of the child to determine whether there were high-risk periods. The influence of African American culture was not considered and would have made a strong addition to this study. Direct observation of mother-son interactions rather than maternal reports of behavior, as well as a longitudinal design, would strengthen subsequent studies.

Karl (1995) conducted a secondary analysis of interactions between 19 high-risk, low-income mothers with depressive symptoms and their 6- to 9-month-old infants from a larger study of high-risk mothers (Lyons-Ruth, Connell, Zoll, & Stahl, 1987). Over half of the sample had not completed high school and were being monitored by child protective services. Using observations of infant elicitation cues and maternal responses, coded as overresponsive, underresponsive, and good enough, Karl found that five of the six "good-enough" mothers scored as "depressed" on the CES-D. This suggested that depressed mothers could adequately interact and that "good-enough" mothering may be a reasonable outcome of parenting interventions with chronically symptomatic mothers. While based on attachment theory, the study did not clearly articulate how it was used. The study did, however, capture the reciprocal nature of the mother-child relationship using naturalistic observational methods. The method was well described, and reliability of the coding schema was reported. A significant limitation was lack of specificity about depression scores. In addition, broader ecological factors, such as family characteristics, support, child gender, level of poverty, and culture, were not considered.

Based on critical social theory, Kneipp (2000) examined whether there were differences in psychosocial health between mothers who made a transition from welfare to employment and those who did not. Consistent with the demographics of the state (Washington), most of the mothers were white. Strikingly, mothers who left welfare for work did not improve their psychosocial well-being scores after 1 year, supporting the notion of the high cost of "self-sufficiency"—namely, bare subsistence coupled with greater uncertainty about income. A strength of the study was the multiple measures of mental health used, including self-worth, self-efficacy, self-esteem, depressive symptoms, and emotional support. The study lacked an ecological framework and therefore did not examine other multiple factors that might affect mental health. Furthermore, there were no links to parenting or child outcomes.

In her program of research on the promotion of mental health in postpartum mothers, Horowitz and colleagues have not focused specifically on mothers living in poverty (Horowitz, Chang, Das, & Hayes, 2001; Horowitz et al., 2001). One exception was a study focused on stressors and satisfactions in 95 postpartum mothers from a health maintenance organization that served an urban, multiethnic population (Horowitz & Damato, 1999). Thirty percent of the women had incomes below $20,000, although detailed information about socioeconomic status was not given. The conceptual framework was not clear, but mental health was measured using the Brief Symptom Inventory, a measure of general mental distress. Stressors included combining maternal roles with work and school, meeting personal needs and child care tasks, and finances. Rewards included loving relationships, sharing a sense of the future, and pride in being a mother. The most highly stressed mothers felt trapped and inadequate and pulled between work and motherhood demands. Notable in this study was an acknowledgement of the satisfactions of parenting and the use of both qualitative and quantitative methods. No specific analysis of culture or ethnicity was done, although the sample was diverse. The cross-sectional design limited the information about what is an evolutionary process.

Special Populations: Women in Prison, Homeless Mothers, and Mothers with HIV

Two investigators focused on mothers who were prisoners, one team focused on homeless mothers, and another focused on mothers with HIV, three comorbid factors in low-income mothers' lives. Crime and incarceration are a harsh reality in many of these mothers' lives. Fogel and colleagues studied the mental health of incarcerated mothers. One study compared imprisoned mothers ($n = 35$) and nonmothers ($n = 11$) on depressive symptoms and anxiety at two time points (Fogel & Martin, 1992). On admission to prison, both groups experienced high anxiety scores; within 6 months, the mothers' scores had fallen while the nonmothers' remained elevated. Depressive symptoms, however, were high at both time points. In a related qualitative study, Fogel (1995) found that mothers were concerned about the loss of the bond with their child(ren), which was aggravated by minimal means of communication with them while incarcerated. Another study explored experiences of pregnant women incarcerated during their third trimester of pregnancy (Fogel & Belyea, 2001). Over 60% had experienced violence, 40% were chemically dependent or smokers, and 70% had high depressive symptoms. Most were low on empathetic awareness of the child and on valuing and recognizing the child's needs. These studies are notable for focusing on a population that is not generally included in research and for contributing a better understanding of the parenting risk in this population. The studies lacked a conceptual model or guiding theory and had small samples. In addition, broader contextual aspects of the mothers' lives and the prison environment were not included.

Using a longitudinal design, Byrne studied mother-infant dyads residing in codetention in a nursery unit of a state maximum security prison (Byrne, 2002). Maternal depressive symptoms were high. However, maternal self-esteem and spiritual well-being were also high, perhaps as a result of being able to live with their infants. Maternal, child, and dyadic scores on the NCAST teaching scale were positive. Some strengths were the consideration of the dyad and of mothering as a developmental process, and the use of interview data to elaborate on quantitative data. Another strength was the longitudinal design.

Wagner, Menke, and Ciccone (1994) studied homeless mothers using a multidimensional self-report inventory designed to screen for a broad range of psychological problems and psychopathology. Paradoxically, while the mothers' self-reported scores were not indicative of mental health problems, 37% reported illegal drug use, 49% used alcohol, and 74% smoked cigarettes. The results were considered in light of ecological factors related to rurality, including stigma, the tendency to underreport illnesses, and values related to self-reliance and "being strong." This study did not have a developmental perspective, and therefore broader ecological factors of homelessness were not considered; there was no focus on parenting.

Guided by ecological, systems theory, Miles, Holditch-Davis, and colleagues conducted a longitudinal study examining depressive symptoms, the quality of parental caregiving, and developmental outcomes in infants seropositive for HIV (Holditch-Davis et al., 2001; Miles, Burchinal, Holditch-Davis, Wasilewski, & Christian, 1996). Participants were primarily low-income African American biological mothers with HIV, but kin and foster mothers were included. Data were collected over the first 24 months of life using a triangulation of methods. Mental health characteristics of the mother included depressive symptoms using the CES-D scale and HIV-related stigma. In a longitudinal examination of depressive symptoms in 54 HIV-infected biological mothers, 35% to 38% of the mothers had at-risk depressive symptom scores. Stigma and perception of health were significantly associated with depressive symptoms over time, whereas the other psychosocial and contextual factors were not (Miles et al., 1996). In another analysis, parental caregivers (63 biological mothers, 13 kin, and 14 foster mothers) were categorized based on their CESD scores over time as nondepressed, episodically depressed, or chronically depressed. Mothers in both the episodic and chronic depressive groups had a lower perception of self as a mother and higher worry about the infant's health than nondepressed mothers. Mothers with episodic depressive symptoms showed decreased positive and increased negative behaviors over time, while mothers in the chronic depressive symptom group exhibited a lower quality of stimulation in the home environment (Miles, Holditch-Davis, & Burchinal, 1998). Quality of parental caregiving, especially positive attention, caregiver consistency, and HIV status of the infant, were related to infant developmental outcomes, but depressive symptoms were not (Holditch-Davis et al., 2001). This study had a strong developmental perspective. An ecological, systems framework was used to examine how parent and family characteristics affected the quality of parental caregiving and developmental outcomes. A longitudinal design explored processes over time, and the data were analyzed longitudinally. While culture and ethnicity were not specifically evaluated, a majority of the participants were African American, and culture was discussed in several of these papers.

SUMMARY AND CRITIQUE

Nursing research with mothers rearing children in poverty began in the 1980s with Barnard's groundbreaking intervention research. Since then, a number of investigators have or are developing programs of nursing research on the mental health and parenting of low-income poverty mothers, perhaps the result of the National Institutes of Nursing Research initiatives to reduce health disparities. Findings provide important information about the stressors and challenges faced by these mothers; about factors that affect maternal mental health, particularly depression; and about the impact of depressive symptoms on parenting. Only a few studies examined the impact of parenting and other aspects of poverty on developmental outcomes in the child. Some studies did identify maternal attributes such as social skills to elicit resources and maternal behaviors, such as positive attention and consistency of parenting, that related to more positive child outcomes. While these findings collectively provide some evidence about ways that strong parenting can compensate for the detrimental effects of poverty, this area of research remains limited. There was great variability across studies regarding the extent to which the studies were designed using principles of developmental science.

No consistent theoretical framework was used in this research. Many of the studies were atheoretical or used an empirically based framework that was not developmental or family focused. Some used stress and coping frameworks (Hall et al., 1985; Hall & Farel, 1988; Murata, 1995) and psychological-social theories such as self-efficacy (Webster-Stratton, 1982, 1987; Gross, Fogg, et al., 1995) and critical social theory (Kneipp, 2000). Many of these frameworks had limited developmental focus, and, as a result, broad aspects of the family and community were excluded. Ecological developmental systems frameworks were used by Barnard and colleagues (Barnard et al., 1988; Barnard & Morisett, 1995) and by Miles and Holditch-Davis and colleagues (Holditch-Davis et al., 2001; Miles et al., 1996, 1998). Webster-Stratton combined self-efficacy into a developmental ecological model (Webster-Stratton & Hammond, 1988), and Kitzman and Olds used a social support and ecological model (Kitzman et al., 1997).

Many of the studies were cross-sectional descriptive designs that did not capture the complex nature of parenting in the context of poverty. Still, consistent with developmental science, there were a significant number of longitudinal studies that allowed for the study of process over time. However, even when longitudinal data were collected, many investigators did not explore the experiences, processes, and outcomes of parenting over time using longitudinal statistical analyses. It is impressive that many researchers have moved toward intervention studies aimed at helping these at-risk mothers improve their mental health, their parenting of their children, and, ultimately, their children's health and development. Several of the well-designed and theory-based interventions showed improvements in parenting and child outcomes.

Few studies addressed the ecology of the "culture of poverty," and, as a result, there was limited attention given to the complex nature of parenting in this context. Kearney's theory of self-salvaging and development of the motherhood role in crack-addicted poor women, which provided an in-depth description of the culture of poverty, was an exception (Kearney et al., 1995). Another limitation was the lack of focus on culture and ethnicity. While some studies tried to view mothers in poverty from a different perspective than the dominant model of white, middle-class families (Tropp, Coll, Alarcon, & Vazquez-Garcia, 1999), little attention was paid to the interaction of culture and poverty. Future research needs to focus on the culture of poverty, ethnicity, and the processes mothers use to protect their children against the effects of poverty.

A major challenge in reviewing this research was determining if the studies met the criteria for focusing on mothers in poverty. Samples were not clearly described in terms of educational level and socioeconomic status, and further, the methods used to assess socioeconomic status were very general and did not have great reliability. Therefore, it is impossible to know how representative the studies were of mothers currently living in poverty. Future studies need to incorporate multiple methods for evaluating the socioeconomic status of participants and compare the participants' income against federal standards for poverty.

Data collection methods in these studies were diverse. The primary tool used to assess mental health was the CES-D, a measure of depressive symptoms. The CES-D has proven valid and reliable with low-income women (Gross et al., 1995; Hall & Farel, 1988). However, it is a measure of only one aspect of mental health. Future research needs to incorporate more in-depth assessments of mental disorders that accompany poverty such as drug addiction (American Psychiatric Association, 2000). Since only a few of the studies addressed maternal development or strengths, future studies should address maternal development and strengths as well as broader characteristics of mental health. Furthermore, future studies should explore the relationship between the mother's developmental processes and those of her child. While some studies included mother-child interaction data and child outcomes, most did not. Some used maternal self-report measures, a method that can be biased by mental symptoms, as the only child outcome measure. Since one ultimate goal of research on mothers rearing children in poverty is to improve the developmental outcomes of children, future research would be strengthened by using observational methods and developmental assessments that provide more precise data.

In conclusion, there is an urgent need for more research using theories and methods grounded in developmental science and testing of theory-based interventions with mothers and their children living in poverty. Since the social landscape has changed for mothers in poverty as a result of welfare reform, new programs of research must revisit questions that were answered prior to welfare reform and integrate new understandings about poverty and the interaction of maternal mental health and child development in light of the work requirements, low wages, and insufficient resources. Finally, the role of fathers in the lives of low-income mothers and their children needs to be examined.

REFERENCES

American Psychiatric Association. (2000). *Diagnostic and statistical manual of mental disorders.* Washington, DC: American Psychiatric Association.

Backer, B. (1993). Lillian Wald: Connecting caring with activism. *Nursing & Health Care, 14,* 122–129.

Barnard, K. E., Booth, C. L., Mitchell, S. K., & Telzrow, R. W. (1988). Newborn nursing models: A test of early intervention to high risk infants and families. In E. Hibbs (Ed.), *Children and families: Studies in prevention and intervention* (pp. 63–81). Madison, CT: International Universities Press.

Barnard, K. E., Magyary, D., Sumner, G., Booth, C. L., Mitchell, S. K., & Spieker, S. (1988). Prevention of parenting alterations for women with low social support. *Psychiatry, 51,* 248–253.

Barnard, K. E., & Morisett, C. E. (1995). Preventive health and developmental care for children: Relationships as a primary factor in service delivery with at risk populations. In H. E. Fitzgerald & B. M. Zuckerman (Eds.), *Children of poverty* (pp. 167–195). New York: Garland Publishing.

Barnard, K. E., Morisset, C. E., & Spieker, S. J. (1993). Preventive interventions: Enhancing parent-infant relationship. In C. Zeanah (Ed.), *Handbook on infant mental health* (pp. 386–401). New York: Guilford Press.

Barnard, K. E., Snyder, C., & Spietz, A. (1991). Supportive measures for high-risk infants and families. In A. L. Whall & J. Fawcett (Eds.), *Family theory development in nursing: State of the science and the art* (pp. 139–175). Philadelphia: F. A. Davis.

Bee, H. L., Hammond, M. A., Eyres, S. J., Barnard, K. E., & Snyder, C. (1986). The impact of parental life change on the early development of children. *Research in Nursing & Health, 9,* 65–74.

Beeber, L. S. (1998a). Social support, self-esteem, and depressive symptoms in young American women. *Image, 30,* 91–92.

Beeber, L. S. (1998b). Testing an explanatory model of the development of depressive symptoms in young women during a life transition. *Journal of the American College Health Association, 47,* 227–234.

Beeber, L. (1998c). Treating depression through the therapeutic nurse-client relationship. *Nursing Clinics of North America, 33,* 153–172.

Beeber, L. S. (2000, May). *Treatment of maternal depression.* Paper presented at the meeting of the NCAST Institute, Seattle, WA.

Beeber, L. S., & Caldwell, C. L. (1996). Pattern integrations in young depressed women: Part II. *Archives of Psychiatric Nursing, 10,* 157–164.

Beeber, L. S., Canuso, R., Holditch-Davis, D., Belyea, M., & Campbell, C. (2002, February). *Intervention for depressive symptoms in low-income mothers of infants and toddlers.* Paper presented at the meeting of the Southern Nursing Research Society, San Antonio, TX.

Beeber, L. S., & Charlie, M. L. (1998). Depressive symptom reversal in a primary care setting: A pilot study. *Archives of Psychiatric Nursing, 12,* 247–254.

Beeber, L. S., Hendrix, M. J., Taylor, C. S., & Wykle, M. L. (1993). The challenge of diversity: The mental health of women. *Journal of Psychosocial Nursing, 31*(8), 23–29.

Booth, C. L., Mitchell, S. K., Barnard, K. E., & Spieker, S. J. (1989). Development of maternal social skills in multiproblem families: Effects on the mother-child relationship. *Developmental Psychology, 25,* 403–412.

Brody, G., & Flor, D. (1998). Maternal resources, parenting practices, and child competence in rural, single parent African-American families. *Child Development, 69,* 803–816.

Bronfenbrenner, U. (1989). Ecological systems theory. *Annals of Child Development, 6,* 5–246.

Brooks-Gunn, J. (1995). Children in families in communities: Risk and intervention in the Bronfenbrenner tradition. In P. Moen, G. H. Elder, & K. Luscher (Eds.), *Examining lives in context* (pp. 467–522). Washington, DC: American Psychological Association.

Brooks-Gunn, J., Kelbanov, P. K., & Duncan, G. J. (1996). Ethnic differences in children's intelligence test scores: Role of economic deprivation, home environment, and maternal characteristics. *Child Development, 67,* 396–408.

Brown, G., & Moran, P. (1997). Single mothers, poverty and depression. *Psychological Medicine, 27,* 21–33.

Buhler-Wilkerson, K. (1991). Lillian Wald: Public health pioneer. *Nursing Research, 40,* 316–317.

Byrne, M. (2002). *Maternal and infant outcomes of a prison nursery: Preliminary study.* Unpublished report submitted to the New York State Department of Health and the Institute for Child and Family Policy at Columbia University.

Campbell, J. C., & Parker, B. (1992). Review of nursing research on battered women and their children. In J. Fitzpatrick, R. Taunton, & A. Jacox (Eds.), *Annual review of nursing research* (Vol. 10, pp. 77–94). New York: Springer.

Campbell, J. C., & Parker, B. (2002). Clinical nursing research on battered women and their children: A review. In A. S. Hinshaw, S. Feetham, & J. Shaver (Eds.), *Handbook of clinical nursing research.* Newbury Park, CA: Sage.

Chase-Lansdale, L., Brooks-Gunn, J., & Zamsky, E. S. (1994). Young African-American multigenerational families in poverty: Quality of mothering and grandmothering. *Child Development, 65,* 373–393.

Coll, C. T. G. (1990). Developmental outcome of minority infants: A process-oriented look into our beginnings. *Child Development, 61,* 270–289.

Duncan, G. J., & Brooks-Gunn, J. (2000). Family poverty, welfare reform, and child development. *Child Development, 71*(1), 188–196.

Duncan, G. J., Brooks-Gunn, J., & Klebanov, P. K. (1994). Economic development and early childhood development. *Child Development, 65,* 296–318.

Eckenrode, J., Ganzel, B., Henderson, C. Jr., Smith, E., Olds, D., Powers, J., Cole, R., Kitzman, H., & Sidora, K. (2000). Preventing child abuse and neglect with a program of nurse home visitation: The limiting effects of domestic violence. *Journal of the American Medical Association, 284,* 1385–1391.

Eckenrode, J., Zielinkski, D., Smith, E., Marcynyszyn, L., Henderson, C. Jr., Kitzman, H., Cole, R., Powers, J., & Olds, D. (2001). Child maltreatment and the early onset of problem behaviors: Can a program of nurse home visitation break the link? *Developmental Psychopathology, 13,* 873–890.

Elder, G. H. (1998). The life course as developmental theory. *Child Development, 69,* 1–12.

Ensminger, M. (1995). Welfare and psychological distress: A longitudinal study of African American urban mothers. *Journal of Health and Social Behavior, 36,* 346–359.

Field, T. (1998). Maternal depression effects on infants and early intervention. *Preventive Medicine, 27,* 200–203.

Flick, S., Cook, C., Homan, S., McSweeney, M., Campbell, C., Nettip, N., Parnell, L., & Gallagher, M. (2001a, October). *Persistent tobacco use in pregnancy: An indicator of psychiatric illness?* Paper presented at the meeting of the American Public Health Association, Atlanta, GA.

Flick, S., Cook, C., Homan, S., McSweeney, M., Campbell, C., Nettip, N., Parnell, L., & Gallagher, M. (2001b, October). *Psychiatric disorder in pregnancy: Preliminary evidence in a WIC sample.* Paper presented at the meeting of the American Public Health Association, Atlanta, GA.

Fogel, C. (1995, February). *Incarcerated mothers: The deconstruction of a social identity.* Paper presented at a meeting of the Southern Nursing Research Society, Lexington, KY.

Fogel, C., & Belyea, M. (2001). Psychological risk factors in pregnant inmates: A challenge for nursing. *MCN: American Journal of Maternal-Child Nursing, 26,* 10–16.

Fogel, C., & Martin, S. (1992). The mental health of incarcerated women. *Western Journal of Nursing Research, 14,* 30–47.

Foss, L. A., Hirose, T., & Barnard, K. E. (1999). Relationship of three types of parent-child interaction in depressed and non-depressed mothers and their children's mental development at 13 months. *Nursing & Health Sciences, 1,* 211–219.

Furstenberg, J. (1993). How families manage risk and opportunity in dangerous neighborhoods. In W. J. Wilson (Ed.), *Sociology and the public agenda* (pp. 231–258). Newbury Park, CA: Sage.

Gennetian, L., & Miller, C. (2002). Children and welfare reform: A view from an experimental welfare reform program in Minnesota. *Child Development, 73,* 601–620.

Goodman, S., & Gotlib, I. (1999). Risk for psychopathology in the children of depressed mothers: A developmental model for understanding mechanisms of transmission. *Psychology Review, 106,* 458–490.

Gross, D., Conrad, B., Fogg, L., Willis, L., & Garvey, C. (1995). A longitudinal study of maternal depression and preschool children's mental health. *Nursing Research, 44,* 996–101.

Gross, D., Conrad, B., Fogg, L., & Wothke, W. (1994). A longitudinal model of maternal self-efficacy, depression, and difficult temperament during toddlerhood. *Research in Nursing and Health, 17,* 207–215.

Gross, D., Fogg, L., & Tucker, S. (1995). The efficacy of parent training for promoting positive parent-toddler relationships. *Research in Nursing & Health, 18,* 489–499.

Gross, D., & Grady, J. (2002). Group-based parent training for preventing mental health disorders in children. *Issues in Mental Health Nursing, 23*(4), 367–383.

Hall, L. A. (1990). Prevalence and correlates of depressive symptoms in mothers of young children. *Public Health Nursing, 7,* 71–79.

Hall, L., & Farel, A. (1988). Maternal stresses and depressive symptoms: Correlates of behavior problems in young children. *Nursing Research, 37,* 156–161.

Hall, L. A., Gurley, D. N., Sachs, B., & Kryscio, R. J. (1991). Psychosocial predictors of maternal depressive symptoms, parenting attitudes, and child behavior in single-parent families. *Nursing Research, 40,* 214–220.

Hall, L. A., Kotch, J. B., Browne, D., & Rayens, M. K. (1996). Self-esteem as a mediator of the effects of stressors and social resources on depressive symptoms in postpartum mothers. *Nursing Research, 45,* 231–238.

Hall, L. A., Sachs, B., & Rayens, M. K. (1998). Mothers' potential for child abuse: The roles of childhood abuse and social resources. *Nursing Research, 47,* 87–95.

Hall, L. A., Sachs, B., Rayens, M. K., & Lutenbacher, M. (1993). Childhood physical and sexual abuse: Their relationship with depressive symptoms in adulthood. *Image: The Journal of Nursing Scholarship, 25,* 317–323.

Hall, L., Williams, D., & Greenberg, R. (1985). Supports, stressors and depressive symptoms in low-income mothers of young children. *American Journal of Public Health, 75,* 518–522.

Halpern, R. (1990). Poverty and early childhood parenting: Toward a framework for intervention. *American Journal of Orthopsychiatry, 60,* 6–18.

Hammen, C. (1991). *Depression runs in families*. New York: Springer-Verlag.

Hanks, C., Kitzman, H., & Milligan, R. (1995). Implementing the COACH relationship model: Health promotion for mothers and children. *Advances in Nursing Science, 18*, 57–66.

Harris, K. (1993). Work and welfare among single mothers in low-income. *American Journal of Sociology, 99*, 317–352.

Hoffman, S., & Hatch, M. (2000). Depressive symptomatology during pregnancy: Evidence for an association with decreased fetal growth in pregnancies of lower social class women. *Health Psychology, 19*, 535–543.

Holditch-Davis, D., Miles, M. S., Burchinal, M., O'Donnell, K., McKinney, R., & Linn, W. (2001). Parental caregiving and developmental outcomes in infants of mothers with HIV. *Nursing Research, 50*, 5–14.

Horowitz, J., Bell, M., Trybulski, J., Munro, B., Moser, D., Hartz, S., McCordic, L., & Sokol, E. (2001). Promoting responsiveness between mothers with depressive symptoms and their infants. *Journal of Nursing Scholarship, 33*, 323–329.

Horowitz, J., Chang, S., Das, S., & Hayes, B. (2001). Women's perceptions of postpartum depressive symptoms from an international perspective. *International Nursing Perspectives, 1*, 5–14.

Horowitz, J., & Damato, E. (1999). Mothers' perceptions of postpartum stress and satisfaction. *Journal of the Association of Obstetric, Gynecological, and Neonatal Nurses, 28*, 595–605.

Huston, A. C., McLoyd, V. C., & Coll, C. G. (1994). Children and poverty: Issues in contemporary research. *Child Development, 65*, 275–282.

Jackson, A., Brooks-Gunn, J., Huang, C., & Glassman, M. (2000). Single mothers in low-wage jobs: Financial strain, parenting, and preschoolers' outcomes. *Child Development, 71*, 1409–1423.

Jarrett, R. (1995). Growing up poor: The family experiences of socially mobile youth in low-income African American neighborhoods. *Journal of Adolescent Research, 10*, 111–135.

Jarrett, R., & Burton, L. (1999). Dynamic dimensions of family structure in low-income African-American families: Emergent themes in qualitative research. *Journal of Comparative Family Studies, 30*, 177–187.

Karl, D. (1995). Maternal responsiveness of socially high-risk mothers to the elicitation cues of their 7-month old infants. *Journal of Pediatric Nursing, 10*(4), 254–263.

Kearney, M. H. (1996). Reclaiming normal life: Mothers' stages of recovery from drug use. *Journal of the Association of Obstetric, Gynecological, and Neonatal Nurses, 25*, 761–768.

Kearney, M. H. (1998). Truthful self-nurturing: A grounded formal theory of women's addiction recovery. *Qualitative Health Research, 8*(4), 495–512.

Kearney, M. H., Murphy, S., Irwin, K., & Rosenbaum, M. (1995). Salvaging self: A grounded theory of pregnancy on crack cocaine. *Nursing Research, 44*(4), 208–213.

Kearney, M. H., Murphy, S., & Rosenbaum, M. (1994a). Learning by losing: Sex and fertility on crack cocaine. *Qualitative Health Research, 4*(2), 142–162.

Kearney, M. H., Murphy, S., & Rosenbaum, M. (1994b). Mothering on crack cocaine: A grounded theory analysis. *Social Science Medicine, 38*(2), 351–361.

Kitzman, H. (1999). Studying the effects of nurse prenatal and early infancy home visitations. *Ambulatory Outreach,* Spring, 10–14.

Kitzman, H., Olds, D., Henderson, C. Jr., Hanks, C., Cole, R., Tatelbaum, R., et al. (1997). Effect of prenatal and infancy home visitation by nurses on pregnancy outcomes, childhood injuries, and repeated childbearing: A randomized controlled trial. *Journal of the American Medical Association, 278*(8), 644–652.

Kitzman, H., Olds, D., Sidora, K., Henderson, C. Jr., Hanks, C. R., Cole, R., et al. (2000). Enduring effects of nurse home visitation on maternal life course: A 3-year follow-up of a randomized trial. *Journal of the American Medical Association, 283,* 1983–1989.

Kneipp, S. (2000). The health of women in transition from welfare to employment. *Western Journal of Nursing Research, 22,* 656–682.

Lutenbacher, M. (2000). Perceptions of health status and the relationships with abuse history and mental health in low-income single mothers. *Journal of Family Nursing, 6,* 320–340.

Lutenbacher, M. (2002). Relationships between psychosocial factors and abusive parenting attitudes in low-income single mothers. *Nursing Research, 51,* 158–167.

Lutenbacher, M., & Hall, A. (1998). The effects of maternal psychosocial factors on parenting attitudes of low-income single mothers with young children. *Nursing Research, 47,* 25–34.

Lyons-Ruth, K., Connell, D., Zoll, D., & Stahl, J. (1987). Infants at social risk: Relationships among infant maltreatment, maternal behavior, and infant attachment behavior. *Developmental Psychology, 23,* 223–232.

Lyons-Ruth, K., & Zeanah, C. H. (1993). The family context of infant mental health: I. Affective development in the primary caregiving relationship. In C. Zeanah (Ed.), *Handbook on infant mental health* (pp. 14–37). New York: Guilford Press.

Magnusson, D., & Cairns, R. B. (1996). Developmental science: Toward a unified framework. In R. B. Cairns, G. H. Elder, & E. J. Costello (Eds.), *Developmental science* (pp. 7–30). New York: Cambridge University Press.

McLoyd, V. C. (1990). The impact of economic hardship on black families and children: Psychological distress, parenting, and socioeconomic development. *Child Development, 61,* 311–346.

Miles, M. S., Burchinal, P., Holditch-Davis, D., Wasilewski, Y., & Christian, B. (1996). Personal, family, and health-related correlates of depressive symptoms in mothers with HIV. *Journal of Family Psychology, 11,* 23–34.

Miles, M. S., Holditch-Davis, D., & Burchinal, P. (1998, February). *Depressive symptoms in foster and biological mothers caring for infants sero-positive for HIV: Relationship to parenting.* Paper presented at the meeting of the Southern Nursing Research Society, Fort Worth, TX.

Mistry, R., Vanderwater, E., Huston, A., & McLoyd, V. (2002). Economic well-being and children's social adjustment: The role of family process in an ethnically diverse low-income sample. *Child Development, 73,* 935–951.

Morisset, C. E., Barnard, K. E., Greenberg, M. T., Booth, C. L., & Spieker, S. J. (1990). Environmental influences on early language development: The context of social risk. *Development and Psychopathology, 2,* 127–140.

Murata, J. (1995). Family stress, mothers' social support, depression, and sons' behavior problems: Modeling nursing interventions for low-income inner-city families. *Journal of Family Nursing, 1,* 41–62.

National Institute of Child and Human Development Early Child Care Research Network. (1999). Chronicity of maternal depressive symptoms, maternal sensitivity, and child functioning at 36 months. *Developmental Psychology, 35,* 1297–1310.

Olds, D. L., Eckenrode, J., Henderson, C. R. Jr., Kitzman, H., Powers, J., Cole, R., et al. (1997). Long-term effects of home visitation on maternal life course and child abuse and neglect: Fifteen-year follow-up of a randomized trial. *Journal of the American Medical Association, 278,* 637–643.

Olds, D. L., Henderson, C. R. Jr., Cole, R., Eckenrode, J., Kitzman, H., Luckey, D., et al. (1998). Long-term effects of nurse home visitation on children's criminal and antisocial behavior: Fifteen-year follow-up of a randomized controlled trial. *Journal of the American Medical Association, 280,* 1238–1244.

Olds, D. L., Henderson, C. R. Jr., & Kitzman, H. (1994). Does prenatal and infancy nurse home visitation have enduring effects on qualities of parental caregiving and child health at 25 to 50 months of life? *Pediatrics, 93,* 89–98.

Olds, D., Henderson, C. R. Jr., Kitzman, H., & Cole, R. (1995). Effects of prenatal and infancy nurse home visitation on surveillance of child maltreatment. *Pediatrics, 95,* 365–372.

Olds, D. L., Henderson, C. Jr., Kitzman, H., Eckenrode, J., Cole, R., & Tatelbaum, R. (1999). Prenatal and infancy home visitation by nurses: Recent findings. *Future of the Child, 9,* 44–65.

Olds, D. L., Henderson, C. R. Jr., Phelps, C., Kitzman, H., & Hanks, C. (1993). Effect of prenatal and infancy nurse home visitation on government spending. *Medical Care, 31,* 155–174.

Olds, D. L., & Kitzman, H. (1990). Can home visitation improve the health of women and children at environmental risk? *Pediatrics, 86,* 108–116.

Olson, S. L., & Banyard, V. (1993). "Stop the world so I can get off for a while": Sources of daily stress in the lives of low-income single mothers of young children. *Family Relations, 42,* 50–56.

Petterson, S., & Albers, A. (2001). Effects of poverty and maternal depression on child development. *Child Development, 72,* 1794–1813.

Radloff, L. S. (1977). The CES-D Scale: A self-report depression scale for research in the general population. *Applied Psychological Measurement, 1,* 285–401.

Reid, M. J., Webster-Stratton, C., & Beauchaine, T. P. (2001). Parent training in Head Start: A comparison of program response among African American, Asian American, Caucasian, and Hispanic mothers. *Prevention Science, 2,* 209–227.

Reutter, L., Neufeld, A., & Harrison, M. (1998). Nursing research on the health of low-income women. *Public Health Nursing, 15,* 109–122.

Reutter, L., Neufeld, A., & Harrison, M. (2000). A review of the research on the health of low-income Canadian women. *Canadian Journal of Nursing Research, 32,* 75–97.

Sachs, B., & Hall, L. (1991). Maladaptive mother-child relationships: A pilot study. *Public Health Nursing, 8,* 226–233.

Sachs, B., Pietrukowicz, M., & Hall, L. A. (1997). Parenting attitudes and behaviors of low-income single mothers with young children. *Journal of Pediatric Nursing, 12,* 67–73.

Samaan, R. (1998). The influences of race, ethnicity, and poverty on the mental health of children. *Journal of Health Care for the Poor and Underserved, 11,* 100–110.

Spieker, S. J., Solchany, J., McKenna, M., DeKlyen, M., & Barnard, K. E. (2000). The story of mothers who are difficult to engage in prevention programs. In J. D. Osofsky & H. E. Fitzgerald (Eds.), *WAIMH handbook of infant mental health* (3rd ed., pp. 173–209). New York: Wiley.

Thelen, E., & Smith, L. B. (1998). Dynamic systems theories. In R. M. Lerner & W. Damon (Eds.), *Handbook of child psychology: Vol. I. Theoretical models of human development* (5th ed., pp. 563–634). New York: Wiley.

Thoman, E. B., Acebo, C., & Becker, P. T. (1983). Infant crying and stability in the mother-infant relationship: A systems analysis. *Child Development, 54,* 653–659.

Tropp, L. R., Coll, C. G., Alarcon, O., & Vazquez-Garcia, H.A. (1999). Psychological acculturation: Development of a new measure for Puerto Ricans on the U.S. mainland. *Educational and Psychological Measurement, 59*(2), 351–367.

United States Department of the Census. (2001, September 25). Current population survey. Poverty 2000: Poverty thresholds in 2000, by size of family and number of related children under 18 years. Retrieved June 17, 2002, from *http://www.census.gov/hhes/poverty/threshld/thresh00.html*

Wagner, J., Menke, E., & Ciccone, J. (1994). The health of rural homeless women with young children. *Rural Health Policy, 10,* 49–57.

Walker, L. O. (1989). Stress process among mothers of infants: Preliminary model testing. *Nursing Research, 38,* 10–16.

Walker, L., Crain, H., & Thompson, E. (1986a). Maternal role attainment and identity in the postpartum period: Stability and change. *Nursing Research, 35,* 68–71.

Walker, L., Crain, H., & Thompson, E. (1986b). Mothering behavior and maternal role attainment during the postpartum period. *Nursing Research, 35,* 352–355.

Walker, L., & Kim, M. (in press). Psychosocial thriving during late pregnancy: Relationship to ethnicity, gestational weight gain and birth weight. *Clinical Studies.*

Webster-Stratton, C. (1982). Teaching mothers through videotape modeling to change their children's behavior. *Journal of Pediatric Psychology, 7,* 279–294.

Webster-Stratton, C. (1987). *The parents and children series leader guide.* Seattle: University of Washington, School of Nursing.

Webster-Stratton, C. (1990). Long-term follow-up of families with young conduct problem children: From preschool to grade school. *Journal of Clinical Child Psychology, 19,* 144–149.

Webster-Stratton, C., & Hammond, M. (1988). Maternal depression and its relationship to life stress, perceptions of child behavior problems, parenting behavior, and child conduct problems. *Journal of Abnormal Child Psychology, 16,* 299–315.

Webster-Stratton, C., Reid, M. J., & Hammond, M. (2001). Preventing conduct problems, promoting social competence: A parent and teacher training partnership in Head Start. *Journal of Clinical and Child Psychology, 30,* 283–302.

Wilson, W. (1997). *When work disappears: The world of the new urban poor.* New York: Alfred A. Knopf.

PART IV

Looking Back: The Last 10 Years

Chapter 12

A Review of the Second Decade of the *Annual Review of Nursing Research* Series

JOYCE J. FITZPATRICK AND JOANNE S. STEVENSON

ABSTRACT

This chapter includes a review of the second decade of *Annual Review of Nursing Research*, Volumes 11–20. The authors analyze the content of these volumes and summarize the significant changes in the nursing scientific community. Also described are the contextual changes related to the development of nursing research.

In volume 10 of the *Annual Review of Nursing Research (ARNR)* series, Stevenson (1992) analyzed the content of Volumes 1–10 and identified the contextual factors that influenced nursing research development from 1982 to 1992. Significant changes in the quality and quantity of nursing research were identified during this time period. In fact, the first decade of the *ARNR* series was consistent with many key developmental changes in the nursing discipline. Establishment of the National Center for Nursing Research in April 1986 was a landmark change during this early period, and the federal budget for nursing research grew from $8 million in 1985 to nearly $45 million in 1992. Other significant changes included the expansion of doctoral programs from 21 in 1982 to 53 in 1992, establishment of regional research societies in nursing and development, and implementation of small research grant opportunities through the American Nurses Foundation and Sigma Theta Tau International. Overall, there was a significant increase in nursing research and the preparation and career development of nurse scientists. The stage was set for the second decade of the *ARNR* series.

LEADERSHIP FOR VOLUMES 11–20

With volume 5 of the *ARNR* series, Joyce Fitzpatrick (Case Western Reserve University) assumed the senior editorship position, a position that she has maintained through the second decade of the *ARNR* series. A decision was made that key members of the Advisory Board would serve as coeditors with Fitzpatrick. Joanne Stevenson (The Ohio State University) served as coeditor for Volumes 11–13 (Fitzpatrick & Stevenson, 1993, 1994, 1995); she had served as a member of the Advisory Board since the inception of the *ARNR* series. For Volumes 14 and 15, Jane Norbeck (University of California–San Francisco) joined Fitzpatrick as coeditor (Fitzpatrick & Norbeck, 1996, 1997). Volumes 16 and 17 were edited by Fitzpatrick alone (Fitzpatrick, 1998, 1999). By the time that the planning was formalized for Volumes 18–20, it was decided that a new model for editorship would be advantageous. Since there was a shift in the content focus of the volumes, such that an entire volume would be focused on a particular theme, the decision was made to have both a series editor (Fitzpatrick) and a volume editor, an expert in the chosen content area. Volume 18, focused on chronic illness, was coedited by Jean Goeppinger (University of North Carolina–Chapel Hill) (Fitzpatrick & Goeppinger, 2000); Volume 19, focused on women's health, was coedited by Diana Taylor (University of California–San Francisco) and Nancy Woods (University of Washington) (Fitzpatrick, Taylor, & Woods, 2001); and Volume 20, focused on geriatric research, was coedited by Patricia Archbold and Barbara Stewart (Oregon Health and Science University) (Fitzpatrick, Archbold, & Stewart, 2002).

A new Advisory Board was appointed with the advent of the second decade. This board included distinguished researchers who had contributed at least one chapter to a volume published in the first decade or who had served previously as a coeditor of a volume. Advisory Board members were appointed for 5-year terms. The Advisory Board for Volumes 11–15 included Violet Barkauskas (University of Michigan), Marie Cowan (University of Washington and UCLA), Claire Fagin (University of Pennsylvania), Suzanne Feetham (National Center for Nursing Research and University of Illinois–Chicago), Phyllis Giovannetti (University of Alberta,

Canada), Ada Sue Hinshaw (National Center for Nursing Research and University of Michigan), Kathleen McCormick (Agency for Health Care Policy and Research and Senior Principal, SRA International), Jane Norbeck (University of California–San Francisco), Christine Tanner (Oregon Health and Science University), Roma Lee Taunton (University of Kansas), and Harriet Werley (University of Wisconsin–Milwaukee). Werley continued to serve as a key advisor to the editors since she was the founding editor of the *ARNR* series. The Advisory Board for Volumes 16–20 consisted of individuals who had played a key role in the first 15 volumes, along with new appointees who would be expected to bring a new perspective in the future. Advisory board members for Volumes 16–20 included Marie Cowan (University of California–Los Angeles), Suzanne Feetham (University of Illinois–Chicago), Terry Fulmer (New York University), Barbara Given (Michigan State University), Margaret Miles (University of North Carolina–Chapel Hill), Jane Norbeck (University of California–San Francisco), Joanne Stevenson (The Ohio State University and Rutgers University), and Roma Lee Taunton (University of Kansas).

CONTENT FOCI FOR VOLUMES 11–20

In conducting the analysis of the content of Volumes 11–20, we decided to use the model developed by Stevenson (1992) for the review of Volumes 1–10. Even though the focus of Volumes 18–20 became more targeted—that is, the entire volume was focused on a content area—the broad categorizations were thought to be useful in delineating the state of the science as reflected in Volumes 11–20. Stevenson (1992) used the six key content themes within the original design for the *ARNR* series to categorize the chapters. These themes included life span development, clinical research, research on nursing care delivery, research on professional issues, educational research in nursing, and international nursing research. The first two categories were further divided into subcategories. Life span development included the following subcategories: maternal-child health, infants, and young children; school-age children and adolescents; adulthood; older adult issues and problems; and family research. Nursing practice research included the subcategories of nursing diagnoses and interventions; symptoms and problems; risk behaviors and forms of abuse; physiologic mechanisms and biologic rhythms; care problems of specific diseases; research in nursing specialty areas; crises, grief, loss, and bereavement; and research on special populations.

Research on a Life Span Developmental Perspective

Volumes 11–20 included a strong and consistent focus on nursing research from a developmental perspective (see Table 12.1). A total of 49 chapters were included in this overall category of Life Span Developmental Perspective. The subcategories that are included in Table 12.1 are Maternal-Child Health, Infants, and Young Children (4 chapters); School-Age Children and Adolescents (16 chapters); Adulthood (7 chapters), Older Adult (Geriatric) Issues and Problems (16 chapters); and Family Research (6 chapters). Many of the chapters included in this section are cross-listed in Table 12.2, Nursing Practice. Thus, chapters are included that are not just focused on a specific age cohort, but also on a specific health problem experienced by persons within that age group, such as diabetes in children or pain in older adults. Included in Table 12.1 in the subcategory of Older Adult are 10 chapters from Volume 20. This entire volume was focused on geriatric nursing research; thus it would be expected that these chapters would be included in this subcategory.

Research on Nursing Practice

Volumes 11–20 included the largest number of chapters that were categorized as Nursing Practice Research (a total of 61 chapters), including those chapters within the subcategories of Nursing Diagnoses and Interventions (18 chapters); Symptoms and Problems (16 chapters); Risk Behaviors and Forms of Abuse (7 chapters); Physiologic Mechanisms and Biological Rhythms (4 chapters); Care Problems of Specific Diseases (4 chapters); Research in Nursing Specialty Areas (5 chapters); Crises, Grief, Loss, and Bereavement (3 chapters); and Research on Special Populations (5 chapters) (see Table 12.2). Many of these chapters were cross-listed in other categories, either within the nursing practice area or in the developmental categories. The amount of cross-listing within the nursing practice subcategories is particularly noteworthy; it is a reflection of the specificity within the development of nursing research from 1993 through 2002, the period reflected in reviews published in Volumes 11–20. Of course, the trend for more specificity in nursing research would have begun earlier, since the reviews most often included research from the preceding 5–10 years.

TABLE 12.1   Life Span Developmental Perspective

Title	Author(s)	Volume
Maternal-Child Health, Infants, and Young Children		
Opiate Abuse in Pregnancy	Lindenberg, C. S, & Keith, A. B.	11
Fatigue During the Childbearing Period	Milligan, R., & Pugh, L. C.	12
Parenting the Prematurely Born Child	Holditch-Davis, D., & Miles, M. S.	15
Prenatal and Parenting Programs for Adolescent Mothers	Hoyer, P. J. P.	16 *
School-Age Children and Adolescents		
Pain in Children	Hester, N. O.	11 *
Psychogenic Pain in Children	Ryan-Wenger, N. M.	12 *
Child Sexual Abuse: Initial Effects	Kelley, S. J.	13 *
The Neurobehavioral Effects of Childhood Lead Exposure	Krowchuk, H. V.	13
Pediatric Hospice Nursing	Martinson, I. M.	13 *
Parent-Adolescent Communication in Nondistressed Families	Riesch, S. K.	15 *
Childhood Nutrition	Kennedy, C. M.	16
Health Care for the School-Age Child	Long, K. A., & Williams, D.	16 *
Childhood Diabetes: Behavioral Research	Brandt, P.	16
Prevention of Mental Health Problems in Adolescence	Kools, S.	16
The Development of Sexual Risk Taking in Adolescence	Jadack, R. A., & Keller, M. L.	16
Motivation for Physical Activity Among Children and Adolescents	Pender, N. J.	16
Prenatal and Parenting Programs for Adolescent Mothers	Hoyer, P. J. P.	16 *
Children with Epilepsy: Quality of Life and Psychosocial Needs	Austin, J. K., & Dunn, D. W.	18

(continued)

TABLE 12.1   *(continued)*

Title	Author(s)	Volume
Interventions for Children with Diabetes and Their Families	Grey, M.	18 *
Family Interventions to Prevent Substance Abuse: Children and Adolescents	Loveland-Cherry, C. J.	18 *
Adulthood		
Physical Health of Homeless Adults	Lindsey, A. M.	13
Sleep Promotion in Adults	Floyd, J. A.	17 *
Management of Urinary Incontinence in Adult Ambulatory Care Populations	Wyman, J. F.	18
Women as Mothers and Grandmothers	McBride, A. B., & Shore, C. P.	19
Women and Stress	Cahill, C. A.	19
Health Decisions and Decision Support for Women	Rothert, M. L., & O'Connor, A. M.	19
Women and Employment: A Decade Review	Killien, M. G.	19
Older Adult (Geriatric) Issues and Problems		
Acute Confusion in the Elderly	Foreman, M. D.	11 *
Elder Mistreatment	Fulmer, T. T.	12 *
Interventions for Cognitive Impairment and Neurobehavioral Disturbances of Older Adults	Cronin-Stubbs, D.	15
Health Promotion in Old Age	Heidrich, S. M.	16
Health Promotion for Family Caregivers of Chronically Ill Elders	Given, B. A., & Given, C. W.	16 *
Cognitive Interventions Among Older Adults	McDougall, Jr., G. J.	17
Introduction: Looking Back and Looking Forward	Archbold, P. G., Stewart, B. J., & Lyons, K. S.	20
Maintaining and Improving Physical Function in Elders	Bennett, J. A.	20

TABLE 12.1 *(continued)*

Title	Author(s)	Volume
Pain in Older Adults	Miller, L. L., & Talerico, K. A.	20 *
Transitional Care of Older Adults	Naylor, M. D.	20 *
Interventions for Family Members Caring for an Elder with Dementia	Acton, G. J., & Winter, M. A.	20 *
End-of-Life Care for Older Adults in ICUs	Baggs, J. G.	20 *
Nursing Homes and Assisted Living Facilities as Places for Dying	Cartwright, J. C.	20 *
Telehealth Interventions to Improve Clinical Nursing of Elders	Jones, J. F., & Brennan, P. F.	20
Hearing Impairment	Wallhagen, M. I.	20 *
Elder Mistreatment	Fulmer, T.	20 *
Family Research		
Family Unit-Focused Research: 1984–1991	Whall, A. L., & Loveland-Cherry, C. J.	11
Parent-Adolescent Communication in Nondistressed Families	Riesch, S. K.	15 *
Health Promotion for Family Caregivers of Chronically Ill Elders	Given, B. A., & Given, C. W.	16 *
Interventions for Children with Diabetes and Their Families	Grey, M.	18 *
Family Interventions to Prevent Substance Abuse: Children and Adolescents	Loveland-Cherry, C. J.	18 *
Interventions for Women as Family Caregivers	Bull, M. J.	19 *

TABLE 12.2   Nursing Practice

Title	Author(s)	Volume
Nursing Diagnoses and Interventions		
Quality of Life and the Spectrum of HIV Infection	Holzemer, W. L., & Wilson, H. S.	13
Delirium Intervention Research in Acute Care Settings	Cronin-Stubbs, D.	14
Smoking Cessation Interventions in Chronic Illness	Wewers, M. E., & Ahijevych, K. L.	14
Quality of Life and Caregiving in Technological Home Care	Smith, C. E.	14 *
Interventions to Reduce the Impact of Chronic Disease: Community-Based Arthritis Patient Education	Goeppinger, J., & Lorig, K.	15 *
Long-Term Vascular Access Devices	Fulton, J. S.	15
Chronic Obstructive Pulmonary Disease: Strategies to Improve Functional Status	Larson, J. L., & Leidy, N. K.	16
Guided Imagery Interventions for Symptom Management	Eller, L. S.	17
Patient-Centered Communication	Brown, S. J.	17
Chronic Low Back Pain: Early Interventions	Faucett, J.	17 *
Sleep Promotion in Adults	Floyd, J. A.	17 *
Music Therapy	Snyder, M., & Chlan, L.	17
Adherence in Chronic Disease	Dunbar-Jacobs, J., Erlen, J. A., Schlenk, E. A., Ryan, C. M., Sereika, S. M., & Doswell, W. M.	18
Interventions for Women as Family Caregivers	Bull, M. J.	19 *
Sleep and Fatigue	Lee, K. A.	19
Pressure Ulcer Prevention and Management	Lyder, C. H.	20
Interventions for Persons with Irreversible Dementia	Burgener, S. C., & Twigg, P.	20

TABLE 12.2   *(continued)*

Title	Author(s)	Volume
Interventions for Family Members Caring for an Elder with Dementia	Acton, G. J., & Winter, M. A.	20 *
Symptoms and Problems		
Acute Confusion in the Elderly	Foreman, M. D.	11 *
The Shivering Response	Holtzclaw, B. J.	11
Chronic Fatigue	Potempa, K. M.	11
Side Effects of Cancer Chemotherapy	Dodd, M. J.	11 *
Pain in Children	Hester, N. O.	11 *
Patient Care Outcomes Related to Management of Symptoms	Hegyvary, S. T.	11
Nursing Research on Patient Falls in Health Care	Morse, J. M.	11
Psychogenic Pain in Children	Ryan-Wenger, N. M.	12 *
Delirium Intervention Research in Acute Care Settings	Cronin-Stubbs, D.	14
Uncertainty in Acute Illness	Mishel, M. H.	15
Acute Pain	Good, M.	17
Chronic Low Back Pain: Early Interventions	Faucett, J.	17 *
Wandering in Dementia	Algase, D. L.	17
Uncertainty in Chronic Illness	Mischel, M. H.	17
Pain in Older Adults	Miller, L. L., & Talerico, K. A.	20 *
Hearing Impairment	Wallhagen, M. I.	20 *
Risk Behaviors and Forms of Abuse		
Opiate Abuse in Pregnancy	Lindenberg, C. S., & Keith, A. B.	11
Alcohol and Drug Abuse	Sullivan, E. J., & Handley, S. M.	11
Elder Mistreatment	Fulmer, T. T.	12 *
Child Sexual Abuse: Initial Effects	Kelley, S. J.	13 *
The Development of Sexual Risk Taking in Adolescence	Jadack, R. A., & Keller, M. L.	16
Intimate Partner Violence Against Women	Humphreys, J., Parker, B., & Campbell, J. C.	19
Elder Mistreatment	Fulmer, T.	20 *

(continued)

TABLE 12.2 *(continued)*

Title	Author(s)	Volume
Physiologic Mechanisms and Biological Rhythms		
Blood Pressure	Thomas, S. A., & DeKeyser, F.	14
Psychoneuroimmunological Studies in HIV Disease	McCain, N. L., & Zeller, J. M.	14
The Chronobiology, Chronopharmacology, and Chronotherapeutics of Pain	Auvil-Novak, S. E.	17
Female Troubles: An Analysis of Menstrual Cycle Research in the NINR Portfolio as a Model for Science Development in Women's Health	Reame, N. K.	19
Care Problems of Specific Diseases		
Side Effects of Cancer Chemotherapy	Dodd, M. J.	11 *
Adherence to Therapy in Tuberculosis	Cohen, F. L.	15
Schizophrenia	Fox, J. C., & Kane, C. F.	16
Cancer Care: Impact of Interventions on Caregiver Outcomes	Pasacreta, J. V., & McCorkle, R.	18
Research in Nursing Specialty Areas		
Rural Health and Health-Seeking Behaviors	Weinert, C., & Burman, M.	12 *
Two Decades of Insider Research: What We Know and Don't Know About Chronic Illness Experience	Thorne, S. E., & Paterson, B. L.	18 *
What We Know and How We Know It: Contributions from Nursing to Women's Health Research and Scholarship	Taylor, D., & Woods, N.	19 *

TABLE 12.2   *(continued)*

Title	Author(s)	Volume
Conceptual Models for Women's Health Research: Reclaiming Menopause as an Exemplar of Nursing's Contributions to Feminist Scholarship	Andrist, L. C., & MacPherson, K. I.	19 *
Genetics and Gerontological Nursing: A Need to Stimulate Research	Frazier, L., & Ostwald, S. K.	20
Crises, Grief, Loss, and Bereavement		
Dying Well: Symptom Control Within Hospice Care	Corless, I. B.	12
End-of-Life Care for Older Adults in ICUs	Baggs, J. G.	20 *
Nursing Homes and Assisted Living Facilities as Places for Dying	Cartwright, J. C.	20 *
Research on Special Populations		
Native American Health	Jacobson, S. F.	12
Health Risk Behaviors for Hispanic Women	Torres, S., & Villarruel, A. M.	13
School-Based Interventions for Primary Prevention of Cardiovascular Disease: Evidence of Effects for Minority Populations	Meininger, J. C.	18
Lesbian Health and Health Care	Bernhard, L. A.	19
Immigrant Women and Their Health	Aroian, K. J.	19

Historical, Ethical, Theoretical, and Philosophic Inquiry in Nursing

Four chapters were included in this content area, two in Volume 18 and two in Volume 19 (see Table 12.3). Two of these four chapters, one each for Volumes 18 and 19, set the stage for a review of the research in the specific content focus of the volume. One of the other two chapters included

TABLE 12.3   Historical, Ethical, Theoretical, and Philosophic Inquiry in Nursing

Title	Author(s)	Volume
Two Decades of Insider Research: What We Know and Don't Know About Chronic Illness Experience	Thorne, S. E., & Paterson, B. L.	18 *
Breakthroughs in Scientific Research: The Discipline of Nursing, 1960–1999	Donaldson, S. K.	18
What We Know and How We Know It: Contributions from Nursing to Women's Health Research and Scholarship	Taylor, D., & Woods, N.	19 *
Conceptual Models for Women's Health Research: Reclaiming Menopause as an Exemplar of Nursing's Contributions to Feminist Scholarship	Andrist, L. C., & MacPherson, K. I.	19 *

in this category was a comprehensive historical review of breakthroughs in nursing research from 1960 through 1999, based on a paper that was presented by Donaldson (2000) at the 25th anniversary celebration of the founding of the American Academy of Nursing.

Research on Nursing Care Delivery

Seventeen chapters focused on nursing care delivery were included in Volumes 11–20 (see Table 12.4). Eight of these chapters are cross-listed in other tables: six are cross-listed in Table 12.2, and five are cross-listed in Table 12.1 (cross-listing of some chapters in more than one table is included). The research on nursing care delivery includes a range of topics. Some of these topics are site specific, such as hospice care, home care, and care in ICUs. Other topics are specific to the type of health problem being addressed, such as heart disease and chronic illness. Others are more general topics that could be applied across a range of settings, such as

TABLE 12.4   Nursing Care Delivery

Title	Author(s)	Volume
The Role of Nurse Researchers Employed in Clinical Settings	Kirchhoff, K. T.	11
Rural Health and Health-Seeking Behaviors	Weinert, C., & Burman, M.	12 *
Nursing Workload Measurement Systems	Edwardson, S. R., & Giovannetti, P. B.	12
Case Management	Lamb, G. S.	13
Technology and Home Care	Smith, C. E.	13
Pediatric Hospice Nursing	Martinson, I. M.	13 *
Quality of Life and Caregiving in Technological Home Care	Smith, C. E.	14 *
Organizational Redesign: Effect on Institutional and Consumer Outcomes	Ingersoll, G. L.	14
Organizational Culture	Mark, B. A.	14
Interventions to Reduce the Impact of Chronic Disease: Community-Based Arthritis Patient Education	Goeppinger, J., & Lorig, K.	15 *
Health Care for the School-Age Child	Long, K. A., & Williams, D.	16 *
Primary Health Care	McElmurry, B. J., & Keeney, G. B.	17
Heart Failure Management: Optimal Health Care Delivery Programs	Moser, D. K.	18
Transitional Care of Older Adults	Naylor, M. D.	20 *
End-of-Life Care for Older Adults in ICUs	Baggs, J. G.	20 *
Nursing Homes and Assisted Living Facilities as Places for Dying	Cartwright, J. C.	20 *
Home Health Services Research	Madigan,, E. A., Tullai-McGuinness, S., & Neff, D. F.	20

TABLE 12.5   Professional Issues in Nursing

Title	Author(s)	Volume
AIDS-Related Knowledge, Attitudes, and Risk for HIV Infection Among Nurses	Turner, J. G.	11
Minorities in Nursing	Morris, D. L., & Wykle, M. L.	12
Nursing Minimum Data Set	Ryan, P., & Delaney, C.	13
The Professionalization of Nurse Practitioners	Bullough, B.	13
Feminism and Nursing	Chinn, P. L.	13
Moral Competency	Cassidy, V. R.	14
Violence in the Workplace	Hewitt, J. B., & Levin, P. F.	15
Health Promotion and Disease Prevention in the Worksite	Lusk, S. L.	15
Nursing at War: Catalyst for Change	Brunk, Q.	15

nursing workload measurement systems, organizational redesign, and organizational culture.

Research on Professional Issues in Nursing

Nine chapters focused on professional nursing issues were included in Volumes 11–15 (see Table 12.5). These included chapters on very specific professional issues, such as AIDS-related knowledge, and very general professional issues, such as minorities in nursing. With the publication of Volume 14, the editors and Advisory Board decided to discontinue the special section of *ARNR* that focused on the profession of nursing. Those chapters on professional issues that were published in Volume 15 were then included under a separate section of "Other Research" in this volume.

Research on Nursing Education

Chapters on nursing education research were included in Volumes 11–14. In each of these volumes there was one chapter on nursing education

TABLE 12.6   Nursing Education and Faculty

Title	Author(s)	Volume
Nurse-Midwifery Education	Andrews, C. M., & Davis, C. E.	11
Research on the Baccalaureate Completion Process for RNs	Mathews, M. B., & Travis, L. L.	12
Faculty Practice: Interest, Issues, and Impact	Walker, P. H.	13
Oncology Nursing Education	Workman, M. L.	14

research (see Table 12.6). A wide range of topics was reflected in these four chapters, from specialty education (nurse-midwifery and oncology) to general issues in nursing education (baccalaureate completion programs and faculty practice). The focus on nursing education research within the discipline had declined considerably in the 1990s. It was becoming harder and harder to identify experts in the area of nursing education research and to identify topics that could be included in the reviews. Thus, the editors and Advisory Board decided to discontinue this section of the *ARNR* volumes beginning with Volume 15. No chapters on nursing education research were included in Volumes 15–20.

International Nursing Research

During the second decade of the *ARNR* series, there were five chapters that included nursing research from other countries (see Table 12.7). These chapters were written by nurse researchers from the country in which the studies were conducted. Chapters focused on research in Korea, Israel, Brazil, Taiwan, and Italy.

Overall Changes in the Content Focus of Volumes 11–20

As mentioned, there was a shift in the focus of categories included in the *ARNR* volumes, beginning with Volume 15. Midway through the decade the plans included a more concentrated emphasis on clinical nursing research. Thus, the decision was made to drop the categories of Research

TABLE 12.7   International Nursing Research

Title	Author(s)	Volume
Nursing Research in Korea	Choi, E. C.	12
Nursing Research in Israel	Golander, H., & Krulik, T.	14
The Evolution of Nursing Research in Brazil	Mendes, I. A. C., & Trevizan, M. A.	14
Nursing Research in Taiwan	Shiao, S. P. K., & Chao, Y. Y.	15
Nursing Research in Italy	Zanotti, R.	17

on Nursing Education and the Profession of Nursing beginning with Volume 15. Three categories were then included in Volumes 15 and 16: Nursing Practice Research, Research on Nursing Care Delivery, and Other Research. For Volume 15, the Nursing Practice Research category had no specific focus; Nursing Practice Research for Volume 16 was targeted toward health promotion across the life span. Volume 17 included chapters in only two categories: Nursing Practice Research and Other Research; Nursing Practice Research included two subcategories: research on complementary therapies and pain research.

After considerable reflection on the development of nursing research, in planning for future volumes (beyond Volume 17) the senior editor decided to begin to develop theme volumes, that is, volumes in which the majority of chapters would be focused on a specific content area. To plan the content themes, the senior editor consulted with staff members of the National Institute of Nursing Research to determine content areas in which there would be a considerable body of knowledge. The three initial content areas identified were chronic illness, women's health, and geriatric nursing. Key content experts were asked to provide leadership as volume editors.

SOME OBSERVATIONS ABOUT THE CHAPTERS OF THE SECOND DECADE

The authorship trends did not change much from the first decade; most chapters had single authors, and about one third were coauthored. Publication of two chapters by three or more authors also occurred. It is interesting that the chapter with five coauthors had significantly more references than any other chapter in the decade; perhaps there is a parallel between number of authors and comprehensiveness of the literature review.

Almost all of the chapter authors had PhDs (93%), and through Volume 19, all coauthors were doctorally prepared; following through on the policy set during the first decade, no one engaged his or her doctoral students as coauthors. The editorial boards continued to enact the policy that senior scientists in the profession should author the integrative reviews. In Volume 20, the rule was relaxed; there were three doctoral student authors, and one was the first author.

In the review of the first decade of the *ARNR*, Stevenson (1992) discussed the variety of definitions of nursing research that she found in the first 10 volumes. In the first decade, the definitions included (a) any topic of research as long as the investigator or author was a nurse; (b) research on a topic in the domain of health care that constitutes nursing's societal mission, restricted to only studies by nurses or to all studies regardless of the investigator or author's discipline; and/or (c) a special way of looking at health-related issues and problems from a nursing perspective. During the second decade, the first of these interpretations was not found. Overwhelmingly, the reviews focused on topics that are important to nursing's health care mission, and authors reviewed all the relevant research regardless of the investigator's discipline or the disciplinary orientation of the journal.

The array of journals from outside of nursing that were included in the references expanded exponentially compared to the first 10 volumes. Interestingly, the number of nurses who were authors in these journals also greatly expanded when compared to the first decade.

Citations from nursing journals ranged from lows of 5% of the reference list for several of the chapters to over 50% for a select few of the chapters. These differences were explainable in relation to the topics of the reviews and to how much history each one had as a traditional or avant-garde nursing research topic. Along the same line, it depended whether there were or were not (usually clinical) nursing journals that focused on that topic. Traditional topics such as maternal-child care, pediatric problems, cardiovascular and cancer care, acute or chronic illness management, pain, sleep, informal caregiver issues, and gynecological-type women's health topics typically contained high percentages of references by nurse authors and were published in nursing journals. Both the nursing journals that only report nursing research and the clinical journals that are specific to the clinical area were frequently cited when the topic was a traditional one that had been of interest to nurse scientists for many years.

On the other hand, newer topics of interest to nurse scientists had few references to nursing journals, and those citations authored by nurses more often appeared in non-nursing journals. Examples included psycho-neuroimmunology, substance abuse, sexual abuse, violence in the work-place, women's health problems that were not gynecologically oriented, health promotion research (such as exercise, nutrition, or smoking cessation), and rural health care. There are not yet clinical journals in nursing that are dedicated to these problems, and even the nursing journals that publish only research may not accept such manuscripts, under the belief that the topic is not of interest to sufficient numbers of readers to justify publication. It will be interesting to watch the trends over the next decade to see if some of the newer research topics, including genetics, move into the mainstream of nursing journalism.

The comprehensiveness and the quality of the reviews improved considerably during the second decade. All topics were much more specific and allowed a more thorough review of the topic, which resulted in more useful reviews. Since the reviews were more specific, their authors were more closely associated with the topic, and generally the first author was the leading nurse scientist expert on that topic. Hence, the conclusions about substantive voids in the corpus of studies, recurrent methodological problems, and recommendations for future research were much more pointed than in the first decade.

CONTEXTUAL CHANGES IN NURSING RESEARCH, 1983–2002

Research Funding at the Federal Level

Beginning in 1955, the Division of Nursing within the United States Public Health Service began funding nursing research projects, but the amount available each year never exceeded $8 million until well into the 1980s. On November 20, 1985, Public Law 99-158 was passed overriding President Reagan's veto, and, as part of this law, the National Center for Nursing Research (NCNR) was created within the National Institutes of Health. Nursing research funding also got a significant increase from $8 million

TABLE 12.8   Growth in NCNR and NINR Budget from 1988 to 2003

Year	Amount ($) (in millions)	Percent increase
1988	23,361	0
1989	29,118	25
1990	33,508	15
1991	39,892	19
1992	44,925	13
1993	48,477	8
1994	51,002	5
1995	52,689	3
1996*	55,676	6
1997	59,551	7
1998	63,531	7
1999	69,851	10
2000*	90,261	29
2001*	105,456	17
2002*	120,751	15
2003	130,809	8

to $16.2 million in the appropriations bill for fiscal year 1986. The new NCNR became operational over the next year; this resulted in significantly increased federal support of nursing research projects. On June 10, 1993, Public Law 103-43 was signed and NCNR was elevated to the National Institute of Nursing Research (NINR). Table 12.8 shows the growth in funding levels for NCNR/NINR from 1988 through the present (Grady, 2002; National Institute of Nursing Research, 1999, 2000, 2001, 2002, 2003).

In addition to regular research grants, having the NCNR and NINR within NIH has made many research training programs, midcareer research training programs, and other developmental mechanisms available to the nursing science community. The NCNR/NINR leadership also have consistently maximized the yield from their budgets by partnering with other institutes and programs to cosponsor and cofund initiatives. Also, during the past several years the number of nurse scientists who have been funded by other institutes within NIH has grown significantly.

NINR remains a very small institute, and the success rates for applications submitted to NINR never match the success rates enjoyed by the larger NIH institutes. This means that a proportionately larger number of applications which have peer review scores in what would be fundable ranges for other Institutes or Centers do not get funded at NINR. This low success rate persists in the face of growth rates in NINR appropriations which have kept pace during the "NIH doubling" period of 1999 through 2003. Nevertheless, NINR has had a significant impact on the quantity and quality of science produced within nursing since the mid-1980s.

Research-Oriented Doctoral Preparation Over the Decade

The number of research-oriented doctoral programs in nursing grew more rapidly from 1990 through 2002 than in any comparable earlier period. There were 25 such programs in 1990, but the number grew to 73 by 2000 and to 79 by 2002 (see Table 12.9). This addition of 54 programs in 10 years, however, did not produce a parallel growth in the number of graduates. Berlin and Sechrist (1999) found that there were only 200 more nurses with doctorates who graduated in 1998 compared to 1989; the doctoral programs were producing fewer than six graduates per year. This meant we were not keeping up with the minimum replacement need for academic teachers and administrators, let alone providing time for academicians to have release time to write grants, do research, and publish the results. Even more alarming, in 1999 the median age of these new graduates of doctoral programs in nursing was 46 years, and 12% of them were over

TABLE 12.9   Trends in Nursing Doctoral Programs, Research Based Only

Decade	Total # of Programs	PhD	DNS/DNSc/DSN
1970	17	14	3
1980	30	25	5
1990	25	22	3
2000	73	64	9
2002	79*	69*	12**

*Includes 6 collaborative programs across more than one university
**Two schools confer both PhD and DNSc degrees

Source: American Association of Colleges of Nursing.

55 (Berlin & Sechrist, 2002). The leadership of the American Association of Colleges of Nursing (AACN, 2002) and the NINR issued numerous statements and warnings about the need to attract more younger students into doctoral programs in nursing.

Growth in Research Resources Within Academic and Practice Settings

During the past several years there has been a significant increase in the resources devoted to nursing science in both academic settings and in large research-oriented practice settings. According to a recent survey by Yoon, Wolfe, Yucha, and Tsai (2002), in the US schools of nursing offering doctoral degrees, about 40% of the 56 research offices have been added in the past decade. These research offices provide a wide range of services to nurse scientists, but in general the goal is to decrease the time the scientists spend on repetitive tasks involved in both the grant application process and in the administrative aspects of conducting the work and reporting the findings in a timely fashion. During the past decade, there also has been a significant increase in the resources supplied to nursing departments and nurse researchers in hospitals, as more of these institutions have moved toward attainment of magnet hospital status with its attendant emphasis on the conduct of nursing research.

Many academic nursing programs have added laboratories for both biological and behavioral research, either as free-standing laboratories in schools of nursing or as cooperative ventures with other health sciences. Such entities significantly enhance both the training of doctoral students and the ability of nurse scholars to conduct state of the art research.

Growth of Regional and National Research Societies

The regional nursing research societies have expanded in membership over the past decade. These societies include the Western Institute of Nursing (WIN), the Midwest Nursing Research Society (MNRS), the Eastern Nursing Research Society (ENRS), and the Southern Nursing Research Society (SNRS). These regional societies hold conferences each year, and they provide other research development efforts and valuable networking opportunities to their members.

COUNCIL FOR THE ADVANCEMENT OF NURSING SCIENCE (CANS)

This is a new national and international organization; its aims are (a) to be a strong voice that supports the development, conduct, and utilization of nursing science; (b) to share research findings with individuals, communities, institutions, and industry; and (c) to facilitate lifelong learning opportunities for nurse scientists (Council for the Advancement of Nursing Science, 2002). Earlier, the ANA Council of Nurse Researchers served the purpose of fostering nursing research at the national level, but it became extinct in the mid-1990s when the American Nurses Association fully embraced the federation model. CANS was the brainchild of Dr. William Holzemer (University of California–San Francisco) and was encouraged and fostered by the President and Board of the American Academy of Nursing (AAN) beginning in 1998 (Dr. Joyce Fitzpatrick was AAN President and Dr. Ada Sue Hinshaw was President-Elect). CANS cosponsored with AAN and NINR an inaugural national meeting in January 2002 on promoting research-intensive environments.

The first Nursing Research State of the Science (SOS) Conference was initiated by the *ARNR* series Senior Editor with support from Springer Publishing Company; that conference was held in Washington, D.C. in 1993. Several nursing organizations cosponsored this first SOS conference (in particular, AACN was instrumental in much of the conference organization). Subsequently, the American Academy of Nursing led the sponsorship of the second State of the Science Conference in Washington in 1999 and the third in 2002 had lead cosponsorship by the AACN and Sigma Theta Tau International. CANS was tied into the 2002 conference and provided information about the organization to attendees. As of 2004, CANS will assume leadership for planning the biennial State of the Science conferences, with continued cosponsorship and participation by several members of the National Nursing Research Roundtable (NNRR).* (W. Holzemer, personal communication, September, 27, 2002).

The CANS organization is quite new, but it fills a critical void that was previously filled by the ANA Council of Nurse Researchers from

---

*The NNRR initially began as a group invited to meet in Washington by the director of NCNR/ NINR. It is convened by the NINR and a rotating cosponsoring organization and is composed of persons representing a number of organizations which have research as a major goal, including the American Academy of Nursing, the American Nurses Association, the American Association of Colleges of Nursing, Sigma Theta Tau International, the National League for Nursing, the National Council of State Boards, the regional research societies, and some specialty nursing organizations.

the early 1970s until the mid-1990s. The ANA Council and the ANA Commission on Nursing Research were largely responsible for the NIH Task Force studies of nursing research at NIH and the eventual legislation that created the NCNR (later the National Institute of Nursing Research). That kind of national constituent voice for nursing science has been largely absent since the early 1990s, as has the networking that occurs when nurse scientists from all over the US and other countries get together to report their research and talk with each other once a year. Cross-fertilization of ideas and collaboration among nurse scientists has flourished within the regional research societies for the past two decades, but there is also a need for systematic intra- and international networking and partnership development.

TriService Nursing Research Program (TSNRP)

This program was established in 1992 to sponsor research conducted by military (army, navy, and air force) nurses. The primary goal of TSNRP is to promote research that will enhance the standards of nursing care throughout all branches of the armed forces, thus improving the health of military personnel and their families. TSNRP-funded nurse researchers include those on active duty and nurse researchers at more than 40 schools of nursing across the country. The initial TSNRP funding level was $1 million. As of 2002, the annual funding has been increased to $6 million; this provided funding for 230 research projects. The TSNRP links military nurse researchers across the country, focuses on disseminating research findings, and integrates research into practice.

Expansion of Research Journals in Nursing

Since 1987 four new research journals have been launched within the nursing scientific community. *Scholarly Inquiry in Nursing Practice* was begun in 1987; this journal was renamed *Research and Theory for Nursing Practice* in 2002. In 1988, *Applied Nursing Research* was launched; it is now in its 15th volume. *Qualitative Health Research* published its first issue in 1991, and *Biological Research for Nursing* began in 1999. These journals join the following established research journals in the field: *Nursing Research* (begun in 1952); *Research in Nursing and Health* (begun in 1978); and *Western Journal of Nursing Research* (begun in 1979). Also, in the past decade we have witnessed an increase in research articles published in the clinical specialty journals and the general scholarly journals in nursing.

FROM THE 20TH ANNIVERSARY INTO THE NEXT DECADE

Dr. Ursula Springer hosted an anniversary reception during the third State of the Science Conference in Washington, D.C., on September 27, 2002. In attendance were many of the nurse scientists who had contributed to the *ARNR* series over the years as editors, board members, or authors, as well as upcoming editors and the young nurse scientists who will be the authors of the future.

The research and research training funded by NINR will continue to be investigator-initiated. An analysis of the current portfolio of NINR shows that most Program Announcements (PAs) or Requests for Proposals (RFAs) for which NINR is the primary sponsor are for training and research intrastructure initiatives: the core center grants, the exploratory center grants, the institutional training grants, and career development. These PAs and RFAs are tied into the NINR Areas of Research Opportunity which generally include an "infrastructure development" thrust. NINR is only occasionally a primary sponsor for PAs or RFAs which solicit research applications for an area of science. The thematic areas for solicitations of research applications embedded in the Areas of Research Opportunity have remained broadly defined since 1998 as: symptom management and self care in chronic illnesses, behavioral changes and interventions in vulnerable populations (e.g., older adults, children/adolescents), health disparities, end of life/palliative care, health promotion, and selected aspects of women's health (O'Neal, 2002). The new announcements for 2002 and 2003 include a focus on chronic pain, long term care needs and interventions, high risk adolescent behaviors, caregiving, mobility disorders, clinical decision making and community partnered interventions to reduce health disparities (NINR, 2002, 2003). NINR cosponsors with other Institutes and Centers a number of PAs and RFAs in other areas of science and has the opportunity to revise those RFAs and PAs to ensure the wording is suitable for potential nurse investigators. In October, 2002, NINR hosted a series of roundtable discussions with leading nurse scientists to prioritize research topics for the future. This assessment will be particularly instructive to future scientists.

A significant challenge facing the nursing science community is the aging of its scientists coupled with the low numbers of students coming into research-focused doctoral programs and the "advanced age" of those who are completing doctorates. The discipline had 73 schools of nursing offering doctoral programs in 2002 and 6 collaborative programs (offered by more than one school of nursing). Yet these programs were graduating about the same number per year as when there were 52 doctoral programs during the later 1980s and early 1990s. To address this issue nursing must convert to the graduate education model of the older disciplines and promote baccalaureate through doctoral education for honor students and others who have the potential to become scientists. NINR has encouraged baccalaureate to PhD programs through research training support. At least thirty-eight schools of nursing now offer these programs.

Another challenge is the disconnect between areas of knowledge development and the lack of implementation in practice settings. *ARNR* can be an intermediary in this process by providing the integrative reviews that inform practitioners about what is ready for research utilization. The disciplinary focus on evidence-based practice as a concept must become a reality in the future. Hopefully, the next decade will provide a major turning point in the multistep process from the development of knowledge to integration, and from synthesis of knowledge to utilization of knowledge, for higher-quality nursing and health care.

REFERENCES

American Association of Colleges of Nursing. (2002). *AACN Position Statement: Indicators of quality in research-focused doctoral programs in nursing.* Washington, DC: Author.

Berlin, L. E., & Sechrist, K. R. (1999). Projecting the shortage of doctorally prepared nursing faculty: A supply problem of International concern. Centennial Conference, International Council of Nurses. London, England. June 28, 1999.

Berlin, L. E., & Sechrist, K. R. (2002). The shortage of doctorally prepared nursing faculty: A dire situation. *Nursing Outlook, 50,* 50–56.

Council for the Advancement of Nursing Science. (2002). Mission, goals, membership, partners, and sponsors. Washington, DC: Author. Retrieved October 8, 2002, from *http://nursingworld.org/aan/council.htm*

Donaldson, S. K. (2000). Breakthroughs in scientific research: The discipline of nursing, 1960–1999. In J. J. Fitzpatrick & J. Goeppinger (Eds.), *Annual review of nursing research* (Vol. 18). NY: Springer.

Fitzpatrick, J. J. (Ed.). (1998). *Annual review of nursing research* (Vol. 16). New York: Springer.

Fitzpatrick, J. J. (Ed.). (1999). *Annual review of nursing research* (Vol. 17). New York: Springer.

Fitzpatrick, J. J., Archbold, P., & Stewart, B. (Eds.). (2002). *Annual review of nursing research* (Vol. 20). New York: Springer.

Fitzpatrick, J. J., & Goeppinger, J. (Eds.). (2000). *Annual review of nursing research* (Vol. 18). New York: Springer.

Fitzpatrick, J. J., & Norbeck, J. (Eds.). (1996). *Annual review of nursing research* (Vol. 14). New York: Springer.

Fitzpatrick, J. J., & Norbeck, J. (Eds.). (1997). *Annual review of nursing research* (Vol. 15). New York: Springer.

Fitzpatrick, J. J., & Stevenson, J. S. (Eds.). (1993). *Annual review of nursing research* (Vol. 11). New York: Springer.

Fitzpatrick, J. J., & Stevenson, J. S. (Eds.). (1994). *Annual review of nursing research* (Vol. 12). New York: Springer.

Fitzpatrick, J. J., & Stevenson, J. S. (Eds.). (1995). *Annual review of nursing research* (Vol. 13). New York: Springer.

Fitzpatrick, J. J., Taylor, D., & Woods, N. (Eds.). (2001). *Annual review of nursing research* (Vol. 19). New York: Springer.

Grady, P. A. (2002). *Fiscal Year 2003 Budget Request.* National Institute of Nursing Research. Retrieved November 8, 2002 from *http://www.nih.gov/ninr/about/budget2003.pdf*

Holzemer, W. (2002). Personal communication.

National Institute of Nursing Research. (1999, 2000, 2001, 2002, 2003). Bethesda, MD: Author. Retrieved August 22, 2002, from *http://www.nih.gov/ninr/research*

O'Neal, D. J. (2002). Personal communication.

Stevenson, J. S. (1992). Review of the first decade of the *Annual review of nursing research.* In J. J. Fitzpatrick, R. L. Taunton, & A. K. Jacox (Eds.), *Annual review of nursing research* (pp. 1–22). New York: Springer.

Yoon, S. L., Wolfe, S., Yucha, C. B., & Tsai, P. (2002). Research support by doctoral-granting colleges/schools of nursing. *Journal of Professional Nursing, 18*(1), 16–21.

Index

Contents of Previous Volumes

ORDER FORM

Save 10% on Volume 22 with this coupon.

____ Check here to order the *Annual Review of Nursing Research*, Volume 22, 2004 at a 10% discount. You will receive an invoice requesting prepayment.

Save 10% on all future volumes with a continuation order.

____ Check here to place your continuation order for the *Annual Review of Nursing Research.* You will receive a prepayment invoice with a 10% discount upon publication of each new volume, beginning with Volume 22, 2004. You may pay for prompt shipment or cancel with no obligation.

Name _____

Institution _____

Address _____

City/State/Zip _____

Examination copies for possible adoption are available to instructors "on approval" only. Write on institutional letterhead, noting course, level, present text, and expected enrollment (include $3.50 for postage and handling). Prices slightly higher overseas. Prices subject to change.

Mail this coupon to:
SPRINGER PUBLISHING COMPANY
536 Broadway
New York, NY 10012

2191